THE PSYCHOLOGY
OF DEAFNESS

Dr. Myklebust is also author of
AUDITORY DISORDERS IN CHILDREN
A MANUAL FOR DIFFERENTIAL DIAGNOSIS

Second Edition

THE PSYCHOLOGY

OF DEAFNESS

Sensory Deprivation, Learning, and Adjustment

HELMER R. MYKLEBUST

Northwestern University

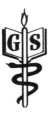

GRUNE & STRATTON
A Subsidiary of Harcourt Brace Jovanovich, Publishers
New York   San Francisco   London

Grune & Stratton, Inc.
111 Fifth Avenue, New York, New York 10003.

Distributed in the United Kingdom by
Academic Press, Inc. (London) Ltd.
24/28 Oval Road, London NW1

Library of Congress Catalog Card Number 64-22056
International Standard Book Number 0-8089-0339-X

Printed in the United States of America

6
7
8 f
9 g
0 h
1 i
8 2 j

TO

THOSE WITH

DEAFNESS

CONTENTS

LIST OF ILLUSTRATIONS

Fig.   *Page*

PREFACE

ONLY A FEW YEARS HAVE ELAPSED since publication of the original edition of this volume, The Psychology of Deafness. During these years we completed an investigation of the development and disorders of written language and a major portion of this work concerned acquisition of the written word by the deaf child. While portions of this material appeared in the original edition, the major findings became available only after its publication. Because we wished to have them included, it was necessary to prepare this revised edition.

Brief discussions of three additional studies of the psychology of deafness, completed at The Institute for Language Disorders, have been provided. Roland Farrant's investigation comprises a major attempt to analyze the ways in which deafness modifies factors of intelligence. An extensive study of the personality attributes associated with good social adjustment in the adult deaf was conducted by Arthur Neyhus. John Brannon performed an experiment to learn more about the neurosensory monitoring processes available to the deaf for the production of intelligible speech. These studies are mentioned as harbingers of swiftly moving events in the area of the psychology of deafness.

The Figures have been redrawn so that they portray greater accuracy and readability, while only minor changes and corrections have been made in other divisions of the volume.

The purposes and objectives of this second edition remain the same as those of the original. It is intended as a textbook for advanced courses in Audiology, Language Pathology, Deaf Education, and Psychology. It is anticipated that it might be useful also to students of Otolaryngology, Psychiatry, Pediatrics, Neurology, and Rehabilitation, as well as in other professional endeavors concerned with the provocative and intriguing ramifications of sensory deprivation.

Many persons have assisted with this work: students, colleagues, friends, and those with deafness. Dean James H. McBurney of the School of Speech, Northwestern University, has made it possible to pursue the necessary research and clinical activities. While indebted to them all, I alone must be responsible for the contents.

The response of professional persons in many lands to the first edition has been gratifying, indeed an inspiration. I can only hope that they will now find the volume more useful.

HELMER R. MYKLEBUST
Evanston, Illinois

Part One
The Nature and Extent of Deafness

Chapter I
THE PROBLEM

MAN IS HIGHLY DEPENDENT on his senses. Through his senses come the sensations which constitute his experience. Upon the information he receives from his senses he builds his world, his world of perception and conception; of memory, imagination, thought, and reason.

A sensory deprivation limits the world of experience. It deprives the organism of some of the material resources from which the mind develops. Because total experience is reduced, there is an imposition on the balance and equilibrium of all psychological processes. When one type of sensation is lacking, it alters the integration and function of all of the others. Experience is now constituted differently; the world of perception, conception, imagination, and thought has an altered foundation, a new configuration. Such alteration occurs naturally and unknowingly, because unless the individual is organized and attuned differently, survival itself may be in jeopardy.

The degree of the sensory impairment, the age at which it is sustained, and other factors, influence the extent and nature of the shift which the organism undergoes. It is not identical for all who have impaired sensory capacities. However, some shift, some reorganization of experience seems imperative and inevitable. Furthermore, the psychological structure which results seems highly characteristic. Apparently sensory deprivation produces an impact which modifies behavior according to a certain pattern. This seems to be true despite the many variables and individual differences which are involved. It is the purpose and objective of psychological study to ascertain the nature of this impact and to foster the best possible learning and adjustment in all so handicapped.

The study of deafness, one type of sensory deprivation, has a long history. During the 16th century there was increasing reference to those who could not hear. Up to this time they were referred to in the same category as the mentally deficient. By the 17th century attitudes were changing. Diderot's letter on the Deaf and Dumb,[7] written in the 18th century reveals that philosophers then were interested in the deaf, especially in terms of speech and its importance in relation to thought. Attempts to instruct the deaf began in Europe in the Middle Ages; by the middle of the 18th century a deaf person's right to education was becoming established. During this period Samuel Heineke started a school for the deaf in Germany, the Abbe' de l'Eppe began such work in France, and Thomas Braidwood initiated the first work in Great Britain. The work of de l'Eppe had considerable influence on the early work with the deaf in America.

The first efforts toward establishing schools for the deaf in the United States date from the beginning of the 19th century. Attempts were first made to establish schools in New York, Virginia, and Connecticut; and the first permanent school for the deaf was founded in Hartford, Connecticut during the period of 1816 and 1817. Since this time much progress has been made. There are now at least ten public day schools and 240 public day classes. There are 72 public residential schools and 16 private residential schools.[3] There are also private day centers. Additional educational, psychological, medical, and audiological facilities are being established every year. Many new understandings have been forthcoming regarding all aspects of impaired hearing. Changes have occurred rapidly in methods of medical treatment, methods of instruction, and in methods of guidance and rehabilitation. Scientific advancement has made possible new vistas in the use of amplification, in diagnosis, in educational management, and in medical and surgical treatment.

Deafness is a broad and inclusive condition which encompasses a wide variety of problems. Therefore, many fields are entailed in its study. Since approximately 1947 all of the educational, clinical and scientific areas most concerned with the problem of deafness have been designated as the field of audiology. A professional person who specializes mainly in diagnostic and rehabilitative procedures and techniques as they pertain to individuals with impaired hearing is referred to as an audiologist. However, each area of specialization, whether it is medicine, psychology, education, physics, or one of several others, has a contribution which it makes in its own way. As one area progresses, it usually benefits all of the other areas; it benefits the individual with deafness in some way. This is illustrated by advancements in physics and electronics making it possible for the educator to inaugurate new programs of auditory training. No one field of specialization can encompass all of the problems entailed in deafness.

DEFINITIONS AND CLASSIFICATIONS

The implications of an auditory impairment vary from person to person and from one circumstance to another. This makes it difficult to define rigorously what is meant by terms such as *hearing loss, deaf,* and *hard of hearing.* Such classifications vary according to the purpose for which they are being made. In medicine frequently a classification is made on the basis of the type of pathology present. In education prime considerations are the degree of deafness and the age at which it was sustained. Because the purpose, the criterion, is different no one set of definitions can be expected to meet all needs. Therefore, it is advantageous to be familiar with the various ways in which hearing losses can be defined and classified. In this way the implications of deafness can be clarified and more fully realized.

One of the long standing, useful definitions of deafness was given by the Committee on Nomenclature of the Conference of Executives of American Schools for the Deaf.[1] This committee defined the deaf as "those in whom the sense of hearing is nonfunctional for the ordinary purpose of life." They classified the deaf into two groups on the basis of the age at which deafness occurred:

a. *The congenitally deaf.* Those who are born deaf.

b. *The adventitiously deaf.* Those who are born with normal hearing but in whom the sense of hearing becomes nonfunctional later through illness. This same committee defined the hard of hearing as "those in whom the sense of hearing, although defective, is functional with or without a hearing aid."

For educational purposes it is necessary to add another factor before suitable classification can be made. This factor is the extent to which the hearing loss has affected language development. During recent years this consideration has become increasingly important. A greater number of individuals can be classified as having *functional,* or useful hearing because they can be benefitted through the use of hearing aids. This being true, it has become more difficult to distinguish between those who have functional hearing with a hearing aid and those who do not. Such a distinction usually is critical in educational planning, so an additional definition has become necessary. It is based on the type of educational problem presented by a specific child. This definition is:

a. *The deaf.* Those whose hearing loss has precluded normal acquisition of language.

b. *The hard of hearing.* Those having a hearing loss but in whom language acquisition has not been precluded.

These definitions are not based directly on the degree of deafness but emphasize the extent to which the deafness has affected the child's acquisition of language. The distinction differentiates between the child who presents a major problem educationally and the one who does not. Any child whose deafness precludes his acquiring language should be given the advantage of specialized training even though he has considerable residual hearing, might wear a hearing aid, and classify as being hard of hearing.

The definitions given by the Committee of the Conference of Executives of American Schools for the Deaf emphasize two of the factors which must be considered in dealing with all types of handicapped people. These factors are the *degree* of the involvement and the *time* factor, or age at which the handicap was sustained. For scientific, clinical, and educational purposes these factors must be viewed separately. To combine them inadvertently leads to confusion of the learning and adjustment problems involved.

Another confusion encountered in studying the various classifications used in the area of deafness is the attributing of causal meanings to terms which refer only to the extent of the impairment, or to the age at which it was sustained. This occurs most often with the terms *congenital* and *adventitious.* These terms refer only to the *time* of onset of the sensory deprivation. Congenital means present at the time of birth and adventitious means that the onset was after birth. In the past confusion has arisen because congenital was used to include hereditary deafness, or more specifically deafness due to causes other than disease or accident. This has resulted in confusion of classification, especially for research purposes because if congenital is used to mean other than disease or accident, much error ensues. A number of diseases cause deafness prenatally. Such deafness is both adventitious and congenital. It is caused by disease, and it is present at the time of birth.

To overcome this confusion and error in classification, Myklebust[8] suggested applying the terms exogenous and endogenous; terms which have been used in the study of mental deficiency and other handicapping conditions.[5] These terms make it possible to classify deafness on the basis of *cause* without reference to the degree, or to the time of its onset. Exogenous refers to all factors *other* than heredity, while endogenous includes *only* the hereditary. The terms deaf and hard of hearing refer to the *extent*, or the degree of deafness.

Other classifications which are necessary, especially in connection with medical diagnosis and treatment, are sensory-neural, conductive, and central deafness. The basis of these classifications is the *site of the lesion*, the site of the defect. *Sensory-neural deafness* includes all hearing loss which derives from trauma, maldevelopment, or disease affecting the normal function of the inner ear. *Conductive deafness* includes all hearing loss which derives from lack of normal function in the middle ear. *Central deafness* includes all auditory impairment which derives from lack of normal function of the auditory pathways leading from the inner ear to the interpretive areas of the brain.

The significance of these classifications is indicated in the discussion of the types and causes of deafness in Chapter III. There are several subdivisions of each of these classifications. Here we emphasize that it is necessary to include a fourth factor in the definition and classification of deafness; the physical origin of the sensory deprivation, usually referred to as the site of the lesion.

Other classifications used in the study, treatment, and educational classification of individuals with impaired hearing are presbycusia and deafened. *Presbycusia* is the term used for deafness which results from the natural loss of hearing which accompanies advancement in age. With the problem of geriatrics growing year by year, the study of presbycusia has become highly important. Because a presbycusic hearing loss is of the sensory-neural type, this term includes three factors; site of the lesion, age of onset, and cause. It is due to inner ear defect, its onset is in later life, and the cause is gradual deterioration due to the aging process.

Deafened is another such term. Used critically it means that hearing was normal, language was acquired and is remembered, and the degree of deafness is so great that no useful residual hearing is retained. This degree of hearing loss can occur only from sensory-neural deafness. Therefore, the term deafened includes the factors of age of onset, site of the lesion, degree of the involvement, and language usage. Whenever the term deafened is used, these criteria should be met.

To summarize the problem of definition and classification of deafness, there are four basic factors or variables which must be considered. These are:

a. *Degree of deafness,* the basis of the classifications deaf and hard of hearing.

b. *The factor of time,* referred to as the age of onset; the basis of the classifications congenital and acquired.

c. *The causal factor,* the basis of the classifications exogenous and endogenous.

d. *The physical origin* of the impairment, referred to as the site of the lesion; the basis of the classifications sensory-neural, conductive, and central deafness.

Two other classifications used in the study of deafness and in educational and psychological work with the hearing impaired are:

a. *Presbycusia,* natural loss of hearing which accompanies advancement in age.

b. *Deafened,* profound sensory-neural deafness occurring subsequent to the age at which the use of language is retained, after approximately five years of age.

It should not be assumed that there is complete agreement as to the use of these terms. For example, there is not uniform agreement as to what constitutes a significant or even a total loss of hearing. It must be remembered that such difference of opinion is common in many areas of scientific study and in clinical and educational work. Often such differences are the bases of progress.

In fact, any consideration of definition and classification must entail analysis of the intent or purpose for which it is made. When the frame of reference and the assumptions are understood, the differences are less confusing and often entirely justified.

Perhaps the best example of the importance of assumptions occurs in connection with the different ways in which the degree of deafness is emphasized. The physician and audiologist frequently view a hearing loss as being severe only when the loss is so great that there is no response on the speech range at maximum levels of amplification. The educator views the degree of deafness as being critical when it impedes language acquisition and necessitates special remedial procedures educationally. The psychologist, on the other hand, emphasizes that a hearing loss is of critical significance as soon as the loss is of sufficient extent to influence development of psychological processes or to affect the adjustment and well-being of the individual. Thus, he might consider even minor hearing losses of importance and of warranting consideration.

When the assumptions and frame of reference are understood, usually there is close agreement as to what constitutes a significant hearing loss as well as on the other factors involved in classification. This is shown by the work of Davis.[2] He established the Social Adequacy Index, a criterion for the degree of deafness affecting social behavior and interpersonal relationships. While the physician, audiologist, educator, and psychologist each have their special needs for emphasis which must be recongnized, there is increasing agreement in the definition of what constitutes a significant loss and in the other aspects of classification.

INCIDENCE OF HEARING LOSS

It is of importance to secure as much information as possible regarding the incidence of impaired hearing. Such information is the basis for anticipating medical, training, and rehabilitative needs. These considerations are urgent because of rapid population increases and a lack of trained workers of all types, especially of trained teachers.

As indicated by the discussion in the previous section, it is not a simple task to define the minimum limits of a significant hearing loss. When the question of incidence is raised, it becomes

evident that it is not possible to use one definition for all professional and scientific purposes. For example, the Committee on the
Conservation of Hearing for the American Medical Association has
recommended that an individual who has a twenty decibel loss on
two frequencies should be referred to a physician for examination
and treatment. Although this practice is important in conservation, such an individual should not be viewed as having a significant loss of hearing from any other point of view. It is consequential only from the point of view of needing medical attention;
he is not in need of special education, speech development, and
he does not present problems of learning and adjustment. His
degree of deafness is not sufficient to interfere with personal or
social well-being.

Nevertheless, much work in hearing conservation consists of
identifying those in school populations who have slight hearing
losses, thus needing attention in order to prevent further loss of
hearing. When this group of children is included with those who
are defined as being in need of special educational procedures, it
has been estimated that approximately five per cent of school age
children have hearing losses which require some type of attention.
The incidence of hearing loss found by the use of screening procedures might vary on the basis of the training and experience of
the personnel, the equipment used, the testing environment, the
socio-economic level of the sample, and the age levels being
screened.

The incidence of impaired hearing also varies by age. This
factor was considered in the study by the Department of Health,
Education and Welfare.[6] They computed the incidence of hearing
loss by sex, by age, and by degree of deafness. Because of factors
such as childhood illnesses causing hearing loss in early life and
presbycusia in later life, this type of estimate of the number with
impaired hearing is most useful. In this study it was estimated
that two and one-half million persons in the United States have
some hearing loss. This figure was based on the 1953 census and
included those referred to as deaf as well as those referred to as
hard of hearing.

As indicated above, the number of individuals requiring only
medical attention is substantially greater than the number requir-

ing special attention or consideration from the point of view of the psychology of deafness. Therefore, this group should be distinguished from those whose sensory deprivation influences development of psychological functions and imposes stress on the processes of learning and adjustment. Even such delimitation does not consider variations from extreme effect to moderate and mild influence.

The number of children enrolled in schools for the deaf and hard of hearing provides a guide to the magnitude of the problem as it appears at one end of the life span. These figures as reported in the American Annals of the Deaf,[4] beginning with the year 1850, are presented in Table 1. There has been continuous increase in the population of hearing impaired children in schools, largely on the basis of increase in the general population. These figures reveal further that the incidence is higher in males than in females, a circumstance prevailing in virtually all categories of handicapped children. Much discussion has ensued as to whether this is a true sex difference or whether it can be attributed to variations in environmental demand between the sexes. Conclusive evidence is not available, but it is increasingly difficult to argue against a true sex difference, especially since the ratio of the difference appears to be remarkably stable. As can be seen in Table 1 this ratio has re-

TABLE 1. The number of children enrolled in schools and classes for the deaf and hard of hearing since 1850

Year	Male		Female		Total
	N	%	N	%	N
1850	651	57	486	43	1137
1858	901	55	743	45	1644
1868	1667	57	1270	43	2937
1878	3629	58	2598	42	6227
1888	4765	57	3571	43	8336
1897–98	5380	55	4369	45	9749
1907–08	6317	54	5331	46	11648
1917–18	6791	53	6001	47	12792
1927–28	8964	54	7701	46	16665
1937–38	10491	54	8787	46	19278
1947–48	9822	54	8494	46	18316
1958–59	13692	54	11833	46	25525
1959–60	14172	54	12271	46	26443
1960–61	14766	54	12823	46	17589
1961–62	15312	54	13217	46	28529
1962–63	15821	54	13577	46	29398
1963–64	16557	54	14242	46	30799

mained essentially unchanged for more than a century. Almost exactly 8% more male than female children have been enrolled in schools and classes for the deaf and hard of hearing during this period. Interpretation of this fact should consider that more male children are born per year. Irrespective of the cause of this greater incidence of hearing impaired males, the ratio seems to be so stable that programs should be planned accordingly. More facilities for male children will be required.

When all types and degrees of hearing loss, at all age levels, are combined it is obvious that the problem is one of considerable magnitude. Although much has been accomplished in regard to this sensory deprivation, much remains to be done, especially in terms of its effects on behavior.

REFERENCES

1. Committee on Nomenclature, Conference of Executives, American Schools for the Deaf, Am. Ann. Deaf, 83, 1, 1938.
2. Davis, H.: Hearing and Deafness. New York, Murray Hill Books, 1947.
3. Doctor, P. V.: Tabular statement of American Schools for the Deaf. Am. Ann. Deaf, 105, 1, 1960.
4. _____: Tabular statement of American Schools for the Deaf. Am. Ann. Deaf. 104, 2, 1959.
5. Doll, E. A.: Practical implications of the endogenous-exogenous classification of mental defectives. Am. J. Mental Deficiency, 50, 503, 1946.
6. Frisina, D. R.: Statistical information concerning the deaf and the hard of hearing in the United States. Am. Ann. Deaf, 104, 265, 1959.
7. Jourdain, M.: Diderot's Early Philosophical Works. London, Open Court Publishing Company, 1916.
8. Myklebust, H. R.: Significance of etiology in motor performance of deaf children with special reference to meningitis. Am. J. Psychol., 59, 249, 1946.

Suggestions for Further Study

Best, H.: Deafness and the Deaf in the United States. New York, Macmillan, 1943.
Ewing, I., and Ewing, A.: The Handicap of Deafness. New York, Longmans Green, 1938.
Farrar, A.: Arnold's Education of the Deaf. London, Francis Carter, 1923.
Goldstein, M.: Problems of the Deaf. St. Louis, The Laryngoscope Press, 1933,
Love, J. K.: The Deaf Child. New York, William Wood, 1911.

Chapter II

THE PROCESS OF HEARING

THE PROFESSIONAL WORKER in the area of deafness must be oriented to the sensory process itself. He must have a basic knowledge of the auditory mechanism, the ear, and of the physics of sound. The otolaryngologist is mainly concerned with the diseases causing deafness, the audiologist with the psychophysiology and psychoacoustics of hearing, while the educator, rehabilitation worker, and psychologist are principally concerned with the effect of the sensory deprivation on learning and adjustment. However, no professional worker can be concerned with only one aspect of the problem to the exclusion of all others. All facets overlap and interact.

The behavioral effects are related to the type and the extent of the impairment. The stress experienced by the individual varies on the basis of whether his deafness is sensory-neural, conductive, or central in type, whether it is moderate or severe in degree, and on the basis of the age at which it occurred. In other words, psychologically there is a relationship between the effect of the deafness and the site of the lesion, the age of onset, and the degree of the involvement.

As far as peripheral deafness is concerned, generally the greatest psychological effect occurs when the deafness is of the sensory-neural type, when onset is in early life, and when the impairment is severe. From these interrelationships of the problem it is clear that understanding the individual with deafness assumes a fundamental knowledge of the process of hearing and the nature of the sensory deprivation.

THE EAR

Sensory receptors, those parts of the body which serve as receivers of stimulation from outside of the body, are called *end-organs*. The ear is the end-organ for hearing. The end-organ is activated by stimuli which are converted into nerve impulses. It is these nerve impulses which are transmitted to the brain where

FIG. 1. Diagram of the ear.

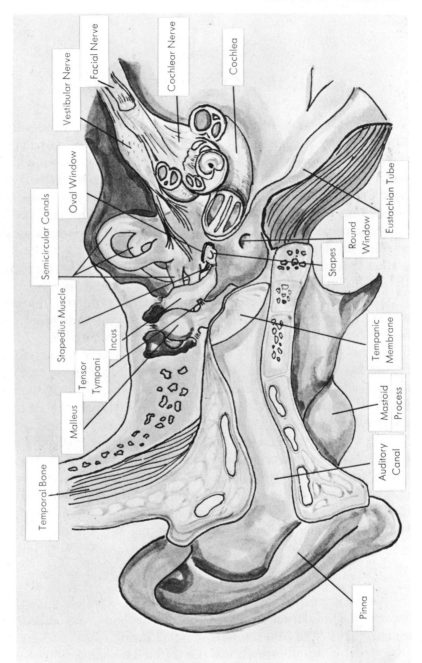

Facial Nerve

Vestibular Nerve

Cochlear Nerve

Cochlea

Oval Window

Semicircular Canals

Eustachian Tube

Round Window

Stapedius Muscle

Stapes

Incus

Tensor Tympani

Tympanic Membrane

Malleus

Mastoid Process

Temporal Bone

Auditory Canal

Pinna

they are interpreted and become meaningful experience. For better understanding of the problem of deafness it is necessary to recognize that hearing is one of Man's major sensory channels.

The Outer Ear

As shown in Figure 1, for purposes of study the ear is divided into three parts: the outer ear, the middle ear, and the inner ear. The outer ear consists of two parts: the pinna and the auditory canal. Some forms of animal life, such as the dog, can move their pinnas and focus them toward the source of sound and thereby hear better. Because Man cannot move his pinnas, he turns his head in order to catch the sounds in his environment more effectively.

The auditory canal is the opening on the side of the head leading inward to the middle ear, an arrangement by nature providing unusual protection for the middle and the inner ear. If these delicate parts of the ear were exposed on the side of the head, they would be subject to much damage and deterioration.

The Middle Ear

The tympanic membrane terminates the outer ear and serves as the beginning of the middle ear. It is a sturdy, thin, fibrous material which stretches tightly across the auditory canal. Attached to it is one of the ossicles, the malleus, and the tensor tympani, a small muscle which helps keep the tympanic membrane tight and flexible. The purpose of the tympanic membrane is to transmit air vibrations to the middle ear by causing the ossicular chain to vibrate; the ossicular chain consists of the malleus, the incus, and the stapes. The function of this chain is to conduct vibrations into the inner ear. The stapes provides a connection between the middle and inner ear and protrudes into the oval window, the avenue through which sound vibrations are transmitted, and into the inner ear. Around the foot-plate of the stapes is the annular ligament which seals the stapes in the oval window but permits vibratory action. The stapedius muscle assists further with making movement possible by pulling the stapes outward as the vibrations press it forward into the inner ear.

There are two other openings in the middle ear whose purpose and function are significant for the understanding of auditory processes: the Eustachian tube and the round window. The Eustachian tube provides a tubular connection between the middle ear and the naso-pharynx. Its purpose is to make possible the equalization of air pressure on both sides of the tympanic membrane. The round window, located just below the oval window, provides another membranous contact between the middle and inner ear. It is an opening covered with a thin, highly elastic, flexible membrane. As the stapes moves, the fluid in the inner ear is forced into the round window in a bulging action.

The function of the middle ear is to conduct the sound vibrations to the inner ear. Hence, it is referred to as the conductive mechanism. When hearing loss results from lesions in the middle ear, it is classified as conductive deafness.

The Inner Ear

The stapes delivers the sound vibrations to the inner ear through the oval window. Up to this point in the process of hearing, these vibrations have been mechanical in nature. The sound waves in the form of air impulses strike the tympanic membrane, causing a vibratory action throughout the ossicular chain; the process of one vibrating mass coming into contact with another. A vibratory type of energy cannot be transmitted via the nervous system and therefore must be converted into another form. This conversion takes place in the inner ear, a process which requires an intricate and delicate mechanism.

The inner ear is found in the temporal bone, which provides a maximum degree of protection. It consists of a series of tubular structures referred to as the *labyrinth*. These are divided into two major parts, the acoustic and the non-acoustic labyrinth. As this division implies, one part is vital to hearing while the other is not. The non-acoustic labyrinth includes the semicircular canals which comprise the end-organ for balance. There are three canals: the superior, posterior, and horizontal. Each canal is at right angles to the others, providing the organism with the necessary sensations irrespective of the position of the body. The brain is informed of the body position at all times, as each canal covers a specific set of positions.[20]

While the vestibular mechanism is the end-organ for balance in the same manner as the ear is the end-organ for hearing, there is an essential difference. The vestibular mechanism is not activated by stimuli originating from outside of the body but rather by movements of the body itself. As movements occur, the fluid in the semicircular canals activates the hair cells which in turn cause nerve impulses to be released. These impulses reach the brain as signals, via the nervous system. Because the vestibular mechanism cannot be stimulated from outside of the body, it is categorized as a proprioceptive sense.

Both the auditory and vestibular nerve impulses reach the brain by way of the eighth nerve. Therefore, in cases of sensory-neural deafness the otolaryngologist may use procedures such as the caloric test to differentiate between acoustic and non-acoustic involvements in the inner ear. The neurologist may use such procedures to distinguish between vestibular and ataxic disturbances. In the psychology of deafness these determinations are of considerable consequence because of the prevalence of deafness due to meningitis. This disease commonly affects both hearing and balance with specific implications for disorders in learning and adjustment.

The acoustic labyrinth is the part of the inner ear which pertains specifically to audition. The central portion of the inner ear is referred to as the vestibule. On one side of the vestibule are the semicircular canals and on the other side is the *cochlea*. It is the cochlea which is the vital organ in the chain of structures comprising the hearing mechanism. The cochlea is divided by a membranous wall into upper and lower scalae. The basilar membrane provides another division. It is on the vestibular side of the basilar membrane that the sensory cells are found which are known as the Organ of Corti. The vibratory energy from the middle ear causes the basilar membrane to bulge, activating the cilia on the Organ of Corti. It is the movement of these cilia which constitutes the specific conversion of vibratory energy into nerve impulses. This process is not fully understood, but much has been learned about it in recent years through the contributions of scientists such as Stevens and Davis,[21] Wever and Lawrence,[24] Davis,[7] and Bekésy.[2] When the nerve impulses are discharged, they proceed to the brain through the eighth nerve. Tests have been developed which in some instances make it possible to differentiate between defects in the cochlea and in the auditory nerve. However, all deafness which results from deficiences in the inner ear, irrespective of the specific site of the lesion, are classified as being of the sensory-neural type.

THE CENTRAL AUDITORY PATHWAYS

Hearing can be impeded by lesions in the middle ear, the inner ear, or in the auditory pathways in the central nervous system. While these pathways have not been fully ascertained, many aspects of their function have been established. As can be seen from Figure 2, nature has provided nerve pathways from each ear to both hemispheres of the brain. Such an arrangement is highly protective to the organism because if the pathways from one ear are damaged, the individual still has usefulness of both ears.

Each ear having connections to both cerebral hemispheres seems to have significance for the psychology of hearing. While conclusive evidence is lacking, studies indicate that both hemispheres are required for maximum effectiveness of audition, for the various psychological dimensions of audition. It is necessary for the individual to distinguish foreground from background sounds, noise from speech, to localize and to differentiate between many other aspects of auditory experience. Some of these more complex facets of auditory behavior seem to be possible only if both ears and both hemispheres of the brain are functioning simultaneously.

As shown in Figure 2, the auditory pathways in the central nervous system pass through connecting or "relay" stations on the way to the temporal lobe, to the auditory cortex. As the nerve impulses leave the cochlea they pass through the first junction in the central nervous system, the Cochlear Nucleus. From this point it ascends through the Olivary Complex, the Inferior Colliculus, the Medial Geniculate Body and then to the Auditory Cortex. It is these nerve connections leading from the Cochlear Nucleus to the Medial Geniculate Body that are known as the Auditory Pathways in the central nervous system. These pathways connect with motor nerves in the brain stem which apparently makes possible reflex actions, such as startle. Further knowledge of the auditory pathways is being gained especially through the studies of Neff,[15] Woolsey,[12] Ades,[1] and Galambos.[10]

In the study of auditory disorders it is necessary to distinguish

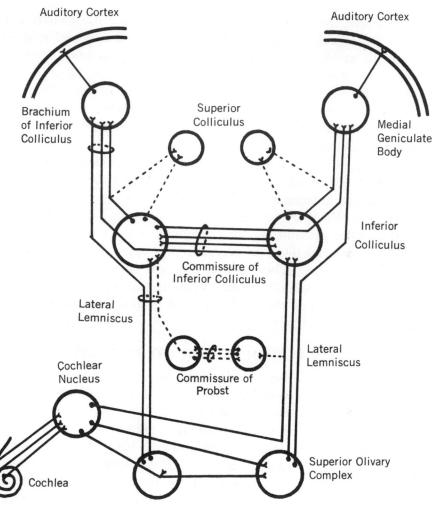

FIG. 2. The auditory pathways in the central nervous system. (Adapted from Neff.)

between deficiences at the level of the peripheral nervous system, the level of the auditory pathways, and those which occur as a result of lesions in the auditory cortex. When the damage occurs in the auditory pathways, it is referred to as *central deafness*. In other words, if the lesion occurs in the pathways, not at the level of the ear or in the interpretive area of the brain, it is classified as central deafness. This distinction or diagnosis cannot be made except inferentially at this time.

For the spoken word to be comprehensible the sounds must reach the superior temporal convolution in the temporal lobe, referred to as Wernicke's Area.[16] Damage to this area results in *receptive aphasia,* not central deafness. When the lesion impedes interpretation, the result is a language disorder, not one of transmission; therefore, the defect is properly designated as an aphasia. If the lesion disturbs perception of all types of sound, it is referred to as an *auditory agnosia.*

While differential diagnosis usually is presumptive, it can be assumed that central deafness varies in nature and in extent. It is apparent that in some instances normal hearing is retained for reflex function, such as startle, while speech is not heard because the lesion precludes the stimulus reaching the level of the cortex. Both end-organ and central deafness may occur in cases due to meningitis, rubella, or anoxia. When central deafness is present, it is of significance psychologically because learning and adjustment problems might ensue both on the basis of neurological deficit and of sensory deprivation.

MATURATION OF AUDITORY PROCESSES

Little study has been made of the maturational aspects of audition. In fact, much work has disregarded this phenomenon and has assumed that audition functions in an all or none manner. It is apparent from the work of Carmichael,[5] Froeschels,[9] and Wedenberg[22] that the infant hears at birth and even before birth. However, his auditory capacities immediately following birth and during early infancy differ in several respects from those of the more mature child and of the adult. For example, Wedenberg has demonstrated that startle reactions are present in the newborn. On the other hand, Piaget[17] has shown that the first *acquired* auditory responses date from the second month. He states further that sight and hearing are coordinated by the third month, as evidenced by scanning behavior such as turning the head in the direction of sound. In the study of hearing it is necessary to separate startle, or involuntary reactions, from listening, or voluntary behavior. Listening behavior must be acquired and is dependent on learning and maturation.

That auditory processes mature in other respects has been demonstrated by Spencer.[19] She investigated the maturation of auditory perception in normal children between two and six years of age. This study revealed that hearing, like vision, has a number of dimensions psychologically. Presumably all of these dimensions have not been studied, but it is apparent that factors such as rhythm, auditory memory span, and auditory discrimination are directly dependent on maturation. The age at which each of these dimensions attains full maturity has not been determined. By comparison, some of the visual processes such as stereoscopic vision, are known not to be matured until approximately eight years of age. (See Chapter XII.) While the maturational aspects of vision and audition may vary, the study of Spencer, the work of Myklebust[14] and of Birch and Mathews[3] suggests that full maturity of auditory functioning does not occur until approximately seven years of age; auditory memory span continues to mature well beyond this age.

The maturational aspects of audition have many implications for the study of deafness and other auditory disorders in making a differential diagnosis of deafness in young children.[14] Although the auditory mechanism is fully developed at the time of birth, the infant's capacity to respond to sound seems to be limited to reflex or to startle reactions. As indicated in Figure 2, this suggests that the infant is able to use only the auditory connections in the brain stem, in the sub-cortical region. Not until he is two or three months of age, has sufficient maturation of the total nervous system been achieved so that higher, more complex auditory functions can be incorporated voluntarily. Only much later does he attain the maturity to make fine auditory discriminations, to follow rhythms, and to achieve other aspects of mature auditory behavior. Presumably, therefore, the hearing mechanism does not mature, but ability to listen, as well as all other integrative uses of sound, does.

A difficult question arises regarding the extent to which a loss of hearing in early life may impede the maturation of auditory processes, although substantial residual hearing is retained. The work of Riesen,[18] discussed further in Chapter XII, may be relevant. He found that 16 months of light deprivation in a chimpanzee, which had been permitted normal development until eight months of age, resulted in irreversible changes in ganglion cells and in the optic nerve. The implication is that unless normal stimulation occurs, maturational development may be seriously reduced, especially as it pertains to sensory functioning. This problem warrants further consideration in relation to those with impaired hearing.

FUNDAMENTALS OF SOUND

Most sound in everyday life is produced by vibrating objects because any vibrating mass produces sound waves. Sound waves are the disturbances of air which are transmitted to the ear and activate the hearing mechanism. The individual learns to associate meanings with the auditory sensations and thereby has the experience referred to as hearing. Wever[23] has related past and present theories of hearing to research findings.

Man's auditory capacities have been well ascertained and his hearing mechanism is known to have certain limitations. For example, it does not respond to as wide a frequency range as does the dog's. Cobb[6] suggests that this is one reason Man has a higher potential for learning. The dog is more dependent on hearing alone, which limits his reactions and his adaptability. Man's hearing mechanism is adequate for his needs because other senses, especially vision, also are highly developed. It is necessary, however, to know the exact capacities and limitations of Man's ability to respond auditorially. Only from such knowledge can hearing loss be determined and interpreted.

To understand hearing requires familiarity with the nature of sound. Sound is the term used to designate the stimuli, usually airborne, which activate the hearing mechanism. It has both psychological and physical dimensions. The psychological dimensions are those which the individual experiences. For example, sounds may be judged as being high or low in pitch and as being loud or faint. Such judgments depend on subjective evaluation, on experience. In contrast, the physical dimensions of sound are objective and are determined and measured only by appropriate instruments; these attributes are defined in terms of physics.

The three primary psychological attributes of sound are *pitch, loudness,* and *timbre.* The three primary physical attributes are *frequency, intensity,* and *complexity.* There are correlates between the physical and psychological attributes which are shown schematically in Figure 3. This illustration shows that the relationships

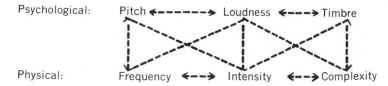

Psychological: Pitch ←-------→ Loudness ←---→ Timbre

Physical: Frequency ←--→ Intensity ←--→ Complexity

FIG. 3. The correlates between the physical and psychological attributes of sound.

between the physical and psychological attributes of sound are intricate and complex, a fact of importance in the study of hearing and deafness.

Frequency and Pitch

Stevens and Davis[21] have defined frequency as "the measure of the number of times per second that a vibrating particle executes a complete cycle." The range of frequencies to which Man can respond auditorially is from 20 to 20,000. The term *high frequency* refers to the upper and *low frequency* refers to the lower range of Man's auditory capacities. Man's hearing mechanism is limited in its response as compared to various forms of lower animal life, such as the dog. Furthermore, the human ear does not respond to all frequencies with equal facility or sensitivity. The band of frequencies to which it is most sensitive is from 500 to 4000 cycles, the range which is essential for hearing speech. Nature has provided the greatest auditory sensitivity for those frequencies which are essential for hearing the spoken word.

From Figure 3 it can be seen that there is a relationship between frequency and pitch. A listener judges high frequency sounds to be high and low frequency sounds to be low in pitch. However, pitch, one of the psychological attributes of sound, varies also on the basis of intensity. The relationship between pitch and intensity has been stated by Stevens and Davis[21] as, "for low tones, the pitch decreases with intensity, but for high tones, the pitch increases with intensity. For certain tones in the middle range, both effects are present to a certain degree."

Intensity and Loudness

Intensity is a physical attribute of sound while loudness is one of the subjective evaluations made by the individual as he receives auditory sensations. Intensity refers to the magnitude or the power of sound, to the energy of the sound waves; this energy is proportional to the amplitude of these waves. The unit of measurement in sound is the *decibel*. This unit can be compared to the foot in measuring distance or to the gallon in liquid measure. However, unlike these measures, the decibel is not a fixed unit. A foot always consists of 12 inches and a gallon of four quarts, but the magnitude of a decibel varies. It expresses a ratio rather than a fixed unit. A decibel expresses the extent to which one sound intensity is greater or less than another. If one sound is ten times greater than another, it is said to be one *bel* greater. This ratio is gross and inconvenient so it is divided into tenths, hence the unit decibel; a decibel is one-tenth of a bel. The bel, and thus the decibel, is based on a logarithmic scale. Therefore, the difference between five and six decibels is vastly less as compared to the difference between 95 and 96 decibels.

Because the decibel is a ratio and not a fixed unit, it is necessary to have a point of reference. To say that one sound is three db greater than another is meaningless since neither may be audible to the human ear. Therefore, a *standard reference* level is used, 0.0002 dynes per square centimeter at the frequency of 1000 cycles. This point of reference is used because, while it is not the exact equivalent, it is comparable to the amount of sound pressure required to make a 1000 cycle tone audible. Using 0.0002 dynes per square centimeter as a reference level, the human ear has an intensity tolerance range of from one to approximately 120 decibels. The 120 db level usually is considered the threshold of pain. This is shown in Figure 4.

There is another significant factor in the measurement of hearing. The faintest 1000 cycle tone detectable by the human ear has a sound pressure level of 0.0002 dyne cm.[2] When this is increased it must be changed by a certain amount before the individual can detect that an increment has occurred, a phenomenon referred to as the *just noticeable difference* (J.N.D.). When hearing is measured by the just noticeable difference method, the increments are called *sensation units*. The decibel and the sensation unit are not identical but they are comparable. When a sound is increased by one db it approximates being increased by one sensation unit.

The experience of loudness is not dependent alone on the in-

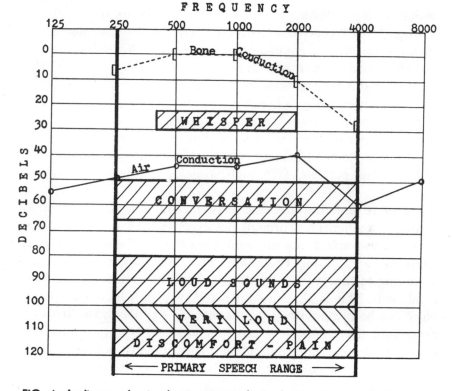

FIG. 4. Audiogram showing hearing test results for bone and air conduction, speech range and sound levels.

tensity of the sound; it varies also on the basis of frequency. A given sound is judged loudest if it falls in the middle frequency range. For a low or high frequency tone to be experienced as being as loud as a middle frequency tone, it must be increased in intensity. When this is done, it provides an *equal loudness contour*. Such calibration is essential in audiometers and in other types of electronic equipment. It is interesting that Man has the greatest ability to respond to loudness in the middle frequency range. Nature has provided most auditory responsiveness in the middle of the speech range where he needs it most.

Complexity and Timbre

Another set of interrelated dimensions of sound is complexity and timbre. Complexity is the objective, physical dimension and timbre is the subjective, psychological attribute to which it is related. Most sounds heard in everyday life are complex sounds, having a mixture of frequencies and intensities. Noise is an example of such sounds but so is speech and a note played on a violin. However, noise differs from speech and music in that it is less ordered in nature. Speech and music have predictable rhythms, intensities, and frequencies. Noise is a conglomeration of many frequencies and intensities without an ordered time sequence. For some purposes in the study of hearing and deafness it is necessary to use a defined noise pattern. One such stimulus is referred to as *white noise*.[13]

Timbre provides tremendously meaningful variations in our auditory experiences. Through the experience of timbre we recognize that two sounds are different even though the frequencies and intensities may be highly similar. The experience of timbre varies according to the ways in which the frequencies and intensities are combined. This is illustrated by the way in which one person's voice can be distinguished from another's. Although the frequency range and the intensity of the human voice is very similar from person to person, each individual's voice quality is unique; it has a quality of its own. It is timbre which gives it this quality and uniqueness.

These attributes of sound, frequency and pitch, intensity and loudness, complexity and timbre are the basis of measurement in hearing. They constitute the foundation for a definition of normal hearing and provide the criteria for evaluation of the extent and nature of a hearing loss, scientifically and clinically. Indirectly these attributes are the fundamental principles from which develops the psychology of deafness.

The Speech Range

The speech range refers to the band of frequencies found in the spoken word. Human speech does not extend from the lowest to the highest frequencies audible to Man. While the actual frequency range is slightly greater, for most purposes the speech range is defined as extending from 250 to 4000 cycles; see Figure 4. The low frequency vowels are found near the 500 cycle band and the high frequency consonants near the 3000 cycle band, with the majority of speech sounds falling between the frequencies of 500 and 2000. Approximately 15 per cent of the speech sounds fall between 250 and 500 cycles, 30 per cent between 500 and 1000 cycles, 40 per cent between 1000 and 2000 cycles, and 15 per cent between 2000 and 4000 cycles.[8] These figures are important in audiogram interpretation. Hearing losses are determined by computing the decibel loss on the speech range. Only through experience can one learn the practical, handicapping significance of a certain degree of deafness. The conversational level of intensity is a critical reference point. As shown in Figure 4, ordinary conversation falls between 50 and 65 decibels. Other common reference points are whisper, which falls at 25 to 30 decibels and traffic noise which may reach an intensity of 75 to 85 db. Psychologically a hearing loss becomes a handicap as soon as it precludes *normal* auditory contact with the environment, especially when it prevents hearing conversation.

TESTS OF HEARING

Hearing tests are of many different types but they can be classified as being formal or informal. For most scientific purposes only formal tests are used but for clinical purposes often it is necessary to use informal, uncalibrated, qualitative tests. The history and development of hearing tests, covering a period of several decades, has been reviewed by Goldstein,[11] Bunch,[4] and Hirsh.[13] Except for young children the most common are those given through the use of tuning forks or the audiometer. The otolaryngolist, in his clinical diagnostic work, administers three principal tuning fork tests, the Weber, Rinne, and Schwabach.[4] While these are of considerable value to the physician, they are mainly qualitative and thus are not used in most scientific work.

The Audiometer

The audiometer is the instrument which was developed specifically for the precise measurement of hearing. The stimulus consists of pure tones, making it possible to control rigidly the frequency and intensity. Because of the cost and portability problems involved, most audiometers are not made to test the entire range of Man's hearing; the typical audiometer includes only the frequencies from 125 to 8000. This frequency band includes approximately one octave above and one octave below the speech range. Likewise, the entire range of Man's ability to respond to intensity is not covered by the typical audiometer. Characteristically the intensity range included is from the threshold of audibility to 100 db, because it has been generally assumed that a loss of 100 db represents a total loss of useful hearing.

For most purposes in the study of impaired hearing it is necessary to do both air and bone conduction tests. The *air conduction test* measures the response capacities of the total auditory system. The receiver is placed on the ear and the stimulus presented at the desired intensities. The tones are airborne through the auditory canal to the tympanic membrane. From there they are conducted through the middle and inner ear to the auditory nerve. All parts of the hearing mechanism are being stimulated and tested simultaneously. This is not true of the *bone conduction test* inasmuch as the sound is transmitted through the temporal bone directly to the inner ear; the middle ear is circumvented. The *bone conduction test* makes it possible to compare the responses of the middle and inner ear.

Administration of both air and bone conduction tests provides a measure of the individual's hearing acuity when the total hearing mechanism is involved and when the middle ear is not taking part, a procedure which is revealing diagnostically. When a hearing loss exists by air conduction but not by bone conduction, there is deafness resulting from a lesion in the middle ear. If the air and bone conduction results are equal, usually it is assumed that the lesion is in the inner ear, although the presence of central deafness cannot be denied. When the bone conduction results reveal better hearing than by air, but do not reach the level of normal, both middle and inner ear factors are assumed.

Audiometric findings have broad implications for medical treatment, educational planning, rehabilitative procedures and for predicting the psychological effects of the deafness. For example, sensory-neural deafness often is not medically treatable and may be total, whereas conductive deafness is treatable medically or surgically, and the degree of loss does not exceed the limits usually referred to as hard of hearing. This illustrates the importance of the classifications discussed in Chapter I.

The Audiogram

When audiometric test results are properly recorded graphically, the composite is an *audiogram*. The responses are recorded at the point where the frequency and intensity meet. Usually bone and air conduction are recorded on the same audiogram, as shown in Figure 4.

REFERENCES

1. Ades, H. W. and Brookhart, J. M.: Central auditory pathway. J. Neurophysiol., 13, 189, 1950.
2. Bekésy, G.: Experiments in Hearing. New York, McGraw-Hill, 1960.
3. Birch J. W. and Mathews, J.: The hearing of mental defectives. Am. J. Mental Deficiency, 55, 384, 1951.
4. Bunch, C. C.: Clinical Audiometry. St. Louis, C. V. Mosby, 1943.
5. Carmichael, L.: Manual of Child Psychology. New York, John Wiley and Sons, 1946.
6. Cobb, S.: Borderlands of Psychiatry. Cambridge, Harvard University Press, 1948.
7. Davis, H.: Biophysics and physiology of the inner ear. Phys. Rev. 37, 1, 1957.
8. _____: Hearing and Deafness. New York, Murray Hill Books, 1947.
9. Froeschels, E. and Beebe, H.: Testing hearing of newborn infants. Arch. Otolaryng., 44, 710, 1946.
10. Galambos, R., Schwartzkopff, J. and Reipert, A.: A microelectrode study of superior olivary nuclei. Am. J. Physiol., 197, 527, 1959.
11. Goldstein, M.: Problems of the Deaf. St. Louis, The Laryngoscope Press, 1933.
12. Harlow, H. F. and Woolsey, C. N.: Biological and Biochemical Bases of Behavior. Madison, University of Wisconsin Press, 1958.
13. Hirsh, I. J.: The Measurement of Hearing. New York, McGraw-Hill, 1952.
14. Myklebust, H. R.: Auditory Disorders in Children. New York, Grune and Stratton, 1954.
15. Neff, W. D.: Auditory Nervous System, in Coates, G. M. (ed). Otolaryngology, Hagerstown, W. F. Prior, Volume I, 1955.
16. Penfield, W. and Roberts, L.: Speech and Brain Mechanisms. Princeton, Princeton University Press, 1959.
17. Piaget, J.: The Origins of Intelligence in Children. New York, International Universities Press, 1952.
18. Riesen, A. H.: Plasticity of behavior: Psychological series, Harlow, H. F. (ed.). Biological and Biochemical Bases of Behavior. Madison, University of Wisconsin Press, 1958.
19. Spencer, E.: An investigation of the maturation of various factors of auditory perception in preschool children. Evanston, Unpublished Doctoral Dissertation, Northwestern Univ., 1958.
20. Spiegel, E. A. and Sommer, I.: Neurology of the Eye, Ear, Nose and Throat. New York, Grune and Stratton, 1944.
21. Stevens, S. S. and Davis, H.: Hearing: its Psychology and Physiology. New York, John Wiley and Sons, 1938.

22. Wedenberg, E.: Auditory tests on newborn infants. Acta Oto-laryng., 46, 446, 1956.

23. Wever, E. G.: Theory of Hearing. New York, John Wiley and Sons, 1949.

24. _____ and Lawrence, M.: Physiological Acoustics. Princeton, Princeton University Press, 1954.

Suggestions for Further Study

Barr, B.: Pure tone audiometry for preschool children. Acta Oto-laryng., Suppl. 128, 1956.

Bocca, E.: Clinical aspects of cortical deafness. Laryngoscope, 68, 301, 1958.

Carhart, R.: Clinical application of bone conduction audiometry. Arch. Oto-laryng., 51, 798, 1950.

_____ and Jerger, J.: A preferred method for clinical determination of pure tone thresholds. J. Speech and Hearing Disorders, 24, 330, 1959.

Hardy, W. G.: Problems of audition, perception and understanding. Washington, D. C., The Volta Bureau (reprint), 1956.

Heller, M. F.: Functional Otology. New York, Springer, 1955.

Jerger, J. (ed.): Modern Developments in Audiology. New York & London, Academic Press, 1963.

Jerger, J. F. et al.: Some relations between normal hearing for pure tones and for speech. J. Speech and Hearing Research, 2, 126, 1959.

Meyerson, L.: Hearing for speech in children. Acta Oto-laryng., Suppl. 128, 1956.

Newby, H.: Audiology: Principles and practice. New York, Appleton-Century-Crofts, Inc., 1964.

Stevens, S. S. (ed.): Handbook of Experimental Psychology. New York, John Wiley and Sons, 1951.

Travis, L. E. (ed.): Handbook of Speech Pathology. New York, Appleton-Century-Crofts, 1957.

Walsh, E. G.: An investigation of sound localization in patients with neurological abnormalities. Brain, 80, 222, 1957.

Watson, L. A. and Tolan, R.: Hearing Tests and Hearing Instruments. Baltimore, Williams and Wilkins, 1949.

Chapter III

TYPES AND CAUSES OF DEAFNESS

SENSORY IMPAIRMENT MIGHT BE DUE to involvements of the peripheral nervous system, of the central nervous system, or of both of
these systems simultaneously. The scientific study of causation in
disease, referred to as *etiology,* is important in all types of disabilities. Deafness is not an exception. The science of etiology is basic
to preventive medicine and furthermore, when etiology is ignored,
the problems resulting from disease usually are oversimplified. This
is true especially in relation to the learning and adjustment problems which often ensue.

In the psychology of deafness it is generally assumed that the
hearing loss has resulted from peripheral nervous system involvement, in which case a reciprocal relationship exists between the
type and the cause of the deafness. If the type, sensory-neural or
conductive, can be established, an inference can be made concerning the cause. Likewise, if the cause can be determined an inference
can be made concerning the type. Moreover, postulations as to the
type of deafness can be made when it has been determined that the
condition is exogenous or endogenous, congenital or acquired, and
when it is known that the person is deaf or hard of hearing. Establishing the eitology also has implications for the psychological
effects which might follow; these are emphasized in the discussion
of Deafness and Psychological Processes in Part Two.

Causes of deafness vary from one geographic area to another
and from country to country. Hence, although some diseases and
hereditary factors are common to all geographic areas, generalizations must be made cautiously. Etiology also varies with age.
Childhood diseases are common contributors in early life and
middle ear infections are characteristic during school age. The most
frequent etiology in early and middle life is otosclerosis, while in
late adulthood it is presbycusia.

Changes occur in the incidence of any particular etiology,
mainly because of new discoveries in the prevention and treatment

of disease. Until recent years mastoiditis was a common cause of impaired hearing but with the advent of antibiotics its occurrence has been greatly reduced. Such developments have been interpreted as indicating that incidence of impaired hearing will decline. Some advances in the treatment of disease do reduce, if not eliminate, a specific cause of deafness. Other advances might cause an individual to survive an illness but not without having sustained a loss of hearing. For example, prior to the introduction of antibiotics tubercular meningitis often was fatal; it was rare to see a child having deafness with this etiology. Now one rather frequently encounters the child who survived the disease but has severe sensory-neural deafness. Contrary to general impressions most surveys, as shown in Chapter I, do not indicate that the incidence of deafness is either increasing or decreasing. Perhaps advancements in treatment prevent deafness as often as they result in survival with deafness. Another factor to be considered is the number having endogenous hearing impairment. This incidence seems not to have changed significantly over a period of years.

As part of our National Study of the psychological effects of deafness we investigated the etiology of hearing loss as reported for children in schools for the deaf. This study covered all geo-

TABLE 2. Incidence of deafness by etiology for children in schools for the deaf

Etiology	Males		Females		Total	
	N	%	N	%	N	%
Day						
Meningitis	28	17.7	21	13.7	49	15.8
Endogenous	25	15.8	34	22.3	59	19.0
Exogenous	41	25.9	36	23.5	77	24.8
Undetermined	64	40.6	62	40.5	126	40.4
Total	158	100.0	153	100.0	311	100.0
Residential						
Meningitis	32	11.8	11	4.6	43	8.4
Endogenous	65	24.1	62	25.7	127	24.8
Exogenous	82	30.4	70	29.0	152	29.8
Undetermined	91	33.7	98	40.7	189	37.0
Total	270	100.0	241	100.0	511	100.0
Day and Residential						
Meningitis	60	14.0	32	8.1	92	11.3
Endogenous	90	21.0	96	24.4	186	22.6
Exogenous	123	28.7	106	26.9	229	27.8
Undetermined	155	36.3	160	40.6	315	38.3
Total	428	100.0	394	100.0	822	100.0

graphic areas of the United States and included Day, Residential, Public, and Private schools. The age range was from seven to 17 years. The incidence found for each type of etiology is presented in Table 2. The etiological classifications used were endogenous, exogenous, unknown, and meningitis. Meningitis was classified separately because of the importance of this disease in the etiology of deafness. The differences by school were analyzed statistically. The only significant difference was for the meningitic females; more females having this etiology were in Day Schools. If a girl sustains deafness from meningitis in early life, she is more likely to attend a Day than a Residential School. On the other hand the incidence of endogenous deafness was higher in Residential Schools, but this difference did not attain statistical significance. These data suggest that in general deafened children more often attend Day Schools, while those with endogenous or congenital deafness may more often attend a Residential School.

When the total etiological groups were compared by sex, a highly significant difference occurred between males and females in the incidence of meningitis; this disease was reported much more frequently for males. Explanation of this finding is difficult. It seems that boys contract meningitis more frequently than females, or they lose hearing more frequently as a result of this disease. It is interesting that the total incidence of children deaf from meningitis seems not to have changed over a period of years. The incidence in this study was 11.3 per cent and Best[2] reported 10 per cent. Frisina[11] studied the etiology of mentally retarded deaf and found that 11 per cent had an etiology of meningitis. This disease has been the most frequent contributor to exogenous deafness for a period of several decades, and it occurs more frequently in males than in females.

The incidence of endogenous deafness also was investigated. Where deafness was reported to be endogenous, information was secured regarding other deaf relatives; this was defined to include parents, brothers, sisters, grandparents, aunts, uncles, and first cousins. The results are presented in Table 3. When these data were analyzed by statistical tests, it was found that the Residential School children reported more deaf relatives than those in Day Schools; the difference was statistically significant. As shown in

TABLE 3.   The relatives reported to be deaf in the families of endogenously
deaf children

Relatives	Day School N	Day School %	Residential School N	Residential School %	Total N	Total %
Fathers	12	12	35	14	47	13
Mothers	12	12	40	16	52	15
Brothers	28	29	58	23	86	24
Sisters	28	29	62	24	90	25
Grandparents	3	3	7	3	10	3
Aunts	2	2	14	5	16	5
Uncles	9	9	23	9	32	9
Cousins	4	4	16	6	20	6
Total	98	100	255	100	353	100

Table 2, the number reporting endogenous deafness in Residential Schools, as compared to Day Schools, fell slightly below the level required for statistical significance. However, on the basis of the finding shown in Table 3, there is little question but that there are substantially more deaf persons in the families of the children in Residential Schools. It is interesting to note that the ratio of each of the the family members who were deaf was highly comparable for the Day and Residential School children. Essentially the same ratio of parents and other relatives were reported to be deaf by the two groups. This has important psychological implications in that other family members being deaf may influence the processes of identification, language development, and other developmental aspects of behavior.

A group of hearing impaired persons, most of whom acquired deafness in adulthood also was included in our study of etiology. All were receiving services at a Hearing Society and classified as being hard of hearing rather than deaf. The incidence of the various etiologies is shown in Table 4. These data derive from a

TABLE 4.   The etiologies reported by a group of hard of hearing adults

	Sensory-Neural N	Sensory-Neural %	Conductive N	Conductive %
Otitis Media			8	8
Otosclerosis			25	26
Endogenous	12	13		
Childhood Illnesses	11	12		
Meningitis	4	4		
Trauma	1	1		
Unknown	35	36		
Total	63	66	33	34

small, select sample and generalizations cannot be made relative to the total population who sustain impaired hearing in adulthood. Nevertheless, in our sample approximately twice as many had sensory-neural deafness as compared to conductive; 26 per cent reported otosclerosis and 13 per cent reported endogenous deafness. This incidence of endogenous deafness is comparable to that found for children in schools for the deaf. Only 4 per cent of the adults reported meningitis as the etiology while 11 per cent of the children were reported to have deafness as a result of this disease, indicating the variations in etiology on the basis of age.

The etiologies for the children and adults are summarized in Table 5. Otosclerosis was classified as endogenous and meningitis was combined with the other exogenous causes. The causations found are similar by school as well as for the children and adults.

TABLE 5. A summary of the etiologies of deafness found for children and adults

	% Endogenous	% Exogenous	% Unknown
Day School	19.0	40.6	40.4
Residential School	24.8	38.2	37.0
Hearing Society	38.5	25.0	36.5

CONDUCTIVE DEAFNESS

Conductive deafness results from deficiency of function in the middle ear. Such deafness may result from disease, trauma, or maldevelopment. One of the most common causes is otitis media, which might accompany any illness but commonly results from colds, sinus infections, and allergies. Both chronic and acute otitis media may result in a loss of hearing. The use of antibiotics and tympanoplastic surgery, however, has facilitated treatment of this condition.[24]

Otosclerosis is another common etiology of conductive deafness. This disease results in a pathological growth of bone tissue around the footplate of the stapes in the oval window. According to Shambaugh[23] clinical otosclerosis occurs in approximately 1 per cent of the population. It is viewed as being due largely to endogenous factors, although it is more common in women than in men. Its onset may be rapid during pregnancy. The mean age at which the hearing loss becomes noticeable is 19 to 21 years.

Fenestration and stapes mobilization surgery have been successful in restoring hearing in favorable cases and in modifying the
degree of hearing loss in less favorable cases of otosclerotic deafness. While such surgery is beneficial, the individual with this
type of deafness often requires other services, such as assistance
in procuring a properly fitted hearing aid, instruction in speech
reading, and vocational guidance. Furthermore, although the degree of hearing loss usually is moderate, it may cause emotional
stress and development of depression, anxiety, or other psychological and psychiatric conditions which require treatment.

Exogenous and Endogenous

Otosclerosis is the main contributor to hereditary conductive
deafness. While this adds to the population of hearing impaired
people, endogeny is a greater problem in connection with sensory-
neural deafness. There are many exogenous conditions which result in conductive deafness; hence, it is these etiologies which contribute the major challenge from the point of view of conservation
and adjustment. In terms of both research and clinical efforts it
is necessary to be aware that middle ear deafness may be either
exogenous or endogenous in type. Also it is the group having conductive deafness which constitutes the major portion of all persons
having moderate hearing loss, and it is this group which adds
greatly to the total population having impaired hearing.

Congenital and Acquired

The classification of congenital or acquired is based on time
of the occurrence of the deafness. Congenital means present at the
time of birth, while acquired means that the onset was after birth.
Conductive deafness is mainly of the acquired type, but can occur
congenitally. For example, clinical otosclerosis might be present
at the time of birth and is then referred to as congenital fixation
of the stapes. Auditory atresia also might be present congenitally.

Conductive Deafness and Degree of Hearing Loss

Conductive deafness does not exceed a maximum of 60 db.[12]
When a hearing loss exceeds 60 db, some deficiency of inner ear
functioning is present irrespective of the middle ear involvement.

Although the middle ear is nonfunctional, vibratory stimulation can reach and activate the inner ear. Therefore, individuals having conductive deafness usually fall in the category of hard of hearing rather than deaf. It follows that the educational and psychological problems derived from middle ear deafness are less severe than those associated with sensory-neural deafness.

SENSORY-NEURAL DEAFNESS

Sensory-neural is the term used to designate hearing losses resulting from inner ear deficiencies. Other terms used for this condition are perceptive, nerve, and inner ear deafness. Sensory-neural hearing impairment, like conductive deafness, results from three main causes: disease, trauma, and maldevelopment; however, another contributing factor is presbycusia. As shown in Table 2, disease is the most common cause of sensory-neural deafness in children.

Meningitis was the most frequently reported illness causing deafness. This disease often destroys both the acoustic and non-acoustic labyrinths of the inner ear. Hence, it may not only cause deafness but also marked disturbance of balance; total loss of hearing and destruction of the semi-circular canals are not uncommon. Depending on the age of onset, a few days to a few weeks might be required for the individual to learn to maintain balance through vision and kinesthetic sensation. Typically such persons continue to have more difficulty in maintaining balance in darkness and have a "lunging" gait; they might reveal in other ways that they have difficulty with equilibrium. Meningitis is etiologically significant for other reasons. It is a disease of the outer membrane covering the brain and sometimes it causes damage to brain tissues; the inflammation includes the brain, not only the meninges. This is referred to as meningo-encephalitis. Usually such sequelae can be identified by neurological and electroencephalographic study. The psychological impact of this disease might be dramatic; the onset of deafness is sudden with emotional trauma being common. Furthermore, other handicaps, such as psychoneurological learning disorders, often are present; these disorders are discussed in Chapter XIII.

Since the work of Gregg,[13] *maternal rubella*, another disease which frequently causes hearing losses of the sensory-neural type, has received increasing attention. The involvements of this condition have been explored by various workers and a number of other congenital conditions have been found to be caused by this prenatal disease. Blindness, cardiac disorders, and mental deficiency frequently are attributed to this etiology.[17] Study of maternal rubella has highlighted the importance of the early months of pregnancy. Deafness results most frequently if the rubella is contracted during the third month. If it is contracted earlier, more widespread involvements may occur.

In our study of etiology for children in schools for the deaf 3.8 per cent reported maternal rubella as the cause. A higher incidence can be assumed as this etiology was not known until recent years. Furthermore, those with slight losses of hearing would not have been included in this study, inasmuch as only those with moderate or greater degrees of impairment would be entered in schools for the deaf. Characteristically rubella results in a degree of deafness which is moderately severe but not total. The greatest loss is for the high frequencies with relatively slight loss for low frequencies. In some instances other conditions are superimposed on the hearing loss. These include aphasia, dyslexia, mental retardation, and motor disorders such as spasticity and ataxia. We can assume that there is a significant number of children with an etiology of maternal rubella in schools for the deaf. Moreover, it is probable that this group presents characteristic problems of learning and adjustment and has special needs in terms of the psychology of deafness.

Sensory-neural deafness also can be caused by *erythroblastosis foetalis*. Lamm[17] has emphasized the importance of this etiology in pediatric neurology. This disease is referred to as Rh because the original study of its effects was made on rhesus monkeys. The pathology derives from the incompatibility of blood type between the mother and the fetus, occurring when the mother is Rh negative and the fetus is Rh positive. It has been estimated that approximately 15 per cent of the population have Rh negative blood type. The erythroblastosis foetalis results from the Rh negative blood developing antibodies against the Rh positive blood, causing anemia, deprivation of oxygen in the blood stream with destruction of cells and nerve tissue. Goodhill[12] has stressed the importance of this condition in the causation of congenital sensory-neural deafness. Masland, Sarason and Gladwin[19] have emphasized this etiology in relation to cerebral palsy and mental deficiency. It is not uncommon to find multiple involvements in Rh children.

Mumps, pertussis, influenza, measles and various other diseases are known to cause sensory-neural deafness.[4, 25] As shown in Table 2, 27.8 per cent of the children studied were reported to have exogenous deafness from causes other than meningitis. With meningitis included, a total of 39.1 per cent were reported to have deafness of this type, constituting a considerable number of the total population of hearing impaired children.

The most common etiologies for sensory-neural deafness other than disease are trauma and presbycusia, the largest group being the presbycusic. As standards of living and scientific knowledge have combined to add to the life span, presbycusia has become very common, the specialized study of which is referred to as geriatric audiology. The loss of hearing which accompanies advancement in age becomes a significant handicap on the average at approximately 65 years of age but the onset of this gradual deterioration can be seen much earlier through audiometric study. A measurable presbycusic loss appears at approximately 40 years of age. Because of Man's reserve of hearing, it does not affect his state of well-being until much later. This is in contrast to vision because the average age for needing refraction as a result of presbyopia is between 40 and 45 years.

The nature of the process of deterioration due to aging is not fully understood. Kaplan[16] has suggested that it is essentially a cellular deterioration. The deterioration is generalized because ability to hear, see, remember, engage in abstraction, and perform motor acts all gradually show a decline. As Carhart[5] has indicated, there are many individual differences with the rate of aging varying from person to person. Nevertheless, most people have significant hearing losses when they reach the age of 65 to 70 years.

The psychological problems peculiar to the aged are manifold. In addition to deterioration of sensory and other physiological functions, there might be marked problems of resettlement, rejection, and loneliness. The psychologist concerned with sensory deprivation frequently encounters the presbycusic and study of the behavioral effects of this type of hearing loss is an essential aspect of the psychology of deafness.

Classifications

Sensory-neural is a diagnostic classification indicating the site of the lesion. Such classification has many implications for learning and adjustment but these problems can be understood more readily if the condition is classified also in other ways; being categorized on the basis of the site of the lesion is insufficient.

The handicap associated with sensory-neural deafness is clarified by the use of the classification of *deafened*. As defined in Chapter I this refers to onset occurring after about five years of age, no useful residual hearing, and memory for language. Most individuals falling into this classification have deafness as a result of disease, notably meningitis. However, some have an etiology of trauma, while others have progressive endogenous nerve deafness with onset after five years of age. The classification of deafened is most consequential in meeting educational and adjustment needs. Because the deafened retain language and memory for speech their educational, psychological, and rehabilitative needs are different from those with congenital deafness, or with onset before five years of age.

Much sensory-neural deafness is *exogenous;* in children often it is exogenous and congenital. This is illustrated by hearing losses due to maternal rubella and erythroblastosis foetalis. The age of onset is prenatal but the causation is exogenous.

Endogenous sensory-neural deafness has been recognized over a period of many years. Studies of the incidence of this condition have been made by Fay,[9] Bell,[1] Day, Fusfeld and Pintner,[7] Hopkins and Guilder,[15] and Wildervanck.[26] Best[2] in reviewing the evidence in 1943 found that 28.7 per cent of the group studied had deaf relatives. In our study (see Table 2) it was found that 19 per cent in Day Schools and 24.8 per cent in Residential Schools reported endogenous deafness. Of the hard of hearing adults, 38.5 per cent reported this etiology. When these three groups are combined the total incidence of endogenous deafness is 27.4 per cent, which is exceedingly close to the figure given by Best. These studies covering a span of from two to approximately eight decades do not indicate a decline or an increase in the incidence of endogenous deafness; about one-fourth of all deafness, not including presbycusia, is endogenous. Otosclerosis has been included in the above figure and therefore it must not be assumed that this total incidence of endogenous hearing loss is of the sensory-neural type. Nevertheless, with the exception of otosclerosis, most endogenous hearing impairment is of this type. While Hopkins and Guilder have shown that endogenous hearing impairment might be associated with other anomalies, it is not uncommon to find this condition in families who are otherwise superior intellectually and culturally, and in which there are no other defects.

Sensory-neural deafness may be either *congenital* or *acquired;* as compared to conductive it is more frequently congenital. Those with acquired inner ear impairment include the trauma and disease entity cases. The congenital group includes the endogenous, maternal rubella, erythroblastosis, and all others having impairment because of prenatal or natal involvements.

Congenital and acquired as a classification refers to the time of occurrence, the age when the deafness was sustained, which is a significant factor in relation to the learning and adjustment problems resulting from hearing impairment. The incidence of these types of deafness was explored in our National Study of the psychology of deafness. The results are given in Table 6. When statistical tests of significance were used, no differences appeared by sex or by type of school. Congenital and acquired deafness was equally common in the males and females and in the Day and Residential population. This is of considerable consequence when these groups are compared on the psychological concomitants of hearing

TABLE 6. The incidence of congenital and acquired hearing losses in children in schools for the deaf

Age	7		9		11		13		15		17		Total	
Sex	M	F	M	F	M	F	M	F	M	F	M	F	M	F
					Residential									
Congenital	26	15	22	24	35	17	19	26	26	20	13	13	141	115
Acquired	22	14	13	17	47	42	16	17	21	24	10	12	129	126
					Day									
Congenital			31	22	17	33	30	22	9	10			87	87
Acquired			19	22	20	15	19	21	13	8			71	66

loss. Although the differences were not significant, 60 per cent of the Day group had congenital and 40 per cent had acquired deafness; in the Residential group 47 per cent had congenital while 53 per cent had acquired. These data revealed that sex and type of school were not significantly related to age of onset when the children were classified as congenital or acquired.

Deaf and Hard of Hearing

All degrees of hearing loss are found in the sensory-neural group. However, in general those with conductive deafness classify as hard of hearing while those with sensory-neural loss include many with profound, or total deafness. Therefore the involvements associated with inner ear defects usually are more severe. In our study of etiology the degree of hearing loss (Better Ear Average) was ascertained for the meningitic, the endogenous, exogenous, and undetermined groups. Audiometric data were not available for the total number studied. This analysis included 777 children and the results are presented in Table 7. When statistical tests of significance were applied, two differences occurred, both for total groups. The females in Day Schools had a greater loss of hearing than the females in Residential Schools. Furthermore, when the sexes were combined, the total group in the Day Schools had a somewhat greater degree of deafness. The difference in decibels was not large but it was significant. It must be concluded that those in Residential Schools had the lesser hearing loss, the greater difference being between the females.

TABLE 7. The mean decibel loss by etiology for children in schools for the deaf

	Males			Females			Totals		
	N	Mean	SD	N	Mean	SD	N	Mean	SD
Meningitic	31	86.2	15.0	11	93.3	10.8	42	88.1	14.3
Exogenous	74	79.8	15.4	64	75.1	29.2	138	77.3	22.9
Endogenous	60	81.1	16.8	58	82.9	16.9	118	82.0	16.8
Undetermined	79	81.1	16.2	85	80.1	17.3	164	80.5	16.8
Totals	244	81.3	16.0	218	80.0	21.5	462	80.7	18.8
Day									
Meningitic	27	86.3	13.5	19	88.2	13.8	46	87.0	13.5
Exogenous	39	84.7	15.3	39	82.5	18.9	78	83.6	17.1
Endogenous	24	83.7	14.5	34	85.7	12.1	58	84.9	13.1
Undetermined	70	83.6	12.8	63	88.1	13.4	133	85.8	13.2
Totals	160	84.3	13.7	155	86.2	14.8	315	85.3	14.3

Residential

It is necessary to use caution when discussing differences between Day and Residential Schools on the basis of degree of deafness. Both groups have a profound loss of hearing. As the data in Parts Two, Three and Four indicate, apparently the differences which exist have little modifying influence on the basic effects of deafness. Perhaps beyond a certain point other factors, such as age of onset or intelligence, are more consequential. The type of school was unrelated to degree of deafness for the specific groups, as well as for those in whom the etiology was undetermined. These data disclose that children in schools for the deaf constitute a group with severe hearing loss of the sensory-neural type.

The discussion in this chapter has emphasized that the determination of etiology is a noteworthy aspect of all scientific study of deafness. It is relevant to the work of the physician, audiologist, educator, and psychologist. The findings that Day and Residential School populations are comparable relative to age of onset, etiology, degree of deafness, and to site of the lesion is pertinent to the data presented in Parts Two, Three, and Four. If these groups differed significantly on any one of these factors, differences in learning and adjustment might be attributed to such variation. This not being the case, any differences which exist must be explained on other bases.

CENTRAL DEAFNESS

Deafness occurs because of three major types of disorders. The one which is most frequent, and to which the data in the following sections pertain, is that which results from peripheral nervous system defects, from end-organ deficiencies. The other types are central and psychogenic deafness. *Central deafness* was defined in Chapter H. It results from dysfunction or maldevelopment of the auditory pathways in the central nervous system. While it can be determined that such deafness is present in certain individuals, the nature and extent of this condition has not been fully established. Most authorities agree that central deafness occurs only when the pathways to both hemispheres are impaired. Relatively little change from normal acuity occurs in lower animals from the severation of the pathways to one hemisphere. The same is true of hemispherectomized humans. However, the degrees of deafness resulting are relatively unexplored in other respects. Differences in the effects might be expected if the damage occurs at the superior olivary nucleus, as compared to the lateral lemniscus, the inferior colliculus, or the medial geniculate body.

In much diagnostic work both peripheral and central deafness must be suspected, especially in children presenting problems of the psychoneurological type. These children often have histories of anoxia, maternal rubella, erythroblastosis foetalis, or of central nervous system diseases such as meningitis and encephalitis. Fiedler,[10] Hardy,[14] and Myklebust[21] have reported studies on children presenting disorders of this type. Whenever central deafness is suspected, intensive study must be made of both psychological and neurological aspects.

PSYCHOGENIC DEAFNESS

A deficiency in hearing which is psychological rather than organic in nature is referred to as *psychogenic deafness*. This condition, found in both children and adults, must be distinguished from malingering. The psychologically deaf person is unaware that he has normal hearing. He is not volitionally trying to make himself appear deaf. His inability to use his hearing is the result of mental illness, and he is firmly convinced that he cannot hear. The malingerer, on the other hand, is aware that he has normal hearing and is volitionally intent on deluding others, usually with some specific purpose in mind. His behavior, too, is abnormal with implications for mental illness. Most psychogenic deafness in adults seems to be associated with psychoneurosis rather than with psychosis. In children it is most often associated with psychotic conditions, such as schizophrenia and infantile autism.[20]

The audiologist frequently suspects psychogenic deafness through the use of tests such as speech audiometry,[6] the Doerfler-Stewart Test,[8] and electro-dermal audiometry.[3] Usually when this condition is indicated, the individual is referred for psychological and psychiatric study and treatment. The incidence of psychogenic deafness is not well known. During the stress of wartime the incidence seems higher than in peacetime. Various workers have stressed the importance of this problem.[18, 22] From the point of view of the psychology of deafness, it must be recognized that this sensory disorder occurs on both organic and nonorganic bases. The discussion and data given in the following chapters pertains only to deafness which is organic.

REFERENCES

1. Bell, A. G.: Graphical studies of marriages of the deaf. Washington, D. C., Volta Bureau, 1917.
2. Best, H.: Deafness and the Deaf in the United States. New York, Macmillan, 1943.
3. Bordley, J. E. and Hardy, W. G.: A study in objective audiometry with the use of psychogalvanometric response. Ann. Otol. Rhinol. and Laryng., 58, 751, 1949.
4. _____: Etiology of deafness in young children. Acta Oto-laryng. 40, 72, 1951.
5. Carhart, R.: Auditory impairment of old age. Evanston, Northwestern University, Unpublished Report, 1959.
6. _____: Speech audiometry. Acta Oto-laryng., 40, 62, 1953.
7. Day, H. E., Fusfeld, I. S. and Pintner, R.: Survey of American schools for the deaf. Washington, National Research Council, 1928.
8. Doerfler, L. and Stewart, K.: Malingering and psychogenic deafness. J. Speech and Hearing Disorders, 11, 181, 1946.
9. Fay, E. A.: An inquiry concerning marriages of the deaf in America. Am. Ann. Deaf, 41, 22, 1896.
10. Fiedler, M. F.: Good and poor learners in an oral school for the deaf. Exceptional Children, 23, 291, 1957.
11. Frisina, D. R.: A psychological study of the mentally retarded deaf child. Evanston, Northwestern University, Unpublished Doctoral Dissertation, 1955.
12. Goodhill, V.: Pathology, diagnosis, and therapy of deafness, in Travis, L. E. (ed.), Handbook of Speech Pathology. New York, Appleton-Century-Crofts, 1957.
13. Gregg, N. M.: Congenital cataract following German measles in the mother. Trans. Ophthalmol. Soc. (Australia), 3, 35, 1942.
14. Hardy, W. G.: Problems of audition, perception and understanding. Washington, D. C., The Volta Bureau, Reprint #680, 1956.
15. Hopkins, L. A. and Guilder, R. P.: Clarke School studies concerning the heredity of deafness. Northampton, Clarke School for the Deaf, Monog. #1, 1949.
16. Kaplan, O. J.: Gerontology, in Brower, D. and Abt, L. (ed). Progress in Clinical Psychology. New York, Grune and Stratton, 1952.
17. Lamm, S. S.: Pediatric Neurology. New York, Landsberger Medical Books, 1959.
18. Martin, N. A.: Psychogenic deafness. Ann. Otol. Rhin. and Laryng., 55, 81, 1946.
19. Masland, R., Sarason, S. and Gladwin, T.: Mental Subnormality, Biological, Psychological, and Cultural Factors. New York, Basic Books, 1958.
20. Myklebust, H. R.: Auditory Disorders in Children. New York, Grune and Stratton, 1954.
21. _____: The deaf child with other handicaps. Am. Ann. Deaf, 103, 496, 1958.

22. Rosenberger, A. S. and Moore, T. H.: Treatment of hysterical deafness at Hoff General Hospital. Am. J. Psychiat., 102, 666, 1946.
23. Shambaugh, G. E.: Fenestration operation for ostosclerosis. Acta Oto-laryng., Suppl. 179, 1949.
24. _____: Surgery of the Ear. Philadelphia, W. B. Saunders, 1959.
25. _____ et al.: Physical causes of deafness. Arch. Otolaryng., 7, 424, 1928.
26. Wildervanck, L. S. Audiometric examination of parents of children deaf from birth. Arch. Otolaryng., 65, 280, 1957.

Suggestions for Further Study

Boies, L. R.: Fundamentals of Otolaryngology, 3rd ed. Philadelphia, Saunders, 1959.

Carhart, R. and Jerger, J.: Preferred method for clinical determination of pure tone thresholds. J. Speech and Hearing Disorders, 24, 330, 1959.

Coates, G. M., Schenck, H. and Miller, M.: Otolaryngology, Vol. 2, Hagerstown, W. F. Prior, 1955.

House, H.: Trends in mobilization surgery. Laryngoscope, 69, 1085, 1959.

Kallman, F.: Expanding Goals of Genetics in Psychiatry. New York, Grune and Stratton, 1962.

Pestalozza, G. and Shore, I.: Clinical evaluation of presbycusis on the basis of different tests of auditory function. Laryngoscope, 65, 1136, 1955.

Proceedings of the International Conference on Audiology. Laryngoscope, Special Issue, 68, #3, 1958.

Rasmussen, G. and Windle, W. (ed.): Neural Mechanisms of the Auditory and Vestibular Systems. Springfield, C. C. Thomas, 1960.

Rosenzweig, M. R.: and Rosenblith, W. A.: Responses to auditory stimuli at the cochlea and at the auditory cortex. Psych. Monog. #363, 1953.

Spiegel, E. A. and Sommer, I.: Neurology of the Eye, Ear, Nose and Throat, New York, Grune and Stratton, 1944.

Chapter IV

SENSORY DEPRIVATION AND BEHAVIOR

IT IS DIFFICULT for those with normal capacities to understand the implications of a sensory deprivation. Perhaps this is the reason for the consequences frequently being over-simplified and viewed only in terms of the obvious. The more subtle, pervasive implications often are not recognized. This is illustrated by the extensive attention given to the effect of deafness on language and communication, without emphasis on its influence on other aspects of behavior. Presumably deafness modifies behavior in many ways. It might be hypothesized that there are generalized effects which are felt irrespective of the degree of the hearing loss, and of the age of onset, if the impairment is sufficient to interfere with normal environmental contact. It might be expected further that the greatest impact on behavior ensues when the loss is extensive, and when it occurs preverbally, before language has been acquired. The data considered in the succeeding chapters are pertinent to these hypotheses. The basic task for the psychology of deafness is to ascertain the ways in which such sensory deprivation alters modes of growth and manners of adjustment.

More generally, in the psychology of sensory deprivation the need is to ascertain the influences on the organism when one, or more, of the senses is impaired. When audition is deficient, this is the function of the psychology of deafness. When vision is impaired, it is the task of the psychology of blindness. When both deafness and blindness are present, the problem embodies a combination of these approaches. Gradually information is forthcoming relative to all types of sensory deprivation and although salient differences exist, as knowledge accrues regarding one of these handicaps, all of the others are benefitted.

It is chiefly through the senses that the organism mediates between inner needs and external circumstances. In the study of sensory behavior, particularly in relation to sensory deprivation, it is advantageous to classify the five senses into *close* and *distance* senses. Thus, hearing and vision are the distance senses, while olfaction, gustation and taction are the close senses.

THE DISTANCE SENSES

When the distance senses, hearing and vision, are compared a number of differences appear. Vision is directional, focusing only on the area immediately in front of the person. Hearing, by comparison, encompasses all directions. In some respect, at some level, hearing persists unceasingly, even during sleep. Nature's plan seems to have been to provide one distance sense which functions uninterruptedly, keeping the organism in contact with its environment at all times. Vision is discontinued during sleep and can be suspended at any time by closing the eyes. Nature did not provide a means for closing the ears, and in recent years Man has been searching for "ear defenders." This comparison accents the scanning, alerting function of hearing, that aspect of audition which is highly relevant to the psychology of deafness. Ramsdell[12] first suggested this basic signaling, warning role of hearing. It provides a mandatory antennae type of contact, constantly warning the organism regarding the stability and friendliness of the total environment. Psychologically audition acts as a background sense while vision is primarily a foreground sense, usually focused on an experience after it has been identified through hearing. Vision is directed to that which is in the foreground of attention. In contrast, even while eating, viewing a painting, or tying one's shoes, audition continues to scan the background and to call attention to changes in the surrounding environment. On the other hand, there are many instances of vision serving background needs and hearing the foreground. For example, when listening intently to what is being said, or to a pure tone during an audiometric test, one looks at the floor, or even closes his eyes. Likewise when listening to beautiful music the eyes are directed away aimlessly, or closed, to force the auditory experience into the foreground as much as possible. This epitomizes listening behavior.

Although hearing serves more as a background sense and vision more as a foreground sense, these distance senses also perform in a reciprocal manner. Cobb[2] has stressed that this equipotentiality, this psychological equality of the distance senses, is characteristic only of Man. He describes the dog as an animal that has only one well developed distance sense, hearing. Thereby, the dog is mainly dependent on hearing and olfaction, with vision being relatively undeveloped. Neff[11] has stated that the cat is essentially an auditory animal with both olfaction and vision being comparatively less developed. Man is unique in having two highly developed and flexible distance senses; one did not develop at the expense of the other. Either distance sense can be used as a *lead* sense for purposes of exploration and acquisition of experience. These considerations have important implications for the psychology of sensory deprivation, and specifically for the psychology of deafness. Apparently a deaf cat or a deaf dog is relatively more deprived than Man because it lacks another equally developed distance sense. This viewpoint stresses that Man's superiority can be explained partially by his not being principally visual or principally auditory. Both distance senses are highly developed and function in a supplementary manner to a marked degree. Harris,[5] who has reviewed the relationships between hearing and vision, stressed the phenomenon of sensory felicitation. Myklebust and Brutten[10] studied the effect of deafness on visual perception and found that when hearing is deprived in early life, visual perception is disturbed. Study of the psychology of deafness provides many other indications of such intersensory reciprocation.

Further evaluation of hearing and vision is revealing particularly when deafness and blindness are compared. In certain respects the stability of what one sees is greater than what one hears. A sound is heard and then it is gone; it cannot be held in time, as a painting is while being viewed. Though sound can be recorded, when reproduced it is heard again only momentarily. This is the main reason for referring to vision as a spatial sense and to audition as a temporal sense. Actually both senses are spatial and both are temporal, but there are fundamental differences in their nature. Auditory experience to be meaningful often assumes temporalness and sequence to a greater extent than vision. The listener must learn to group properly the speech sounds of his language in order for meaning to occur. Some auditory disorders impede this "grouping," and the individual hears a sequence of speech sounds, rather than groups of sounds which constitute words. This highlights one of the differences between hearing and vision. Most visual experience is predetermined and thus more stable; written words have been "grouped," and remain so on the page, a phenomenon which holds for most visual experience. The fluidity of audition is of critical importance in behavior. Only such a sense can effectively serve in a nondirectional, signaling manner and constantly inform the organism of changes in the environmental field. After the organism has been alerted to the change, a sense such as vision is needed to explore it in detail. Often then it can be viewed for an indefinite period.

The permissive and mandatory nature of hearing, its susceptibility to all sound, becomes a limitation as well as an advantage. If part or all of a visual experience becomes irrelevant or unduly threatening, it can be avoided by turning the head, or by closing the eyes. This cannot be done with hearing. It becomes a victim of circumstances, resulting in a problem of considerable magnitude in science and in every day life because it is essential that over-exposure to sound be avoided. Despite these limitations imposed by the mandatoriness of audition, it is difficult to conceive of an organism's attaining the level of function found in Man without a sense which provides constant environmental contact. *Only when one is fully cognizant of this uniqueness of hearing can one understand the extreme isolation which occurs from deafness.* Study of the psychology of deafness increasingly indicates that as auditory sensation is reduced, alteration of the use of the other senses, and altered perceptual organization, is imperative in order for the person to maintain an adequate homeostatic relationship between his inner needs and external circumstances.

THE CLOSE SENSES

The close senses are olfaction, gustation, and taction. Less scientific knowledge is available concerning these senses than for the distance senses. Ostensibly many factors are involved, one of which might be, despite their importance, they do not serve as *lead* senses in Man. Phylogenetically and ontogenetically the close senses are more primitive and immature as compared to the distance senses. Therefore, primitive Man was more dependent on the close senses than modern Man. Moreover, psychologists have revealed that infants in early life are dependent essentially on the close senses, gradually attaining maximum use of hearing and vision. Harlow[4] has demonstrated the important role of taction, body contact, in the infant chimpanzee. It can be presumed that in the immature organism developmentally touch, taste, and smell are used more than hearing or vision for environmental exploration and satisfaction of needs. In some forms of life, such as in the cat, vision does not even become functional until some time after birth.

A basic implication is that when a distance sense is deprived, the individual naturally is forced into greater dependence on the close senses. In the psychology of deafness a chief concern is the extent to which this type of alteration of sensory behavior is affected, irrespective of the age of onset or other variables. Before considering this problem further, it is pertinent to recall that other conditions also might result in greater dependence on the close senses. Severe emotional disturbances, in both children and adults, occasionally result not in impairment, but in relinquishment of the use of hearing or vision. Distance sense performance then is impeded by marked regressions, and the individual again uses his close senses much as he did in early infancy. This is manifested by the schizophrenic child who often uses olfaction as a lead sense, as a basic exploratory sense. His behavior is characterized by sniffing. Nothing is eaten or used in other ways except as it is explored through olfaction.

Hebb,[6] Lily,[7] and Shurley[14] have studied the effect of sensory isolation on normal persons. These experiments involved multisensory deprivation and hence are not comparable to having one sensory impairment such as deafness. Nevertheless, these studies have revealed Man's marked dependence on environmental contact. The subjects could not tolerate long periods of sensory isolation. To maintain feelings of well-being, it seems, Man requires constant assurance from his environment. He needs continuous indication that he is accepted, and that his needs will be met. His dependency in this regard has been shown in other ways by investigators such as Bowlby[1] and Spitz,[15] who have demonstrated the effects of deprivation of maternal contact and affection. In relation to these investigations we must emphasize that all types and degrees of deafness, at any age, bring about isolation and detachment from the environment, especially from easy, normal contact with other people. Psychologically a hearing loss is consequential as soon as it reduces the individual's contact with the outside world. Audiometrically the loss might be mild, but as soon as environmental contact has been disturbed, as soon as the background function of audition has been impaired, the individual is in need of altering the typical means whereby Man maintains homeostatic equilibrium.

THE BEHAVIORAL EFFECTS OF SENSORY DEPRIVATION

Some of the effects of sensory deprivation are conspicuous; observable behavioral effects of deafness in young children have been described by Gesell[3] and Myklebust.[8] Many of the involvements of impaired sensory capacities can be revealed only by appropriate scientific procedures and effort. It is through such effort that a psychology of deafness must ascertain the basic ways in which hearing loss alters modes of perceptual organization and manners of adjustment.

Characteristically the close and distance senses function in the manner of intersensory perception, through the process of *synesthesia*. Although all sensory avenues are not being stimulated simultaneously, a specific sensory experience is interpreted on the basis of what has been learned from all sensory experience. When a certain sensory input is lacking, however, the experience gained from the remaining senses is structured differently. Loss of information from a given sensory channel must result in reduced perceptual reciprocation. Furthermore, when a distance sense, hearing, is impaired the remaining distance sense, vision, and the close senses, take on different roles. In Man, both hearing and vision take a *lead* role according to the primary purposes they fulfill by nature. When deafness is present the remaining distance sense, vision, must serve a *dual* lead role. It must serve a more inclusive purpose, fulfilling both foreground and background needs. The role of the close senses also shifts; they become more supplementary and more critical to the individual's learning and adjustment.

In Figure 5 an attempt is made to illustrate the shift in the roles of the remaining senses when one or both of the distance senses is impaired. To some extent this represents an hypothesis because much research must be accomplished before definite conclusions

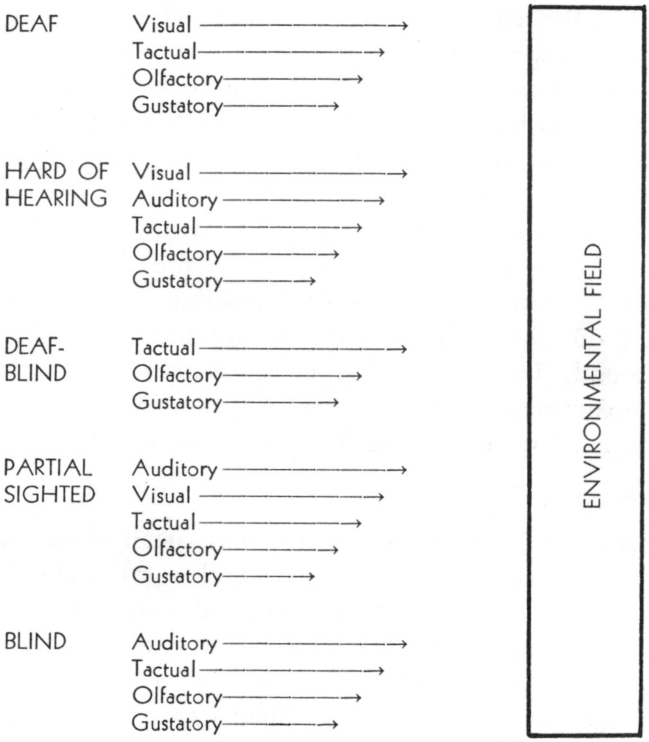

FIG. 5. The hierarchy of sensory organization resulting when distance senses are impaired.

can be made regarding the alterations of psychological processes which derive from sensory deprivation. Nevertheless, the findings of various workers and the data given in the succeeding chapters denote that such alterations do occur. It is essential that these shifts be understood if we are to assist those with sensory losses to actualize their potentials more successfully.

As illustrated by this figure even the hard of hearing, with a moderate impairment must use vision as the principal contact and exploratory sense, with audition serving a significant supplementary role. Comparatively the partially sighted use audition as the lead sense, with vision as the basic supplementary sense. When profound deafness is present, audition is of minor consequence in the patterning of psychological structures, hence it is included after gustation, or left out, according to the residual capacities in a given individual. The deaf use vision as the lead sense, with the tactual sense serving the main supplementary role. The blind use audition in the lead role, with the close senses following the order of tactual, olfactory and gustatory. Compared to the deaf, the blind use olfaction more as a distance sense. The deaf-blind, when both distance senses are lacking, use taction for basic contact and exploration of the environment. They, too, use olfaction in a vital scanning, antennae-like manner. The sensory-psychological organization shown in Figure 5 emphasizes that when a distance sense deprivation occurs, the individual by natural shift maintains a background-foreground relationship with his environment through the best means at his disposal. To illustrate further the ways in which those with sensory impairment use their remaining sensory channels, characteristic behavior of a deaf, blind and deaf-blind child is described.

The Deaf Child

The deaf child playing with a toy periodically looks up to scan the environment to assure himself that changes occurring in the environment are not unduly threatening, also to ascertain whether such changes mean increased pleasure and feelings of well-being. He scans periodically even though there are no cues to environmental change. In addition he scans whenever there are minor changes in the visual field, such as changes in light caused by shadows. Because he has only one distance sense, used for both foreground and background, he must look up and explore essentially all changes in the visual field. Only thus can he maintain psychological equilibrium, maintain adequate monitoring of external circumstances.

The deaf child learns through startling, frightening experiences early in life that environmental changes occur that cannot be monitored visually. Through such experience he develops a unique dependence on his close senses. He learns that another way in which to maintain contact environmentally is through taction. Vibratory sensations become signals in a unique manner. Whenever he feels vibrations, usually through the floor, again, he looks up to explore the occurrence. After identifying the circumstance through the visual or tactual channels, he might explore it further by taking it in his hands, or by smelling and tasting it. It follows that to provide situations conducive to learning for the deaf child, unnecessary visual and vibratory sensations should be avoided. Predominantly he is alerted and scans when light changes occur, when he glimpses even minor movement, and when he feels vibratory sensations. These behavioral consequences of deafness have many implications for learning and adjustment.

The Blind Child

In the study of the psychology of sensory deprivation comparison of the various types of impairments adds to our knowledge and understanding. For example, it is beneficial to compare the behavioral shifts of the deaf and blind. The blind child uses audition, his remaining distance sense, and he uses it in a dual role for both foreground and background purposes. Hence, although he might be speaking to someone, if he hears a background sound, he interrupts his conversation and attends, at least momentarily, to the background sound. When the background sound has been identified, when the environment has again been structured satisfactorily, he resumes his play and conversation. Often the circumstance requires further exploration in order to avoid threat, to appease curiosity, and to increase general satisfaction. To secure the further information needed, the tactual sense, the primary supplemental sense is used. If the background sound is that of a speaker who cannot be identified through audition alone, the child uses his hands to feel the person's face, or clothes. He might also use olfaction in a more direct lead manner as compared to a deaf child. Because audition extends in all directions, and is effective for scanning in the distance, the blind child is less dependent on vibratory sensation than is the deaf child.

The Deaf-Blind Child

There are few more interesting and challenging ways to learn about sensory deprivation than through study of those who are both deaf and blind. These individuals, having no use of the distance senses, are dependent on the close senses alone. Myklebust[9] has indicated procedures which may be used in the diagnostic study and training of deaf-blind children. Salmon[13] has reported on the rehabilitation of deaf-blind adults.

As illustrated in Figure 5, when both distance senses have been deprived, the tactual sense assumes the *lead* role. Supplemental experience is provided by olfaction and gustation. When the deaf-blind child is playing with a toy, he maintains background, scanning contact with the environment through tactual-vibratory sensations. In the deaf child, use of vision is altered to fulfill both foreground and background purposes. In the blind child, it is use of audition which is altered to fulfill this dual role. In the deaf-blind child it is taction, the tactual sense, which assumes this altered function. Thus, when the deaf-blind child is playing with a toy and feels vibratory sensations, or when he is touched by someone, he must drop the toy and use his hands to explore the circumstance that has occurred. He uses olfaction as a scanning, distance sense as much as possible; it serves a significant supplementary role. However, olfaction is not highly developed in Man and is limited as an avenue through which the organism can be alerted. Furthermore, it quickly adapts to a stimulus and then ceases to signal the organism. Another factor which assumes importance is Cobb's view that olfaction is a non-symbolic sensory channel.

This discussion has been given as a frame of reference for the study of sensory deprivation and its effect on learning and adjustment. Such an emphasis does not deny that an individual with impairment of sensory functioning is in most respects like a person with normal sensory capacities. Nevertheless, this position stresses that to understand sensory loss, to understand people with deafness, it is necessary to understand how their handicap makes them different. The point of view that a person with deafness is just like everyone else, except that he has impaired hearing, is unsatisfactory as a frame of reference from which to progress in the study of the psychology of deafness.

In addition to emphasizing that the hearing impaired person is like the person without deafness in most respects, it is beneficial to stress that his problems are different, that he has different sensory experience, and hence a different basis for all experience. In conjunction with the psychology of *similarity*, there is a psychology of *difference* which must be studied in order to understand more fully the significance of a sensory loss. In the following chapters data are presented which indicate some of the differences between hearing impaired and normally hearing individuals. While scientific evidence still is limited, it is on this type of information that the psychology of deafness must be founded. Through the attainment of such knowledge the problems of learning and adjustment which are associated with hearing loss might be alleviated more effectively.

REFERENCES

1. Bowlby, J.: Maternal Care and Mental Health. New York, Columbia University Press, 1952.
2. Cobb, S.: Foundations of Neuropsychiatry. Baltimore, Wilkins and Wilkins, 1958.
3. Gesell, A. and Amatruda, C. S.: Developmental Diagnosis. New York, Paul B. Hoeber, 1947.
4. Harlow, H.: The Nature of Love. American Psychologist, 13, 673, 1958.
5. Harris, J. D.: Some Relations Between Vision and Audition. Springfield, C. C. Thomas, 1950.
6. Hebb, D. O.: A Testbook of Psychology. Philadelphia, Saunders, 1958.
7. Lily, J. C.: Mental effects of reduction of ordinary levels of physical stimuli on intact healthy persons. Psychiat. Research Reports, 5, 1, 1956.
8. Myklebust, H. R.: Auditory Disorders in Children. New York, Grune and Stratton, 1954.
9. _____: The deaf-blind child. Watertown, Perkins School for the Blind, Pub. #19, 1956.
10. _____ and Brutten, M.: A study of the visual perception of deaf children Acta Oto-laryng., Suppl. 105, 1953.
11. Neff, W. D.: Behavioral studies of auditory discrimination. Ann. Otol. Rhinol. and Laryng., 66, 506, 1957.
12. Ramsdell, D. A.: The psychology of the hard of hearing and deafened adults, in Davis, H. (ed.), Hearing and Deafness, New York, Murray Hill Books, 1947.
13. Salmon, P. J.: Rehabilitation of Deaf-Blind Persons. Brooklyn, Industrial Home for the Blind, 1958.
14. Shurley, J. T.: Some findings from experimental sensory isolation research and their possible value for psychiatric theory and practice. Chicago, Northwestern University, Lecture Jan. 28, 1959.
15. Spitz, R.: Infantile depression and the general adaptation syndrome, in Hoch, P. and Zubin, J. (ed.), Depression. New York, Grune and Stratton, 1954.

Suggestions for Further Study

Bartley, S. H.: Principles of Perception. New York, Harper and Brothers, 1958.
Buddenbrock, W.: The Senses. Ann Arbor, University of Michigan Press, 1960.
Geldard, F. A.: The Human Senses. New York, John Wiley and Sons, 1953.
Hebb, D. O.: The Organization of Behavior. New York, John Wiley and Sons, 1949.
Hebb, D. O., Heath, E. S. and Stuart, E. A.: Experimental deafness. Canadian J. Psychol., 8, 152, 1954.

Huizinga, E.: The sense of hearing—its significance in human beings, in Proceedings of International Course in Paedo-Audiology. Groningen, University of Groningen, 1953.

Keller, Helen.: The Story of My Life. New York, Doubleday, 1905.

Snijders, J. Th.: Psychology of hearing and non-hearing, in Proceedings of International Course in Paedo-Audiology. Groningen, University of Groningen, 1953.

Stevens, S. S. (ed.): Handbook of Experimental Psychology. New York, John Wiley and Sons, 1951.

Vernon, J. and Hoffman, J.: Effect of sensory deprivation on learning rate in human beings. Science, 123, 1074, 1956.

Wheeler, R. H. and Cutsforth, T. D.: Synaesthesia, a form of perception. Psychol. Rev., 29, 212, 1922.

Worchel, P.: Space perception and orientation in the blind. Psychol. Monog. #332, 1951.

_____ and Berry, J. H.: The perception of obstacles by the deaf. J. Exper. Psychol., 43, 187, 1952.

_____ and Dallenbach, K. M.: "Facial Vision," perception of obstacles by the deaf-blind. Am. J. Psychol., 60, 502, 1947.

Zahl, P. A. (ed.): Blindness; Modern Approaches to the Unseen Environment. Princeton, Princeton University Press, 1950.

Part Two

Deafness and Psychological Processes

Chapter V

DEAFNESS AND MENTAL DEVELOPMENT

MAN MATURES in three primary ways: physically, emotionally, and mentally. There is a body of knowledge regarding each of these aspects of maturation but more is known about physical and mental maturation than about the emotional. Mental growth has been studied extensively by workers such as Binet,[9] Terman,[90] Thurstone,[92] Piaget,[69] and Wechsler.[98] Factors which affect the development of mental ability have been investigated by Benda,[6] Doll,[18] Masland,[55] and Strauss.[87] Physical maturation has been studied by Baldwin,[5] Meredith,[56] Jones,[40] and Tuddenham and Snyder.[94] While comparatively less specific knowledge is available regarding emotional growth, notable contributions to this area have been made by such workers as Bowlby,[12] Spitz,[85] Kanner,[41] Jersild,[39] and Hall.[30]

It is interesting to note that study of the abnormal, of the handicapped, has been an important source of information regarding the nature of intelligence and how it develops. It is the task of the student of the psychology of deafness to ascertain the extent and the nature of the relationships between loss of hearing and each of these basic ways in which Man matures. We can assume that such study will add to the understanding of psychological processes in both the normal and the abnormal.

Because influences on the growth of psychological processes can best be studied in the developing organism, a fundamental need is to study the effects of deafness in the child. Nevertheless, possible relationships also must be sought in the adult who sustains a hearing loss after maturity has been attained. It might be expected that the effects of a sensory loss will be different if it occurs in adulthood as compared to childhood. It also might be expected that each of the ways in which Man matures is not equally vulnerable to an impact from sensory deprivation. For example, it seems unlikely that deafness would affect physical maturation. In support of this presumption, Myklebust[62] found no difference between deaf and hearing children in ages of sitting and walking. On the other hand, Macmillan and Bruner[54] found differences in some aspects of the physical development of normal and deaf children. There is a possibility that their findings can be explained by socio-economic and other such factors. Here it is necessary to differentiate between physical maturation and motor behavior. As discussed in Chapter VII, there does seem to be a relationship between deafness and motor function. Psychologically, if impaired hearing has an impact, it would be expected to be greater in the areas of mental functioning and personality.

Gradually, more attention is being given to possible relationships between sensory deprivation and growth of intellectual capacities. Hayes[32] first explored this possibility in the blind while Pintner[71] first indicated such a relationship in the deaf. As might be expected, this early work was limited to quantitative comparison with the normal in attempts to ascertain the influence of sensory deprivation on general intelligence. More recently Heider,[34] Oléron,[66] Fiedler,[20] and Myklebust[61] have pursued the question of more specific effects of deafness on mental processes such as abstraction, memory, and learning.

The principal question considered in this chapter is whether deafness influences mental development. This is the area of the psychology of deafness which has been studied most extensively. Such study began around the year 1900. The early work was done mainly by Pintner and by his students and associates; for this reason he is referred to as the father of the psychology of deafness. From his studies he concluded that children deaf from early life were below average in mental capacity. In other words, one of his major conclusions was that the general intellectual level of deaf children was below that of normal children. His explanation of these findings was that diseases causing deafness also affected the brain and caused mental retardation. That such a relationship exists in some instances can readily be verified. Both children and adults who have deafness from meningitis sometimes also sustain cerebral damage to the extent that they are mentally retarded. Such a dual involvement can derive from any disease causing loss of hearing. On this basis, a higher incidence of mental retardation might be expected in a random population of deaf and hard of hearing individuals than in the normal.

Other possibilities must be considered. Some workers have suggested that if endogenous deafness is present, other defects such as mental retardation, will be present more frequently than in families without a history of such deafness.[71] The presumption is that endogenous deafness and endogenous mental retardation will occur in the same person at a certain given rate or frequency. This presumption has not been completely verified nor denied. To accept such generalizations uncritically is to minimize the problem. The nature of the relationship between deafness, mental capacity, and intellectual functioning is more complex. Experienced educators, psychologists, and physicians recognize that there are individuals who have both deafness and mental retardation. They also realize that it is of considerable importance to ascertain whether deaf children as a group have the dual handicap of inferior intelligence and hearing impairment. Such a conclusion would be of major consequence to the deaf and hard of hearing as well as to those who work with them. Generalizations regarding the intellectual capacities of this group cannot be made only on the presumption of relationship to etiology, only on the basis of exogenous and endogenous factors. Perhaps disease and hereditary factors cause mental retardation without deafness with the same frequency that they cause mental retardation with deafness. Then the incidence of mental subnormality would be equal.

Actually the question of relationship between deafness and intelligence raises fundamental issues concerning the nature of mental development and intellectual capacity. To illustrate, we consider the child who has marked deafness from birth, or from the pre-language age. Such a child's experience and opportunity for mental growth must be compared to those of the normal child. If this deaf child's mental development parallels that of the normal child, the significance of auditory experience in growth of intellectual processes can be denied. That auditory experience is unrelated to such psychological development is unlikely.

Many workers have emphasized the importance of stimulation and experience in the mental development of children with normal sensory capacities. Schilder,[82] Soddy,[84] Spitz,[85] Kanner,[41] and Bowlby[12] have shown relationships between early life experience and intellectual behavior. Piaget,[69] especially, has stressed the significance of hearing, vision, and symbolism as the foundations of intelligence. The child having deafness from infancy lacks auditory experience and verbal symbolism. Presumably non-verbal auditory experience is of importance in mental development. However, the question raised most frequently concerns the connection between intelligence and language. A philosophical position commonly held is that without language, there is no thought and inferentially there is no intelligence of the type associated with the human being. This implies that if language development is precluded, mental development will be affected. If normal language development is necessary for normal development of psychological processes and learning, then the mental growth and intellectual functioning of the deaf child will not parallel that of the hearing child. On a broader basis, even the preverbal experience of the child deaf from infancy is different from the hearing. His experience does not include audition, hence his non-verbal behavior, such as perceptual processes, is established and structured differently.

When both the verbal and the non-verbal experiences of the child with early life deafness are considered, one cannot avoid the probability that such a handicap might preclude actualization of true intellectual potential. Important as such a conclusion might be, it is significantly different from the assumption that deafness *and* mental retardation are present as separate and distinct entities. If mental development varies mainly as a reciprocal of the limitation in language acquisition, it follows that if the language limitation can be alleviated, more normal development of mental capacities will ensue. It is in terms of this probability that the data presented in this chapter are considered.

The problem of cause and effect, of poor language acquisition as a result of inferior intelligence, or inability to actualize mental potential because of limited language, is of major concern in the study of the psychology of deafness. This is a basic question when the deafness is of great extent and when it occurs in early childhood. Except as disease, accident, aging, or hereditary factors also cause mental retardation, there is no reason to assume a conjunction between deafness and mental capacity when the hearing loss occurs in adulthood. This does not preclude some effect on thinking processes, even when the sensory deprivation occurs later in life.

DEAFNESS AND INTELLIGENCE

The question of relationship between deafness and intelligence involves other considerations. One of the more important of these is the way in which the mental ability is measured. Discussion of intelligence must include analysis and criticism of the means and techniques whereby it has been ascertained. Such consideration is critical when the study concerns those having deafness. The difficulties in measuring intelligence nonverbally is a complex and involved problem in itself. Non-language mental tests must be used with those whose deafness dates from the pre-speech age if the deafness precluded the use of hearing in acquiring language. This is true irrespective of the age of the individual being studied because this type of hearing impaired person characteristically continues to have a language handicap throughout his lifetime. In some instances it is necessary to use nonverbal tests even with those whose deafness dates from later life, after language has been firmly established and used normally for a period of years. The assumption that such persons can comprehend instructions by speech reading and reading, and that they can express themselves with equal facility in speech and by writing, does not hold in many instances.

Inasmuch as nonverbal tests usually must be used, the problem of similarities and differences between verbal and nonverbal tests must be critically evaluated. Although these tests correlate significantly, it is apparent that they measure different aspects of intelligence. Tests requiring verbal facility correlate most closely with those abilities required for learning academic materials. Nonverbal tests are not as useful for predicting this type of learning. This limitation has presented complex problems for the psychologist who is working with deaf and hard of hearing individuals; it is considered in the discussion of the test results given below.

There is an even more critical problem in the use of psychological tests, not only mental tests, with the deaf and hard of hearing who have language limitations. This is the question of the *assumptions* made in the use of a given test. For example, a common assumption is that all nonverbal tests are equally nonverbal. It is becoming increasingly obvious that this is not true. Some mental tests classified as nonverbal involve considerable ability of the type commonly referred to as verbal ability. Furthermore, there is the problem of the extent to which identical or similar test scores for those with deafness and for the normal can be interpreted as having the same meaning, the extent to which such scores can be used to predict the same type of success or failure in learning and adjustment. This question is confronted in all psychological test study with persons having extensive deafness from early life and to a certain extent with the hard of hearing.

In some instances, although the hearing impaired earn the same test scores as the hearing, they require specialized interpretation; interpretation on the basis of the test manual does not lead to the expected outcome. A common example is the lower correlation between intelligence test scores and academic achievement for the deaf as compared to the hearing. Apparently the individual with marked limitations of language solves the test problem by different psychological processes even though he earns the same score. Although both individuals are presented with the same problem, *the mental task becomes a different problem* on the basis of the abilities available for solving it. This means that the assumptions of the test, derived from its standardization and use with the hearing, do not necessarily hold when the same tests are used with the hearing impaired. This generalization seems to apply to both verbal or nonverbal tests. Therefore, psychological tests should be standardized also on the deaf and the hard of hearing to be most effective. Moreover, the psychologist using these tests in this specialized area needs specific training and experience if he is to do work which is scientifically and clinically valid.

Another comment seems indicated before considering studies of the mental abilities of the deaf and hard of hearing. The *range* of the intelligence levels of the hearing impaired does not differ from the hearing. This is true irrespective of the degree of deafness or of the age of onset. Variations and individual differences must be considered. There are brilliant, average, dull, and mentally retarded deaf and hard of hearing individuals just as there are in the population of the normally hearing.

Early Studies

With the exception of the study by Macmillan and Brunner,[54] most of the early studies of the intelligence of the deaf and hard of hearing were done by or in collaboration with Pintner.[73, 74, 79] It was characteristic of his era to use group tests. In his investigations Pintner used mainly his own group test, the Pintner Non-Language Mental Test.[70] This is one of the important differences between these early studies and those done in more recent years. The later work has been done chiefly through the use of individual performance type tests. While the individual tests are preferred clinically and scientifically, the group tests made it possible to use large samples. Many of the studies using individual tests have entailed small samples from single schools, which in itself has been a source of error and confusion regarding the mental capacity of hearing impaired children.

The most extensive survey of the mental and educational capacities of hearing impaired children was accomplished by Pintner and Reamer.[73] This study included 2,172 children in 26 schools for the deaf throughout the United States. It is this study which most critically raised the question of the relationship between intelligence and deafness. The foremost conclusions were that deaf children on the average are two years retarded mentally and five years educationally. Also, that inasmuch as there is a two-year mental retardation, two of the five years of educational retardation can be attributed to mental inferiority. The three years of educational retardation remaining were attributed to the language handicap resulting from deafness with onset in early life. These conclusions have been debated ever since, with increasing evidence that the basic problem is not mainly that of mental inferiority. It is necessary to reconsider the evidence and to indicate factors which seem more critical to the total capacities of the deaf and hard of hearing.

Soon after Pintner's work gave impetus to psychological study
of hearing impaired children, he and others realized that other test
techniques were necessary. It was at least partially through the
need for individual nonverbal tests to study deaf children that nonverbal performance tests were developed. Pintner and Paterson[72]
devised the first battery of such tests in the United States, and it was
this test which was used to study the mental capacities of the deaf
and hard of hearing for a number of years. Concurrently in England
Drever and Collins[19] devised a similar test. By 1930 the Grace
Arthur Point Scale of Intelligence, another performance scale, was
devised in the United States.[3] Because the work of Drever and
Collins indicated that deaf children were not inferior mentally on
the basis of their test, MacKane[51] made a study using the three
nonverbal performance tests then available, the Pintner-Paterson,
the Grace Arthur, and the Drever-Collins. His results showed that
the Pintner-Paterson and Grace Arthur Scales yielded highly comparable results with the deaf falling about 12 points below the
hearing. The scores on the Drever-Collins scale were higher for
both the deaf and the hearing. MacKane concluded that the Drever-
Collins scale was inadequately standardized and resulted in spu-
riously high scores. This was further demonstrated in a study by
Schick.[81]

Another performance test of intelligence is the Ontario School
Ability Examination.[1] This test was devised by Amoss of the Ontario
School for the Deaf and was standardized on children at that school.
A further study using this test, also on children at this school, was
done by Morrison.[58] While in certain respects an ingenious test and
of use in differential diagnosis, it has not been standardized on hearing children.

Brown[14] devised the Chicago Non-Verbal Examination, a group
test, which has been used in a number of studies of deaf children.
He also did a study correlating the results from selected tests in the
Grace Arthur battery with the Pintner Non-Language Test.

A number of the early workers used a single test such as the
Draw-a-Man[27] and the Porteus Maze Test[75] to appraise the intelligence of deaf children. Such studies are in contrast to those in which
batteries of tests were used. Peterson and Williams[68] first used the
Draw-a-Man Test and this Test has been used by several investiga-

tors. The results from an extensive study using this test with deaf and hard of hearing children, are presented on page 90. This test has gained in usefulness clinically and scientifically in recent years. However, varying results have been reported when used with hearing impaired children. Peterson and Williams reported an I.Q. level of 80, Shirley and Goodenough[83] 88, and Springer[86] 96. It is now evident that the samples used in these studies were too limited and cannot be considered as indicating the general mental level of a random sample of children in schools for the deaf. This criticism pertains to many of the studies on intelligence, as it is not uncommon for them to have been made in a single school. At the time of these early studies, there was considerable variation from school to school in the admission standards, which had an obvious bearing on the results secured. While this variation in standards persists, making it necessary to use wider sampling in research, uniformity of admission procedures and requirements now is much more common.

Zeckel and Van der Kolk[104] used the Porteus Maze Test in a study comparing the congenitally deaf with the normally hearing. They concluded that deaf children were mentally retarded and that deaf girls were more inferior than boys. Their explanation was that deafness from birth had an impact on psychological processes in general, and that the marked language limitation resulted in a permanent effect on mental development. It is interesting that these early workers emphasized this conjunction between deafness and intelligence. They did not say that both inferior mentality and deafness were present, but attributed the intellectual deficit to a reciprocal effect of the deafness itself. This is significant in view of more recent work in which this type of relationship seems predominant.

Pintner and Paterson[71] did a different type of study which should not be overlooked. This was an investigation of learning ability in which they used the Digit-Symbol and Symbol-Digit Tests. These tests measure the rapidity with which one learns to associate a symbol with a digit and then the reverse, a digit with a symbol. This was the first study of its kind with hearing impaired children, and few studies of this type have been made since. The importance of such investigation is suggested by the results which they obtained. Their sample included 992 children for the digit-symbol test and 1,049 children for the symbol-digit test. They found the deaf to be two or three years below the average for hearing children. Although they stated that this test "can be considered as a type of intelligence test," to view these results only in terms of general intelligence seems unwarranted. The Chicago Non-Verbal Examination includes two symbol-digit tests, which have been used to study further this type of learning in deaf children. As indicated by the discussion of these results it does not seem that scores on these tests can be taken as evidence of generalized retardation in deaf children (see page 70). Rather, these tests are a measure specifically of symbolic, verbal learning and with the child who has a severe hearing loss from early life, can be used with confidence in predicting this ability.

More Recent Studies

The implications of sensory deprivation for learning and adjustment have intrigued an increasing number of workers in recent years. Through such study more will be learned about all human behavior, as well as about the complex involvements of sensory deprivation.

Prior to the wide use of the Wechsler Adult Intelligence Scale[99] and the Wechsler Intelligence Test for Children,[100] the most commonly used performance tests were the Grace Arthur Point Scale of Intelligence, Form I,[3] the Leiter International Performance Scale,[47] and the Wechsler-Bellevue.[98] Other performance tests are the Grace Arthur Point Scale of Intelligence Tests, Revised Form II,[4] and the Nebraska Test of Learning Aptitude in Young Deaf Children, by Hiskey.[37] The Hiskey was standardized on children in schools for the deaf, and, more recently, norms for normal children have been made available. It is significant that performance tests now are used in all clinical psychological work. Also, in contrast to the early work in mental testing, the gross average I.Q. score is not viewed as the all important result. The work of Rapaport[77] and Wechsler,[98] revealed the significance of sub-test analysis and interpretation. This emphasis has been applied to study of the mental capacities of deaf and hard of hearing children. When batteries of performance tests first came into use with hearing impaired children, the emphasis continued to be placed on general I.Q. levels because it was necessary to explore further the general mental level of deaf children. Psychologists continued to study the possibility that the child with severe hearing loss was mentally retarded. Such studies were made by Schick,[81] Streng and Kirk,[88] and by Myklebust and Burchard.[63] Results indicated that when individual performance tests were used, children in schools for the deaf were of average intelligence. These findings were in contradiction to those of Pintner.

With the indication that deaf children were not inferior intellectually, other questions arose. Educators became concerned about children who were found to have average or above average mental ability, but who often did not show corresponding ability to learn and to achieve academically. Gradually it became clear that, although the deaf child may be quantitatively equal to the hearing child, significant qualitative differences in his mental functioning had to be considered. Furthermore, the question of what was measured by performance tests as compared to verbal tests became critical. It was evident that batteries of tests, such as the Grace Arthur, Form I, which included several of the formboard type of tests, were not highly useful in predicting academic achievement. In addition, it appeared that children could score within the average range on such tests but fall below average on tests which required more complex intellectual behavior. This was evidenced especially in a study by Birch and Birch.[10] They revealed that deaf school children who presented marked limitations in academic learning, scored within the average range on the Grace Arthur, Form I, the Hiskey, and the Wechsler. However, these children fell below average on the Leiter Scale and on the Goodenough Draw-a-Man Test; there was close agreement between the scores for these two tests.

Varied findings for deaf children on different types of mental tests presented a salient problem to the psychologist and to the educator. It caused some investigators to conclude that the tests on which deaf children fall below average are inadequate measures for this type of child, which may be true in terms of degree of mental ability. Other investigators, however, have emphasized that varying results might be expected if deafness affects development of certain psychological processes more than others. Then children with marked deafness from early life would be expected to show inferiority on those tests which measure the psychological processes that are most affected. Heider and Heider,[34] Oléron,[65] Templin,[89] and Myklebust[61] have shown that deaf children fall below average mainly on tests which require a type of abstraction and reasoning processes. This is considered further in connection with the results presented on page 71.

The Primary Mental Abilities Test

Group tests of intelligence are useful for screening and can be used in research to indicate group trends. When such tests are used, it is revealing to analyze the subtest scores, as is commonly done on individual tests. The Primary Mental Abilities Test,[92] devised and standardized by Thurstone, has been used extensively with normal school children. It is based on Thurstone's factor theory of intelligence. The factors measured are verbal meaning, spatial ability, reasoning, perceptual speed, and number ability. Except for the factor of verbal meaning, this test can be used largely as a nonverbal test. Treacy[93] used it in this manner in a study of deaf and hard of hearing children. The results are presented in Table 8. The children studied were in attendance at a large Day School. The classifications of deaf and hard of hearing were made by the school authorities, the children having been so classified educationally when they entered the school.

TABLE 8.   Intelligence quotients on the Primary Mental Abilities Test for deaf and hard of hearing school children

	Deaf			Hard of Hearing		
	N	Mean	SD	N	Mean	SD
Total quotient	30	94.70	15.3	36	97.25	12.7
Verbal meaning	31	80.19	14.2	36	90.30	10.6
Space ability	37	106.86	24.6	36	100.33	23.7
Number ability	31	98.38	20.2	35	93.48	14.8
Reasoning	25	94.84	19.4	28	106.85	19.5
Perceptual speed	22	104.22	21.5	22	115.68	25.2

These results show that the total intelligence quotients for the deaf and the hard of hearing are slightly below average but are within the normal range. Statistical tests revealed significant differences between the groups on verbal meaning and reasoning, the hard of hearing being superior to the deaf on these abilities. It is evident that the hard of hearing had acquired more language facility and thus were able to achieve a higher level of verbal meaning. Reasons for the hard of hearing scoring higher on reasoning are not so obvious. However, it may be that the mental processes involved in this test entail more abstract ability than do the other nonverbal tests in this battery. It appears that this type of mental process, like that required on the Progressive Matrices,[78] assumes verbal-symbolic functioning. Thus, the hard of hearing, having less language limitation, scored higher than the deaf.

The Chicago Non-Verbal Examination

The Chicago Non-Verbal Examination has been utilized in a number of studies of deaf children.[46] One reason for its use is that it was standardized on both deaf and hearing children. Although some of the items are now outdated and in need of revision, it has proved to be a useful test. The results from one of our studies using this test with a group of deaf children in a public Residential School are given in Table 9.

TABLE 9.   Results for deaf children on the Chicago Non-Verbal Examination

Group	N	C.A. Mean	SD	I.Q. Mean	SD
Males	52	15.9	1.14	104.0	16.7
Females	36	15.5	1.24	99.2	11.9
Total	88	15.7	1.20	102.0	15.1
Acoustic	38	15.6	1.17	98.4	13.8
Oral	31	15.7	1.20	107.3	14.7
Manual	19	16.2	1.12	100.3	16.0

From these results we see that the deaf fell at the average level of intelligence. Furthermore, there were no differences by sex or by educational classification. Children in the acoustic, oral, and manual departments were equivalent in mental ability as measured by this test.

If we take these results from the Chicago Non-Verbal Examination literally, we would assume that the intellectual capacities of deaf children are comparable to the hearing, and that their thought processes as well as other aspects of their mental functioning are comparable. While such a conclusion may be warranted in certain respects, in other ways it might be misleading. This was shown in

TABLE 10. Comparison of sub-test results for deaf and normal children on the Chicago Non-Verbal Examination

| | Deaf | | | | | | Hearing | | | | | |
| | Males N-32 | | Females N-21 | | Total N-53 | | Males N-32 | | Females N-21 | | Total N-53 | |
Test	Mean	SD	Mean	SD	Mean	SD	Mean	SD	Mean	SD	Mean	SD
1	4.09	1.77	3.81	1.75	3.98	1.75	5.13	1.72	4.67	1.78	4.94	1.74
2	10.19	4.29	7.24	2.41	9.02	3.91	11.06	3.90	9.71	3.18	10.53	3.66
3	5.09	1.92	4.33	1.56	4.79	1.81	5.97	1.43	4.71	1.55	5.45	1.59
4	8.56	3.30	7.71	2.92	8.23	3.15	9.81	3.42	8.95	2.33	9.47	3.04
5	7.53	2.12	7.33	1.42	7.45	1.87	8.31	1.12	8.14	1.31	8.25	1.19
6	8.06	5.59	7.45	2.86	7.83	4.71	8.38	4.78	5.81	2.68	7.36	4.24
7	10.20	6.13	8.21	4.71	9.43	5.66	11.31	4.50	9.05	4.59	10.46	4.62
8	9.59	5.22	9.19	3.82	9.43	4.68	11.31	4.43	10.29	3.62	10.91	4.12
9	6.72	1.69	5.57	2.04	6.26	1.90	6.31	2.01	6.05	1.28	6.21	1.75
10	15.28	6.08	13.86	5.28	14.72	5.77	14.97	5.58	15.05	5.42	15.00	5.46
Total:	97.44	15.04	94.62	9.80	96.32	13.18	98.53	14.39	94.48	8.89	96.92	12.56

a study by Blair.[11] He matched 53 deaf with 53 hearing children on the basis of standard scores from the Chicago Non-Verbal test. Sex, socio-economic factors, chronological age, and educational experience all were equated. The total IQ scores for the deaf and for the hearing were highly similar. However, a sub-test analysis of the scores for each of the ten tests on the Chicago Non-Verbal battery revealed additional information. These results are given in Table 10. Even though the deaf and hearing had been matched on IQ scores a number of significant differences occurred from the sub-test analysis. A summary of these findings are given as follows:

Test	Difference Between	Group Superior
1	total groups	hearing
2	deaf males and females	males
	deaf and hearing females	hearing
	total groups	hearing
3	hearing males and females	males
	deaf and hearing males	hearing
	total groups	hearing
4	total groups	hearing
5	total groups	hearing
6	hearing males and females	males
7	no difference	none
8	no difference	none
9	deaf males and females	males
10	no difference	none

From this analysis it is clear that although there are no differences between the groups by total scores, they are not comparable on several of the tests in this battery. This suggests differences quali-tatively, differences on the basis of mental processes used. There-fore, it is advantageous to classify each of the sub-tests according to the intellectual processes involved, albeit this can be done only tentatively until further research can be accomplished on this com-plex problem. Rather arbitrarily, the primary mental task involved in each of the ten sub-tests of the Chicago Non-Verbal may be described as follows:

Test	Task involved
1	rate of learning
2	categorizing—sorting behavior
3	abstracting—inducting
4	synthesizing geometric forms
5	noting details of geometric forms
6	synthesizing meaningful material
7	conceptualizing sequence of events
8	noting absurdities in picture
9	relating detail to a situation
10	rate of learning

The deaf showed inferiority on the first five tests. With the exception of Test 2, these tests in some manner involve geometric form and design, which must be considered a significant factor in these results. On a test which seemingly involves a high level of abstract behavior, Test 7, the deaf were not inferior. This test en-tails *meaningful* material, whereas Test 3, also involving abstraction, entails geometric form or *meaningless* material. Other such com-parisons can be made. To generalize, when the problem consists of situations or circumstances with which the deaf are familiar, such as pictures, they are not inferior. When the test consists of meaningless material, such as geometric form, they show inferiority. Therefore, they are not comparable to the hearing in noting dif-ferences between geometric forms, a relatively concrete task, but they are comparable even in a highly abstract function, such as conceptualizing a sequence of experiential events. We cannot ex-plain this qualitative aspect of their intellectual functioning by simply classifying it on the basis of abstract-concrete behavior. The issue is more complex. As knowledge accumulates regarding the specific relationships between deafness and mental processes, the learning problems of deaf children will eventually be greatly clarified.

The Wechsler-Bellevue Intelligence Test

In recent years standard performance tests have been the common means for studying the intelligence of hearing impaired children. Perhaps the most extensively used tests of this type are the Wechsler-Bellevue Scale,[98] the Wechsler Intelligence Scale for Children,[100] and the Wechsler Adult Intelligence Scale.[99] These tests consist of two parts, verbal and nonverbal, with each part made up of five sub-tests. It is the performance part of these tests which has been used most extensively with hearing impaired children. Murphy[60] has shown that deaf children fall within the normal range of intelligence as measured by the WISC.

The results secured on the Wechsler-Bellevue Scale with deaf pupils in a public Residential School are given in Table 11. Both the

TABLE 11.   Intelligence quotients for deaf children on the Wechsler-Bellevue Scale

Age	N	Verbal		Performance	
		Mean	SD	Mean	SD
12	18	64.6	14.3	102.2	15.1
13	16	60.6	11.4	104.8	13.2
14	16	62.6	14.7	98.5	14.8
15	15	69.9	12.0	102.0	14.5
16	10	73.5	13.6	100.5	12.1
17	10	70.9	10.8	103.0	9.9
Total	85	66.5	13.7	101.8	14.5

Verbal and Performance Scales were administered. In the administration of the Verbal Scale the method of communication was adapted to the need of the child, speech-reading, writing, and gestures being used. These results show that the deaf children fell at the average level on the performance section; this was true of each age group and for the total sample. In contrast, all age groups fell much below average on the verbal part of the scale. These subjects had profound deafness from early life. It is significant psychologically and educationally that there was little growth in verbal facility as they increased in age. In general, these data indicate that the group achieved a level of verbal facility equal to about two-thirds of the normal and that this ratio of achievement showed little change as they progressed through school. Perhaps this indicates that after they attain a degree of verbal usage, they reach a plateau beyond which further language growth is negligible.

Further analysis of these results is given in Table 12. There were no differences by sex or by etiology, indicating that for this group it is deafness itself which is the consequential factor, not sex or etiology. Wechsler[98] reported no sex differences for normals on the Wechsler-Bellevue so in this respect the deaf are comparable. Etiologically, both the endogenous and the exogenous had onset of deafness in early life, therefore the benefit of language acquisition does not appear.

TABLE 12.   Results on the Wechsler-Bellevue Scale for deaf pupils by sex and etiology

		Verbal		Performance		Full Scale	
	N	Mean	SD	Mean	SD	Mean	SD
Males	46	67.3	14.0	104.5	13.6	83.6	13.2
Females	39	66.8	13.5	99.2	14.9	81.0	14.7
Total	85	65.5	13.7	101.8	14.5	82.3	14.1
Endogenous	39	67.2	14.0	103.2	10.4	85.2	12.6
Exogenous	46	64.7	12.9	99.1	12.5	81.9	12.4

TABLE 13.   Mean weighted scores for deaf children on the sub-tests of the Wechsler-Bellevue Scale

Age	14–15	15–16	16–17	17–18	18–19	19–20	Total
Verbal							
Information	6.45	7.31	7.90	7.84	8.91	9.72	8.02
Comprehension	5.63	6.50	7.40	7.52	8.75	9.94	7.62
Arithmetic	4.00	6.23	6.27	4.94	7 25	7.94	6.10
Digit Span	5.54	5.68	7.00	5.78	6.66	6.94	6.26
Similarities	7.00	7.18	7.00	7.15	7.91	7.76	7.33
Performance							
P. Completion	8.81	10.12	12.18	10.31	11.25	12.61	10.88
P. Arrangement	10.55	10.31	12.00	10.36	11.58	10.66	10.91
Object Assembly	9.81	11.06	11.45	10.89	11.08	12.61	11.15
Block Design	8.72	10.12	11.90	10.36	12.00	13.77	11.14
Digit Symbol	7.63	8.75	10.18	9.05	10.58	10.72	9.48
Total	7.41	8.33	9.33	8.42	9.60	10.27	8.89
IQ	84	90	97	90	99	103	93
N	11	16	11	19	12	18	87

In Table 13 are the findings of another of our analyses of results for deaf children on the Wechsler-Bellevue Scale. The subjects, ranging in age from 14 to 20 years, were in attendance at a public Residential School. The weighted scores are given by sub-test and by age. As a group the deaf were inferior on the five verbal tests. However, it is interesting to note that the mean weighted scores by age showed progression and that by 20 years of age, there was no inferiority on the total scale score. At this age level they scored sufficiently above average on the performance scale to obviate the inferiority on the verbal scale. On the verbal scale most growth occurred in the areas of Information and Comprehension. Virtually no growth occurred on memory for digits, arithmetical reasoning, or reasoning by similarities. Presumably the mental functions involved in the abilities measured by these tests are rather directly related to verbal symbolism. That symbolic factors are related to memory in deaf children is shown by the discussion of memory below (see page 77). Both the Arithmetic and Similarities tests can be viewed as types of reasoning tests. The Similarities test especially requires conceptualizing and abstracting ability. Such mental functions have been shown to be vulnerable to modification by various factors, including mental illness and neurological disorders.[7, 62] Increasing evidence suggests that a sensory deprivation such as deafness from early life, also has a modifying influence on this type of behavior. It is noteworthy, as indicated by the subtest results of the Chicago Non-Verbal Examination, that such modification apparently is not generalized but pertains to a type of abstracting process which is dependent on verbal symbols.

The scores on the Performance section of the Scale show that this group of deaf children was not inferior on these tests. In fact, by 20 years of age, they tended to score above the norm on Picture Completion, Object Assembly, and Block Design. This trend for the deaf to score above average on certain mental tests requires consideration in terms of the psychological effects of deafness and is discussed further below under Deafness and Abstract Abilities.

Neyhus[63a] found that a sample of socially well adjusted adult deaf scored above average on the performance section of the Wechsler Adult Intelligence Scale. Subtests on which they characteristically fell above the norms were Digit Symbol and Block Design. He concluded that in order to make a successful adjustment vocationally and socially, it was necessary for the deaf to have higher than average intelligence.

The Grace Arthur Point Scale of Performance Tests, Form I

The Grace Arthur Test[3] has been used in study of the mental abilities of deaf children and the results have shown that they fall at the average level of intelligence.[63, 88] This is indicated also by the data in Table 14, which summarizes a study of a group of children in attendance at a Residential School. The Arthur Scale, Form I consists of more formboards than the Wechsler Scales and the Leiter International Scale. The inclusion of formboards may account for the findings of Birch and Birch[10] showing that deaf children who were academic failures scored at the average level on both the WAIS and the Arthur Scale. Their results suggest that neither of these scales is highly effective for predicting academic success for this group of children, an implication which is in agreement with clinical experience. The Leiter Scale and certain selected tests, such as the Digit Span and Digit-Symbol often are more reliable in predicting academic success in deaf children.

TABLE 14.   The mean intelligence score for a group of deaf children on the Grace Arthur Performance Scale

N	Mean C.A.	SD	Mean I.Q.	SD	Mean M.A.	SD
68	10.77	1.77	101.50	21.20	11.05	2.98

Arthur Point Scale of Performance Tests, Revised Form II

Arthur published a revision of her Form II Scale in 1947.[4] This battery consists of the Knox Cube Test, Seguin, Stencil Design, Porteus Maze, and Healy Picture Completion II. Frisina[23] used this battery in a study of mentally retarded deaf children. The population included 82 children in attendance at three Residential Schools. The mean chronological age was 13.65 years and the mean mental age on the Arthur battery was 7.96 years. A significant sex difference favored the males. In addition to this battery, Frisina used the Healy I, Kohs, and the Goodenough Draw-a-Man Tests. The sub-test results were revealing in that the mean mental age scores ranged from 9.50 to 7.26. The order of the test scores from highest to lowest was Knox Cube, Healy I, Seguin, Goodenough, Kohs, Healy II, Stencil Design, and Porteus Maze. No differences occurred by etiology.

The scores on the Knox Cube and Healy I tests were significantly higher than the scores on the other tests used. This finding warrants consideration as a basic indication of the influence of deafness on mental development and on mental functioning. It is discussed further under studies of memory and of abstract ability.

The Nebraska Test of Learning Aptitude for Young Deaf Children

This test was designed first as a test to be used with deaf children. More recently, Hiskey[36] has provided comparative norms for hearing children, extending from three to 11 years six months. Kirk[42] and MacPherson and Lane[52] have studied the relationship between scores on this test and on other performance tests, and both reported high correlations. To explore further the reliability and usefulness of this test we studied 125 children in a Residential School for the deaf. The results by age and by sub-test are presented in Table 15. The mean scores by age level show progression and agreement with Hiskey's standardization, with some exceptions probably attributable to the small samples. However, there is an indication that this test is most useful for children below ten years of age.

TABLE 15.   Mean M.A. scores for deaf children on the sub-tests of the
Nebraska Test of Learning Aptitude

Age Level	5–6	6–7	7–8	8–9	9–10	10–11	11–12
Object memory	6.03	6.68	8.50	9.33	6.95	9.73	10.00
Bead stringing	5.89	6.32	7.47	9.22	7.95	9.07	8.92
P. associations	5.28	6.44	6.92	8.88	8.12	9.53	9.19
Block patterns	5.54	6.88	7.84	8.50	8.25	9.00	9.15
Digit memory	5.52	6.23	8.26	9.24	9.45	9.80	10.38
P. completion	6.60	8.23	6.72	9.96	10.20	10.07	10.15
* P. identification	6.00	6.56	6.40				
* Paper folding	5.59	6.09	6.50				
Attention span	5.61	6.25	7.12	8.50	7.91	9.84	9.34
Puzzle blocks	5.42	6.75	7.76	9.61	8.41	9.53	9.11
P. analogies	6.00	6.87	7.92	9.87	8.00	10.11	9.76
Mean	5.77	6.66	7.40	9.34	8.36	9.63	9.56
N	33	26	19	9	12	13	13

* Item not included above eight years.

Hiskey's comparative study of deaf and hearing children adds substantially to the understanding of the relationship between deafness and intelligence. He found the deaf most inferior on analogy and memory, whereas on block patterns and paper folding, the deaf were equal or superior. The findings given below in the discussion of memory and abstract ability indicate the same type of variation in the mental abilities of deaf children, suggesting a modification of mental development on the basis of deafness from infancy.

DEAFNESS AND MEMORY

Early workers in psychology were intrigued with memory but in recent years psychologists have given little attention to this problem. This is in contrast to investigators in the field of neurology. Penfield,[67] Nielsen,[64] Cobb,[16] and Brain,[13] testify to the interest which neurologists have shown in this aspect of human behavior. One wonders why this basic function of the mind has not continued to receive the attention it warrants from psychology. Perhaps it is related to the meagre interest which has been shown in symbolic behavior. Study of language and language pathology leads directly to considerations of memory as does the study of sensory deprivation.

Virtually all behavior entails memory; learning and memory can be regarded as being closely allied. *Memory* is the ability to associate, retain, and recall experience. Penfield has indicated that the temporal lobes may be the areas of the brain in which much experience is retained, especially experience which is gained through audition. When he stimulated these areas during neurosurgery, the patient reported having auditory experiences which long had been forgotten. Nielsen emphasizes the importance of time and sequence in all memory; *one remembers in time*. Memory inherently assumes awareness of time and the ability to sequentialize experience.

Memory can be affected by various conditions. Freud[22] first suggested the relationship between memory and emotional conflicts. Rapaport[76] also has considered this problem in regard to both the normal and abnormal. The condition of amnesia often can be attributed to psychogenic factors. However, Nielsen has shown how it also can be caused by organic brain disease. Dramatic memory disorders are manifested by the aphasic, especially the patient with amnestic aphasia. He knows the word he wants to use; he knows he knows it, but he cannot recall it. The word, the experience is associated and retained, but it is not available to him. He cannot recall it through his own volition. As soon as the word is said for him, he recognizes it and can use it, but in a few moments it again is unavailable to him.

Another striking memory disorder is that which accompanies advancement in age. Ability to recall is less facile even at the age of 50 years. By the age of 65 to 70 years, many persons have difficulty even in recalling the names of friends. In the aged it is recent experience that is most affected; memory for the distant past may be recalled more easily. Apparently day by day experience is understood and "recorded," but the "storing" function has deteriorated with age. Therefore, in a few days or a few weeks it is as though the experience had not occurred. An example is the 85 year old man, who, though unusually self-competent otherwise, would read a book and within a few weeks, would read it again as though he had never read it before. The most severe memory disorder of this type is seen in the individual with senile dementia. He is unable not only to recall names but often does not recognize members of his own family. He might converse rationally but has no recollection of the experience even a moment later. Experience is received and there is rationality, but because "recording" is lacking, he has no knowledge of the event. He is devoid of memory.

Study of the effect of sensory deprivation on memory has intriguing possibilities but unfortunately knowledge of such effect is most inadequate. That a relationship might exist between sensory loss and memory seems logical on the basis of intersensory facilitation and perception. Nielsen[64] has indicated ways in which one sensory experience is used to recall another. For example, an amnestic aphasic can be helped to recall the word *orange* by smelling an orange. The individual with deafness lacks not only a channel through which to receive and "record" experience; he lacks a sensory avenue through which to associate, and, thereby to recall experience. In the psychology of deafness this leads to the interesting question of whether deafness, especially from early life, leads to a generalized deficit in memory. As indicated by the discussion below, such a conclusion seems unwarranted. Although it appears that deafness affects memory, apparently certain aspects of memory develop normally.

A possibility which must be considered is that when sensory deprivation exists, memory functions may vary in quality and nature. Because alerting mechanisms and perceptual organization are different, specific memory functions may be superior as compared to those with normal sensory capacities. The studies discussed below provide experimental evidence to this effect. These findings also substantiate the observation that when deafness is present, vision must be used differently; it is the primary basis of the perceptual organization which occurs naturally. Studies of the blind have manifested a similar phenomenon. Hayes[32] has reported that blind children exceed the seeing on auditory digit span ability.

Memory must be sub-divided for purposes of study. One possibility is to divide it on the basis of sensory channels: auditory, visual, tactual, olfactory, and gustatory memory. Such classification is essential when studying the sensorially deprived. Another division commonly used in psychology is immediate versus delayed recall. Binet[9] was one of the first to use tests of this type for diagnostic purposes. To study immediate recall he devised the Digit Span tests as well as other tests involving isolated words and sentences. These tests have proved unusually useful in many ways, including the diagnosis of language disorders in children and adults having normal hearing.

Currently one of the most common ways to measure memory is according to span and non-span ability. *Span* assumes that the stimuli are presented in a series, usually one at a time. In *non-span* the stimuli are presented simultaneously. Blair[11] used this non-span procedure in the Object Location Test in his study of the memory abilities of deaf children, as did Hiskey in his Memory for Colored Objects and Visual Digit Span Tests. These considerations are of importance because experimentation has disclosed that different results will be obtained according to whether the span or non-span approach is used. This may be especially true of digit span tests. A four digit test, for example, using the digits 1-7-6-8, when viewed simultaneously, can be instantly combined into 1768. Whereas when these digits are presented one at a time with each digit removed before the next one is presented, the individual must remember the total sequence in order for such mental organization to occur. Moreover, when the stimuli, digits, objects, or pictures are presented as a group, ability to localize in space becomes an important factor of the memory function.

Much discussion has centered around the question of whether

memory is an integral part of intelligence. Rapaport[76] suggests that it probably is not. Correlations between memory functions, as measured by digit span and other measures of intelligence, characteristically are lower than for other mental tests.[99, 100] On the other hand it is difficult to conceive of intelligent behavior without memory, as illustrated by many cases of senile dementia. Perhaps all behavior, human and non-human, is dependent on memory to some degree. The relationship between learning and retention has been emphasized by Hovland[38] who has summarized the experimental work pertinent to the problem. An obvious approach to the study of the psychology of sensory deprivation is to ascertain whether the sensory loss influences memory. Such studies have been undertaken with deaf children. Although this work is not extensive, it provides a basis for further investigation. There is evidence that additional study would be fruitful and enlightening, not only to the psychology of deafness, but to the study of memory in general.

Memory for Patterns of Movement

Hiskey[37] found the deaf child inferior to the hearing on memory abilities. He explained this as a limitation in symbolic behavior. He observed that the hearing children who were studied often verbalized the names of colors or of numbers while performing memory tests. Presumably such verbalizing, which the deaf children could not do, enhanced their performance on this task of memory. If this is true, then on a memory task in which verbalizing is difficult or impossible, but which can be performed solely through visual observation, the deaf should show no inferiority. To examine this hypothesis, we suggested the Knox Cube Test,[43] which was used by Frisina,[23] Blair,[11] and Costello.[17] Their results are highly interesting and provocative. First, we shall consider the nature of this test in relation to the sensory deprivation of deafness. It measures an individual's ability to observe, organize, retain, and reproduce patterns of movement. It is a test of immediate recall because the pattern must be reproduced as soon as the examiner has completed demonstration of it. In addition to vision, the next most important sensory associations seem to be tactual-kinesthetic, although normal persons may count the movements in attempting to reinforce their memory. Characteristically such reinforcement attempts are not used by deaf children. Hence, at least for them it may be described as a visuo-motor-kinesthetic problem. The response from the subject requires his taking a cube and imitating the movements which he has seen.

Frisina found that one of the tests on which the mentally retarded deaf children scored highest was the Knox Cube Test; they scored significantly higher on this test as compared to six other mental tests. These results were corroborated by Blair, who has made the only extensive study of memory functions in deaf children. He compared deaf and hearing children in an investigation using matched pairs. The age range of the subjects was from seven to 13 years. All children had intelligence levels within the normal range. He found a statistically significant difference between the deaf and the hearing on the Knox Cube Test, in favor of the deaf. Costello used this test in a study of deaf and hard of hearing children and she, too, found a significant difference with the deaf being superior.

These studies disclose that on memory functions, such as those measured by the Knox Cube Test, the deaf are highly successful. A generalized memory deficiency did not exist. Why did deaf children show superiority, even to hearing children, on this test? It was suggested in Chapter IV that when a sensory deprivation such as deafness is present from early life, the organism must modify its means for maintaining adequate environmental contact. A shift in perceptual organization must take place in order for the organism to sustain contact with reality and thereby assure the degree of psychological equilibrium required for adjustment. This is accomplished primarily through vision, the remaining distance sense. The individual with deafness from early life is of necessity dependent on visual clues which are irrelevant when hearing is normal. Therefore, his visual perceptual processes develop differently according to his organismic needs. When these processes do not entail verbal symbolic behavior, they may develop to an extent not required when sensory capacities are normal. In other words, if the psychological process involved conforms to the basic monitoring mechanisms of the individual but not to those of the person with normal hearing, the deaf may show superiority.

From Costello's study it seems that this specific type of shift in psychological organization does not occur in the hard of hearing. The mean db hearing loss for her deaf group was 96.67; for the hard of hearing it was 71.38. The alteration of visual perceptual behavior indicated through use of the Knox Cube Test apparently does not transpire unless the deafness is profound. Further research is necessary before the importance of factors such as the degree of deafness and age of onset can be fully understood. However, other studies discussed below support the findings of these studies in which the Knox Cube Test was used. This is not the only means whereby difference in memory abilities between deaf and hearing children have been demonstrated.

Memory for Designs

Binet[9] first used memory for designs as a test of intelligence. Benton[8] and Graham and Kendall[28] have devised extensive tests of this type and have shown their usefulness in diagnosis of organic brain involvements. The problem involved in this type of test can be compared to the Knox Cube Test; both require seeing, observing, organizing, retention, and reproduction by visual-motor processes. Furthermore, both are highly dependent on ability to revisualize and both test immediate recall. There is an obvious difference, however, because in the Knox Cube the primary cues are movement, while in the memory for designs there is no movement. Another important difference is that the Designs Test is not a test of memory span. A sequence of stimuli is not involved. On the other hand, as in the Knox Cube Test, it can be assumed that tactual-kinesthetic associations are used in recall of the designs. While viewing the design, the subject often makes minor movements of the head or of the hands, indicating use of kinesthetic sensation in a supplementary manner.

Blair, employing the matched pair technique, used the Graham-Kendall Test to study this ability in deaf children. He found the deaf to be superior to the hearing. Interestingly, he observed that the hearing attempted to make associations such as, "This looks like a box" or "This looks like a letter." Behavior of this type was not observed in the deaf, who simply observed and reproduced. Perhaps this is a clue to reasons for the deaf clearly exceeding the hearing in such mental functioning. Apparently the hearing found it necessary to try to generalize to past experience, while the deaf performed the task without such attempts. Although complete explanation is difficult, it may be presumed that the deaf performed the task more concretely, their performance being at a more perceptual level. These results provide additional evidence that deafness from early life does influence mental development and the use of intelligence.

Motor Memory

Motor memory has not been studied extensively in either the deaf or the hearing. This type of study offers possibilities for broader understanding of human behavior, emphasized by the work of Van der Lugt.[95] In her Psychomotor Test Series for Children she included a test of motor memory. It consists of raised mazes which the subject traces with his finger while blindfolded. The examiner assists him in tracing the correct path once, then the subject must retrace it without assistance. Fuller[24] used this test in his study of the growth of intelligence in deaf children. He found the deaf superior to the norm for hearing children as provided by Van der Lugt. These norms were established on European children so direct comparison may be tenuous. Nevertheless, this study indicates that deaf children rely more on tactual-motor organization psychologically and hence, perform at a higher level of ability as compared to the hearing. This is in agreement with various other findings in the psychology of deafness. Motor memory is an area in which extensive study seems warranted because it should provide evidence relevant to the psychology of learning in children with profound deafness from early life.

Memory for Object Location

Morsh[59] first studied the ability of the deaf to remember the position of objects in space. This is not a span test as the objects are viewed simultaneously. Blair used the method of allowing the child to observe the objects for twenty seconds then requiring him to place his set of identical objects in the same positions in which he had viewed them on a board. He found the deaf comparable to the hearing, but not superior. These results were in agreement with those of Morsh; however, in Morsh's study, there was a trend for the deaf to be superior. Apparently alteration of memory processes, which might result from deafness, does not affect the functions measured by this test. The deaf child observes, localizes, organizes, retains, and reproduces the position of objects in a given space with equal facility as compared to the hearing.

Span Tests on Which the Deaf Show Inferiority

In the discussion of deafness and memory we have noted that on certain memory functions the deaf are superior or equal to the hearing. We shall now consider memory functions in which they are inferior. Memory span tests are some of the oldest tests in psychology. Binet experimented with several such tests when devising the famed Binet Scale. The most commonly used memory test for measuring this aspect of intelligence is the Digit Span Test. Hiskey[36] observed that the deaf were inferior to the hearing on visual digit span. Blair[11] used three types of span tests in his study of memory in deaf and hearing children. These were Picture Memory Span, Domino Span, and Digit Span. In each test one item was presented at a time; the memory task was to remember the specific series. The digit span was presented visually, each digit on a card, using the digit series which is given auditorially on the Wechsler Intelligence Scale for Children. In the Domino Span this same series of digits was used but instead of presenting numbers, cards with dots were utilized; the dots were organized as they are on dominoes. The Picture Span Test consisted of pictures of objects, such as a kite, boy, house, and squirrel.

The deaf were inferior to the hearing on all three measures: Picture, Domino, and Digit Span. The differences between the deaf and the hearing were statistically significant. These results, together with those for the Knox Cube and Memory for Designs Tests, reveal that deafness influences retention and recall abilities but that the influence varies from one type of memory function to another. Apparently auditory experience is not necessary for retention of design and object location, nor for retention of movement patterns, such as on the Knox Cube Test. On the other hand, when auditory associations are deprived, it is not possible to remember numbers, dot patterns, or pictures with equal facility as compared to those who can rely on auditory associations. It seems that the inferiority of the deaf on specific memory functions cannot be explained only on the basis of verbal-symbolic limitation.

Fuller[24] also studied visual digit span and his results are in close agreement with those of Blair. Moreover, both Blair and Fuller noted an unusual characteristic of the performance of deaf children on the Digit Span Test. The deaf did almost equally as well on digits reversed as they did on digits forward. Blair found that the mean score on reversed digits actually was higher than the mean score for digits forward. The normal individual remembers digits forward substantially better than digits backwards. Why should there be this difference in the memory function in the deaf? It seems that the processes of "recording," organizing, and retaining might be different neurologically and psychologically. The implications for the psychology of learning in children having deafness from early life are not clear at this time; that such implications are of importance is evident. The close relationship between memory and learning suggests that when more is known regarding the ways in which deafness influences memory, a milestone will have been passed in the long history of attempting to expedite learning in those with profound deafness from infancy.

Summary of Deafness and Memory

Seven types of memory have been studied in deaf children: memory for design, tactual-motor memory, memory for movement patterns, object location, dot patterns, picture span, and digit span. The results, comparing deaf and hearing, are presented graphically in Figure 6. As this figure illustrates, on some memory functions the deaf were found to be superior, on some equal, and on others they were inferior to the hearing. The highest level of memory ability was for designs while the lowest was for digits. Further study of the relationship between sensory deprivation and memory would enhance the knowledge of all aspects of memory and add to the psychology of learning and adjustment.

DEAFNESS AND ABSTRACT ABILITIES

Psychologists have been interested in abstract behavior for decades. Goldstein and Scheerer[26] have studied abstraction as it relates to brain disease. A number of workers have investigated the relationship between abstract thought and language. This work covers a number of fields as illustrated by the noteworthy contributions of Cassirer[15] and Langer[45] in philosophy, of Whorf[102] in linguistics, of Vigotsky[96] and Oléron[66] in psychology, and of Arieti[2] in psychiatry. There is general agreement that Man's ability to behave abstractly is one of his unique achievements. However, there has not been uniform agreement as to the definition of the nature of this ability. Likewise, there has been confusion regarding the specific role of language in abstract behavior. Perhaps philosophers more than other professional workers have emphasized the interdependence of language and abstracting ability. In some instances there has been an opinion that abstract behavior is not possible except through the use of language. Study of those with marked limitation of language can be expected to help clarify this question, one of the most consequential questions in all study of human behavior.

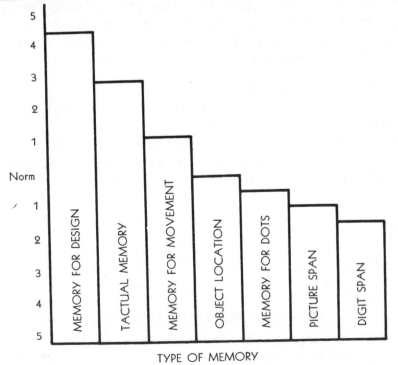

FIG. 6. Memory abilities of deaf children in comparison with the normal.

McAndrews[49] studied concrete-abstract functioning in deaf, blind, and normal children. He concluded that the deaf engaged in more concrete behavior than either the blind or the normal. Furthermore, he suggested that this behavior in the deaf was like that described by Goldstein[25] in the brain damaged. Oléron,[65] who has given considerable attention to this problem as manifested by the deaf, has taken a different point of view. He states that the concreteness found in the deaf is not comparable to that found in those having psychoneurological disorders. His conclusion is that the psychology of deafness and the psychology of brain damage are not identical and research evidence is increasingly substantiating this position.

Templin[89] also has studied the abstract reasoning processes of deaf children and found them to be significantly inferior to the hearing. Her work, and that of others, indicates that as in the case of memory, it is not possible to generalize to the extent of saying that deafness influences all types of abstract behavior. Rather, the type of abstraction involved becomes a critical consideration. Oléron has emphasized that the deaf are inferior on abstract functions which require deduction, on tasks in which the clues are not entirely observable. Examples are the Kohs Block Test[44] and the Progressive Matrices Test.[78] All aspects of the problem presented by the Kohs Test are observable whereas the Progressive Matrices problem cannot be solved without deducing a principle. On this basis the Kohs Test is the more concrete.

Inasmuch as research has shown that the deaf are not inferior on the Kohs Test but seem to be inferior on the Progressive Matrices, this explanation is demanding of consideration. Can we conclude that the deaf are inferior on all tasks which require deduction of a principle, on all tasks in which the clues needed for solution are not observable? This question must be studied further because the findings on the sub-test analysis of the Chicago Non-Verbal Examination suggest that the deaf are not inferior on certain tests of conceptualization, on a type of abstract test in which all the clues are not observable (see table 10). Studies in psychoneurology are revealing in this connection. Halstead,[31] Reitan,[80] Hebb,[33] Milner,[57] Teuber,[91] and McFie[50] have shown that certain psychological functions correlate with specified areas of the brain. Psychological functions requiring language, that is, psycho-linguistic abilities, are localized in the left cerebral hemisphere for right sided individuals. Moreover, psychological functions such as spatial perception and other nonverbal abilities, are localized in the right hemisphere, making it possible for some psychological processes to function irrespective of verbal function. Nature seems to have differentiated neurologically in terms of verbal and nonverbal processes. In the normal person both are used interchangeably and supplementarily. Deafness in infancy impedes development of language and thereby limits the verbal reasoning processes characteristically localized on the left cerebral hemisphere. Such a handicap would not directly preclude development of the nonverbal psychological processes characteristically localized on the right hemisphere. Further study is required to determine whether this explains some of the findings of abstract behavior in deaf persons.

Wright[103] studied the abstract reasoning ability of deaf college students. He matched the deaf and hearing on intelligence, socioeconomic level, and years in college. The Progressive Matrices,[78] the Geometric Design and the Arithmetical reasoning items of the Henmon-Nelson,[35] and the Long and Welch Test of Abstract Reasoning[48] were administered. No differences between the groups were found on the Progressive Matrices or on the Geometric Designs. However, significant differences favoring the hearing were found on Arithmetical Reasoning and on Abstract Reasoning.

These results support the point of view that deafness does not exert a uniform influence on all abstract processes. In Wright's study the deaf were inferior on those tests requiring verbal symbols, words, or numbers but they were not inferior on those using nonverbal stimuli. In contrast to the findings of studies using the Progressive Matrices with children, the deaf adult college student was not inferior on this test as compared to the hearing college student. Perhaps, because this was a select sample, it does not mean that the average person deaf from early life will not be below the average for hearing on this type of abstract function. Murphy[60] and Costello[17] have reported such inferiority for deaf children. Costello found this to be true also of the hard of hearing.

It is clear that some types of abstract abilities and conceptualizing processes are not influenced by deafness. Nevertheless, it must be assumed that deafness is related to the development of abstraction. This relationship seems closely associated with the verbal language limitation which deafness imposes. Therefore, it is logical to conclude that at least to some degree this inferiority in abstraction is a secondary, reciprocal condition to the language limitation and is not a true mental retardation. If the verbal-symbolic function were to be increased the abstract level would be raised concomitantly.

A study using Factor Analysis

The first major study of the mental abilities of the deaf using factor analysis was done by Farrant[19a]. He used a variety of verbal and nonverbal tests in a rigorously defined study comparing deaf and hard of hearing children with the hearing. His findings for the Draw-a-Man Test were supportive of the results reported below. It is of importance that Farrant's study clearly illuminated the differential effect of deafness on intellectual abilities. Some tests factorized differently for the hearing than for the hearing impaired. Because the mental abilities of the deaf and the hard of hearing were less correlated with each other, he concluded that deafness hampers the integration of certain factors of intelligence and distorts others. Studies of this type hold much promise for clarifying the intricate manners in which sensory deprivation in early life modifies or alters intellectual processes.

INTELLECTUAL ABILITIES AND THE DRAW-A-MAN TEST

Review of the studies on the intellectual abilities of hearing impaired children reveals that much of the work has been done on small samples, often from the population of one school. With the exception of Pintner and Reamer's survey,[73] use of a wide geographic distribution, children from different types of schools and of various age ranges have not been customary. In an attempt to overcome some of these hazards in research, a study was planned in which the Draw-a-Man Test played a significant role. This was a National Study designed to investigate certain aspects of the psychology of deafness.

The drawing of the human figure was included because it provides two types of information. As the work of Goodenough[27] demonstrated, it can be used as a measure of mental growth and mental capacity. The work of Machover,[53] Witkin,[101] and Fisher and Cleveland[21] has shown that this test also can be used as a projective test of personality. Therefore, in addition to drawing a man, each subject was asked to draw his mother, his father, and himself. The Draw-a-Man results according to the Goodenough Intelligence Scale are considered here; the projective test results are presented under Personality in Chapter VI.

Other considerations led to the inclusion of the Draw-a-Man Test. Birch and Birch[10] have shown that results from this test correlate with scores on the Leiter Scale[47] and hence may be a valid indication of learning ability in deaf children. In addition, in an extensive study it was necessary to have a test that could be given in small groups. To accomplish this the United States was divided into six geographic areas: southwestern, northwestern, north central, south central, northeastern, and southeastern. Representative Day and Residential Schools, both public and private, were selected from each of these areas; a total of 41 schools participated.

The stratified sampling technique was employed and the age group was from seven through 17 years for the Residential Schools and from nine through 15 years for the Day Schools. This difference in age was determined by the fact that only a small number of seven and 17 year old children was available in Day Schools. There were 511 Residential and 311 Day School children, a total of 822 in the study. Data on the degree of deafness and age of onset for this sample was presented in Chapter III. The Day and Residential groups can be considered comparable in age, degree of deafness, and age of onset. Moreover, the males and females in each group were equal in chronological age.

To add to the study, a sample of normal children was included. This sample was drawn from eight schools in a large metropolitan school system, covering various socio-economic levels. The Draw-a-Man intelligence quotients by age and sex for the total deaf and normal children are presented in Table 16.

As can be seen from these data, the scores for the deaf and normal are similar. The results for both groups show intelligence levels

TABLE 16. Intelligence quotients on the Draw-a-Man Test by age and sex for deaf and normal school children

	Deaf			Normal		
	N	Mean	SD	N	Mean	SD
Age seven						
Males	48	100.14	15.88	43	105.88	17.96
Females	29	108.10	15.34	29	113.79	15.39
Total	77	103.14	16.05	72	109.07	17.29
Age nine						
Males	84	100.87	17.80	20	101.30	19.03
Females	85	98.55	16.86	24	106.25	9.08
Total	169	99.70	17.32	44	104.00	14.50
Age eleven						
Males	119	96.30	14.47	33	94.30	13.04
Females	107	92.28	16.36	27	98.37	12.29
Total	226	94.40	15.49	60	96.13	12.77
Age thirteen						
Males	85	87.22	13.17	24	83.96	9.56
Females	86	86.71	10.83	27	88.56	8.25
Total	171	86.96	12.15	51	86.39	9.10
Age fifteen						
Males	69	89.25	9.23	22	92.45	13.88
Females	62	87.61	10.82	25	93.24	7.28
Total	131	88.47	10.01	47	92.87	10.76
Total group						
Males	405	94.60	15.36	142	96.76	16.95
Females	369	92.89	15.67	132	100.21	14.28
Total	774	93.78	15.53	274	98.42	15.79

within the normal range from seven through eleven years. A difference between the total groups in favor of the hearing was found at the seven year level and at the nine year level, there was a difference between the deaf and normal females, again favoring the hearing. There is a decline in scores for both groups at the 13 and 15 year levels. Apparently ability to Draw-a-Man varies to some extent on the basis of age. These lower scores may be related to the period of adolescence represented by the 13 and 15 year age groups. Moreover, at the 15 year level the hearing scored from five to ten points higher than at the 13 year level, whereas the scores for the deaf 15 year olds showed little change from those for the 13 year group. Despite this slight variation in the mental growth curve for the deaf and hearing at the 13 and 15 year levels, no statistically significant difference was found for the male groups. Such a difference did occur for the females and for the totals at this age, the hearing being superior.

When all ages were combined and total groups compared,

highly significant differences appeared again for the females and for the total groups. No differences appeared for the total male groups which again presents the provocative circumstance of the deaf female falling below the average for hearing females. This difference has been noted by a number of workers and was initially indicated by Pintner.[71] In general, as far as school children are concerned, these data disclose no difference in intelligence between deaf and hearing males, but a significant difference between deaf and hearing females, the deaf being inferior. This difference seems consistent with other findings and must be considered a factor in the psychology of deafness. However, its actual importance remains obscure because, as seen in Chapter VI, the deaf females seem not to be inferior to deaf males in adjustment. Likewise, as indicated in Chapters X and XI, the females are not inferior to the males in language or academic achievement.

Comparison by School

It is of some consequence in the psychology of deafness, particularly to educators, to ascertain whether selective factors are operative in school placement. For this reason in our National Study considerable attention was given to the comparison of results from Day and Residential Schools. The intelligence quotients by school, age, and sex are given in Table 17. No statistically significant differences by school appeared at the nine year level. At 11 years the total Day population was superior to the total Residential and the Day females exceeded the Residential females. In the comparison of the 13 year olds the Residential males scored higher than the Day males but this order was reversed at the age level of 15 years.

These data show no consistent trend for the children in one school to be superior to those in the other, although the Residential School males were superior to the males in the Day Schools. While this must be considered as far as these intelligence test results are concerned, Day versus Residential School placement is not of major consequence. For most purposes of comparison, such as in language development, these groups can be considered of equal mental capacity. Moreover, both groups were within the range of average intelligence as compared to a control group of hearing children.

TABLE 17. Comparison of intelligence quotients for deaf children in Day and Residential Schools by age and sex

	Day			Residential		
	N	Mean	SD	N	Mean	SD
Age nine						
Males	49	98.00	15.56	35	104.88	20.07
Females	44	100.20	13.81	41	96.78	19.23
Total	93	99.04	14.72	76	100.51	20.12
Age eleven						
Males	37	96.62	13.16	82	95.71	15.07
Females	48	98.85	12.74	59	86.93	17.11
Total	85	98.32	12.86	141	92.03	16.48
Age thirteen						
Males	50	84.38	13.67	35	91.28	12.10
Females	43	88.44	9.69	43	84.97	11.72
Total	93	86.26	12.11	78	87.81	12.23
Age fifteen						
Males	22	92.86	6.99	47	87.55	9.72
Females	18	85.89	8.07	44	88.32	11.77
Total	40	89.72	8.19	91	87.92	10.70
Total group						
Males	158	92.89	14.67	199	94.62	15.56
Females	153	94.79	13.11	187	88.97	15.99
Total	311	93.82	13.93	386	91.88	16.00

Comparison by Sex

In the Day School population the males were superior to the females at the 15 year age level. In the Residential School group the males were superior to the females at the 11 and 13 year age levels and in the comparison of the total sex groups. The finding of a difference in intelligence between deaf males and females, as noted previously is not new. The trend has been observed since the early work of Pintner and suggests a selective involvement of deafness by sex.

Comparison of Congenital and Acquired

The importance of age of onset was discussed in Chapter III. The effect of deafness organismically varies to some degree according to the age at which it is sustained. To explore whether differences in intelligence were present on this basis, the congenital were compared with the acquired. These data are given in Table 18. Statistical analyses revealed only a few differences, mainly in the Residential population, where the males with acquired deafness exceeded the females with acquired deafness and the congenital were superior to the acquired. In the comparison by schools the females with acquired deafness in Residential Schools were inferior to the females with acquired deafness in Day Schools. These findings show that when sex differences were present, they were in the Residential group. It is of importance, too, that the congenital were superior to the acquired in the Residential sample and that the Residential females with acquired deafness were inferior to the females in Day Schools having this type of deafness. This suggests that the sex difference in the Residential group may be attributed to the brighter females being in Day Schools. This, however, would apply only to the acquired inasmuch as this difference was not found for the congenitally deaf. The total comparison by age of onset revealed more similarities than differences. When profound deafness is sustained in early life, it is the fact of deafness rather than variations in age of onset which is of major consequence.

TABLE 18.   Intelligence quotients for children with congenital and acquired deafness by sex and school

| | | Congenital | | | | |
| | | Residential | | | Day | |
	N	Mean	SD	N	Mean	SD
Males	142	96.77	15.51	86	92.62	16.40
Females	115	93.43	17.11	86	94.46	13.26
Total	257	95.28	16.30	172	93.54	14.90
				Acquired		
Males	102	94.90	15.42	51	93.84	11.54
Females	93	89.45	14.29	52	96.86	13.60
Total	195	92.30	15.10	103	95.37	12.65

Comparison by Etiology

Consideration of the effects of deafness on learning and adjustment entails exploration of possible varying influences on the basis of etiology. The implications of etiology were discussed in Chapter III. For purposes of this analysis in order to have larger samples, the Day and Residential etiological groups were combined. The data are presented in Table 19.

Significant differences emerged from these comparisons. There were no sex differences *within* the groups; for example, there was no difference between the males and females within the endogenous group, and the same was true for each of the other groups, suggest-

TABLE 19. Intelligence quotients for deaf children by etiology

	Endogenous			Exogenous			Meningitic			Undetermined		
	N	Mean	SD	N	Mean	SD	N	Mean	SD	N	Mean	SD
Males	90	98.69	15.94	123	93.24	16.20	60	94.37	13.43	155	93.74	14.01
Females	96	97.44	15.72	106	89.31	15.55	32	93.72	11.92	160	92.56	15.18
Total	186	98.04	15.80	229	91.42	15.99	92	94.14	12.86	315	93.14	14.61

ing that the etiological agents had no selective effect on the sexes. However, sex differences did appear *between* the groups classified on the basis of etiology. Both males and females in the *undetermined* group were inferior to the males and females in the *endogenous* group. This was true also of the males and females in the *exogenous* group. Stated differently, the endogenous males exceeded the undetermined and the exogenous males, but did not exceed the meningitic males and these same differences occurred for the females.

When the total groups, sexes combined, were compared the findings substantiated those found on the basis of sex. Significant differences appeared in favor of the endogenous; in no instances were the scores in favor of any other group. Although sex differences were not found when the endogenous and meningitic groups were compared, a difference did appear when these comparisons were made on the basis of total groups.

Because of the findings for the undetermined group, there was a presumption that many in this classification had exogenous deafness of prenatal origin. Therefore, for further analysis the meningitic, exogenous and undetermined were combined into one group. This seemed justified by the fact that all in the endogenous classification had deafness in the family. This procedure made it possible to compare those without familial deafness with those having familial deafness. The results are shown in Table 20.

TABLE 20. Comparison of intelligence quotients for children having endogenous and exogenous deafness

	Endogenous			Exogenous		
	N	Mean	SD	N	Mean	SD
Males	90	98.69	15.94	338	94.70	15.11
Females	96	97.44	15.72	298	93.04	15.37
Total	186	98.04	15.80	636	93.91	15.25

Statistical tests disclosed significant differences when analyzed by sex and by total groups. In all instances the endogenous were superior to the exogenous in intelligence. These results corroborate those given in Table 19 for all the etiological classifications. Both the endogenous and the exogenous fell below the actual level of the average intelligence quotient of 100, but both groups fell within the range of normal.

On the basis of intelligence quotients from the Draw-a-Man Test, etiology cannot be considered unrelated to intelligence. Those having hereditary deafness were superior to those having non-hereditary deafness. This denotes that when deafness is caused by disease factors, there is some effect also on mental capacity. As indicated previously, children with neurological deficits are more likely to be exogenous. Therefore, this difference in intellectual capacities may reflect that the exogenous have sustained involvements of the central nervous system in addition to deafness. It is noteworthy that the lowest mean score found was for the exogenous females.

From the data in Chapter III, it is apparent that the exogenous and endogenous did not differ in degree of deafness. It can be assumed that a substantial number of the exogenous sustained their sensory loss after birth, whereas the endogenous were congenitally deaf. This means that a difference in age of onset must be assumed and if there were an advantage in having greater verbal facility, this would have favored the exogenous, not the endogenous.

To consider these differences further and to relate the total findings of this study to other aspects of the psychology of deafness, it is necessary to evaluate what is measured by the Draw-a-Man Test. There has been ample verification through many workers of Goodenough's dictum that the "individual draws what he knows, not what he sees."[27] This emphasizes the importance of this test as a measure of intelligence. Furthermore, most of the investigations using this test with the deaf, including that of Birch and Birch,[10] indicate that it is a measure of general intelligence rather than of a specific aspect of intelligence, such as memory. If the Draw-a-Man Test is a test of general intelligence for normal children, can it be so used with deaf children? Some workers have concluded that it is not a valid measure for predicting academic learning in deaf children. As the correlations given in Chapter XII reveal, this is not true for the present study. In some instances the correlations between the Draw-a-Man scores and scores on the Picture Story Language Test are significant. Apparently, depending on the way in which academic achievement is measured and on the size of the sample, this test can be used to predict verbal, academic learning.

This does not resolve the more difficult question of whether this mental test, as well as others, can be used to predict general learning or brightness in deaf children in the same way as for hearing children. The findings of Blair's study[11] are pertinent. He studied the relationship between Chicago Non-Verbal and Draw-a-Man scores. Correlation between these scores was significant for hearing children but not for the deaf, despite the fact that the hearing and deaf had been matched on scores from the Chicago Non-Verbal Test. For the hearing the Chicago and Draw-a-Man Tests could have been used in selecting much the same children; these tests agreed on indications of brightness and slowness. There was no such agreement for the deaf. This reveals that a risk is involved in concluding that because a deaf child scores as being of normal mental capacity on a given test, his mental functioning, the way in which he uses his intelligence, his mental processes, can be equated with those of the hearing. The relationships between measures of intelligence for deaf and for hearing children cannot be assumed to be identical. While many questions remain unanswered, there is accumulating evidence that different mental processes can result in equivalent scores. Perhaps the drawing of a Man with and without auditory experience results in a different "Man," although the scores are equal. It is the task of the psychology of deafness to ascertain the meaning of scores on psychological tests when used with the deaf. Routine interpretation in terms of findings for the hearing cannot be considered adequate for either clinical or research purposes.

Comparison Between Drawings of a Man and Father

In this chapter we have suggested that equality of quantitative results does not necessarily assure equality of psychological processes. To explore this question further an item analysis was made comparing the Man and Father drawings; the Chi Square technique was used.[97] First, however, the Day and Residential populations were compared by IQ, using the Goodenough scoring procedure for each of the drawings. The results are presented in Table 21.

The scores for the drawing of Father were remarkably similar to those for the drawing of a Man. No statistically significant differences were found between these scores by sex or by school. We had hypothesized that the problem of drawing a Man was more abstract and, therefore, more difficult. These findings did not confirm this postulation. Rather, the scores, scatter, and variations by age level were essentially identical for both drawings and for both School groups.

Before evaluating the qualitative differences a statistical check was made of the similarity between IQ scores on the Man and on the drawing of Self. The sample for this analysis consisted of the males in the nine and 11 year age groups in the Day School population. The results are given in Table 22. These scores, like those for the Man and Father drawings, were remarkably similar. On the basis of these findings it seems that the task of drawing a Man, Father and Self is of equal complexity intellectually. This is interest-

TABLE 21.   The intelligence quotients by school for the Draw-a-Man Test and for drawings of Father

	Day					Residential				
	Man		Father			Man		Father	
	N	Mean	SD	Mean	SD	N	Mean	SD	Mean	SD
Age nine										
Males	49	98	15.56	96	15.67	35	104	20.07	104	15.30
Females	44	100	13.81	100	15.42	41	96	19.23	100	17.03
Total	93	99	14.72	98	15.55	76	100	20.12	102	16.28
Age eleven										
Males	37	96	13.16	95	13.76	82	95	15.07	93	15.10
Females	48	98	12.74	97	12.81	59	86	17.11	87	16.88
Total	85	98	12.86	96	13.81	141	92	16.48	90	16.09
Age thirteen										
Males	50	84	13.67	82	12.96	35	91	12.10	92	11.12
Females	43	88	9.69	86	9.11	43	84	11.72	85	11.49
Total	93	86	12.11	84	11.46	78	87	12.23	88	11.70
Age fifteen										
Males	22	92	6.99	91	7.79	47	87	9.72	89	9.74
Females	18	85	8.07	85	9.51	44	88	11.77	87	11.46
Total	40	89	8.17	89	9.02	91	87	10.70	88	10.64
Total group										
Males	158	92	14.67	91	14.80	199	94	15.29	94	14.47
Females	153	94	13.11	93	13.75	187	88	16.67	89	16.31
Total	311	93	13.93	92	14.31	386	91	16.01	94	15.44

TABLE 22. Comparison of intelligence scores (raw scores)
on drawings of a Man and of Self

	C.A.	N	Mean	SD
Man	9	49	25.90	6.13
Self	9	49	24.96	6.32
Man	11	37	34.19	6.10
Self	11	37	32.44	6.00

ing and manifests that these drawings can be used as a projective test of personality without confounding the results with the factor of intelligence. These drawings were used to study the personality of deaf children and the results are presented in Chapter VI.

Because there were no differences quantitatively between the deaf and the normal, can we conclude that the drawings were equal qualitatively? Likewise, can we assume that because there were no differences between the Day and Residential groups, they drew figures that were otherwise comparable in all respects? The purpose of the item analysis was to pursue this question in greater detail. The results from this analysis comparing the deaf and normal children are given in Table 23. There are 51 items scored on the Draw-a-Man Test as standardized by Goodenough.[27] There was no difference between the deaf and hearing males on 28 of these items; on the 23 items shown in Table 23 significant differences were found. Of these differences, all were in favor of the deaf except two; the deaf scored more often than the hearing on these items. These data reveal that the deaf and hearing males scored differently on 40 per cent of the total number of items. Although there was considerable equality between these groups, although the total points earned were very similar, the deaf and hearing males drew figures that were different in many essential respects.

On the analysis made for the females significant differences between the deaf and the hearing appeared on 18 items, representing 35 per cent of the total number of items scored on this test. These results are given in Table 24. It is noteworthy that 13 of these items also showed significant differences between the males which suggests that there are critical items showing differences between deaf and hearing children, irrespective of sex. Of these items three are on proportion, two on motor coordination, and the remaining pertain to facial features, fingers, or details of clothing. There is some indi-

TABLE 23. Comparison of deaf and normal males on items of the Draw-a-Man Test (Goodenough)

Item	Description	In Favor of
4c	Shoulders definitely indicated	Deaf
6a	Neck present	,,
7d	Both nose and mouth shown in two dimensions; two lips shown	,,
7e	Nostrils shown	,,
8a	Hair shown	,,
8b	Hair present on more than the circumference of the head; better than a scribble; non-transparent	,,
9b	Two articles of clothing non-transparent	,,
9d	At least four articles of clothing definitely indicated	,,
9e	Costume complete without incongruities	,,
10a	Fingers present	,,
10c	Detail of fingers correct	,,
10e	Hand shown as distinct from fingers or arm	,,
11b	Leg joint shown; either knee, hip, or both	,,
12a	Proportion: Head	,,
12b	Proportion: Arms	,,
12c	Proportion: Legs	,,
13	Heel shown	
14d	Motor coordination. Trunk outline	Hearing
14e	Motor coordination. Arms and legs	,,
15a	Ears present	Deaf
15b	Ears present in correct position and proportion	,,
16b	Eye detail. Pupil shown	,,
17b	Projection of chin shown; chin clearly differentiated from lower lip	,,

cation that the deaf gave somewhat more attention to details of the head and face.

The results for the females cannot be viewed as being identical to those for the males. For example, the highest level, from the point of view of intelligence, is attained through profile drawings. For the males no differences appeared on these items, whereas the deaf females drew significantly fewer figures of this type, in agreement with the finding that the deaf females were inferior to the normal. This analysis, like that for the males, indicates that deaf and hearing children draw figures that are different in several details.   The sensory deprivation of deafness seems to shift perceptual-intellectual processes to the extent that what the deaf and hearing *know* about a man is different. This is not revealed by the total quotient scores, which might obscure real differences in the mental processes being used.

It was hypothesized that type of school experience also may be influential on intellectual processes as measured by drawings of the human figure. To examine this hypothesis, the Day and Residential groups were compared by sex on both the Man and Father drawings. The findings for the males are shown in Table 25. Significant differences were found at all age levels as well as for the total groups when all ages were combined. When the age groups were compared, differences appeared on 19 items; the results favoring the Residential males in 15 instances and the Day in four. Two of the four items favoring the Day group pertained to motor coordination. It seems, therefore, that at all the age levels studied, there were ways in which these drawings differed and that the Residential group gave more attention to certain features of the drawing as compared to the Day group.

When the total groups were compared, differences were found for 11 items, seven of these favoring the Day group. Eight of the items which showed differences by age level also showed differences between the total groups. This cannot be taken to indicate complete consistency because in the case of item 17a, *both chin and forehead shown*, the Day exceeded the Residential in the total group comparisons, while at the 11 year level this was scored most frequently for the Residential. A genuine consistency, however, does appear and certain items seem to distinguish between deaf children on the basis of their school experience.

TABLE 24.   Comparison of deaf and normal females on items of the Draw-a-Man Test (Goodenough)

Item	Description	In Favor of
4c	Shoulders definitely indicated	Deaf
7a	Eyes present	Hearing
7e	Nostrils shown	Deaf
8b	Hair present on more than circumference of the head; better than a scribble; non-transparent	''
9b	Two articles of clothing non-transparent	''
9d	At least four articles of clothing definitely indicated	''
9e	Costume complete without incongruities	''
10a	Fingers present	''
12a	Proportion: Head	''
12b	Proportion: Arms	''
12c	Proportion: Legs	''
14c	Motor coordination. Head outline	Hearing
14d	Motor coordination. Trunk outline	''
14e	Motor coordination. Arms and legs	''
16b	Eye detail. Pupil shown	Deaf
17a	Both chin and forehead shown	Hearing
18a	Profile A	''
18b	Profile B	''

TABLE 25.   Comparison of Day and Residential males on items of the Draw-a-Man Test (Goodenough)

Age	Item	Description	In Favor of
9	6b	Outline of neck continuous with that of head, of trunk, or of both	Residential
	9b	At least two articles of clothing non-transparent	,,
	10c	Detail of fingers correct	Day
11	4c	Shoulders definitely indicated	Residential
	5b	Legs attached to trunk. Arms attached to trunk at correct point	,,
	9b	At least two articles of clothing non-transparent	,,
	10c	Details of fingers correct	,,
	17a	Both chin and forehead shown	,,
13	6b	Outline of neck continuous with that of head, of trunk, or of both	,,
	7d	Both nose and mouth shown in two dimensions; two lips shown	,,
	9e	Costume complete without incongruities	,,
	13	Heel shown	,,
	14c	Motor coordination. Head outline	,,
	14f	Motor coordination. Features	,,
	17b	Projection of chin shown; chin clearly differentiated from lower lip	,,
15	6b	Outline of neck continuous with that of head, of trunk, or of both	,,
	8b	Hair present on more than circumference of the head; better than a scribble; non-transparent	Day
	14d	Motor coordination. Trunk outline	Day
	14e	Motor coordination. Arms and legs	,,

All Ages Combined

	4c	Shoulders definitely indicated	Day
	5b	Legs attached to the trunk. Arms attached to the trunk at the correct point	,,
	6b	Outline of neck continuous with that of the head, of the trunk, or of both	Residential
	8b	Hair present on more than circumference of the head; better than a scribble; non-transparent	Day
	9e	Costume complete without incongruities	Residential
	10c	Detail of fingers correct	Day
	11a	Arm joint shown. Either elbow, shoulder, or both	,,
	11b	Leg joint shown. Either knee, hip, or both	,,
	14f	Motor coordination. Features	Residential
	17a	Both chin and forehead shown	Day
	17b	Projection of chin shown; chin clearly differentiated from lower lip	Residential

More variations appeared for the females than for the males. On the age level comparisons there were 27 items on which significant differences were found and only in five instances did they favor the Residential. This suggests substantially more attention to details of the figure on the part of the females in Day schools. However, it must be stressed that the Day females exceeded the Residential females in intelligence at the 11 year level. (See Table 17.)

TABLE 26. Comparison of Day and Residential females on items of the Draw-a-Man Test (Goodenough)

Age	Item	Description	In Favor of
9	5b	Legs attached to trunk. Arms attached to trunk at correct point	Day
	8a	Hair shown	,,
	10c	Detail of fingers correct	,,
	17a	Both chin and forehead shown	,,
11	5b	Legs attached to trunk. Arms attached to trunk at correct point	,,
	8b	Hair present on more than circumference of the head; better than a scribble; non-transparent	,,
	9b	At least two articles of clothing non-transparent	,,
	9d	At least four articles of clothing definitely included	,,
	10c	Detail of fingers correct	,,
	10d	Opposition of thumb shown	,,
	10e	Hand shown as distinct from fingers or arm	,,
	11a	Arm joint shown. Either elbow, shoulder, or both	,,
	12b	Proportion: Head	,,
	12d	Proportion: Feet	,,
	13	Heel shown	,,
	14d	Motor coordination. Trunk outline	,,
	15a	Ears present	Residential
	16b	Eye detail. Pupil shown	Day
	16c	Eye detail. Proportion	,,
	17a	Both chin and forehead shown	,,
13	6b	Outline of neck continuous with that of the head, of the trunk, or of both	Residential
	9b	At least two articles of clothing non-transparent	Day
	10c	Detail of fingers correct	,,
	10d	Opposition of thumb shown	,,
	14d	Motor coordination. Trunk outline	,,
15	6b	Outline of neck continuous with that of the head, of the trunk, or of both	Residential
	12d	Proportion: Feet	,,

All Ages Combined

Age	Item	Description	In Favor of
	4c	Shoulders definitely indicated	Day
	5b	Legs attached to the trunk. Arms attached to trunk at correct point	,,
	6b	Outline of neck continuous with that of the head, of the trunk, or of both	,,
	7d	Both nose and mouth shown in two dimensions; two lips shown	Residential
	8b	Hair present on more than circumference of the head; better than a scribble; non-transparent	Day
	9b	At least two articles of clothing non-transparent	,,
	10c	Detail of fingers correct	,,
	11a	Arm joint shown. Either elbow, shoulder or both	,,
	12d	Proportion: Feet	,,
	12e	Proportion: Two dimensions	,,
	14c	Motor coordination. Head outline	,,
	14d	Motor coordination. Trunk outline	,,
	17a	Both chin and forehead shown	,,

It is interesting that 16 of the 27 items on which differences were found in this comparison fall at the 11 year level. Thus, we cannot conclude that there necessarily were more qualitative differences between Day and Residential females as compared to the Day and Residential males. The greater number of variations for the females can be attributed to dissimilarities in intelligence per se, at least for the 11 year olds.

When the total female groups were compared, the number of differences was 13, which is very similar to the males. It is of im-

TABLE 27.   Items showing difference on drawings of Man and of Father
by sex and by school (Goodenough)

Item	Residental	Group	In Favor of
4b	Length of trunk greater than breadth	Females	Father
		Total	"
6b	Outline of neck continuous with that of head, of trunk, or of both	Females	Man
		Total	"
7d	Both nose and mouth in two dimensions	Males	"
		Total	"
8a	Hair shown	Males	Father
		Total	"
8b	Hair better than a scribble	Males	"
		Total	"
9c	Free from transparencies	Females	Man
		Total	"
10b	Correct number of fingers shown	Males	"
		Total	"
10c	Detail of fingers correct	Males	"
		Females	"
		Total	"
12d	Proportion. Feet	Total	"
14a	Motor coordination	Total	Father
14d	Motor coordination. Trunk outline	Males	"
		Total	"
14f	Motor coordination. Features	Total	Man
15a	Ears present	Total	"
	Day		
9d	At least four articles of clothing definitely indicated	Males	Man
		Total	"
10b	Correct number of fingers shown	Males	"
		Total	"
10c	Detail of fingers correct	Males	"
		Total	"
12b	Proportion. Arms	Total	"
14d	Motor coordination. Trunk outline	Females	"
		Total	"

portance also that seven of these items are identical to those which appeared in the total group comparisons for the males. Furthermore, in all instances these seven items show differences in the same direction. For example, only one of the seven items favors the Residential. This is item 6b, *outline of neck continuous with that of head, of trunk, or of both,* which favors the Residential in the comparison of both males and females. The remaining 6 items which appear for both sexes favor the Day group. These items are 4c, 5b, 10c, 11a, and 17a. All of these items pertain to details of the body, face, or fingers; not clothing, proportion, or motor coordination. This suggests that the children in the Day Schools gave more attention to body contour, fingers, and facial features than those in Residential Schools.

In addition to drawing a Man, the deaf children drew Father. The intelligence quotients derived from these two drawings were remarkably similar, as shown in Table 21. However, the item analysis revealed a number of significant differences. These results for the Day and Residential groups are presented in Table 27. The Residential showed differences on 13 items, while for the Day differences appear on five items. Only on one of them, 14d, did the females in Day Schools show any difference between their drawings of a Man and of Father. The same trend was found for the Residential, the males showing more variations than the females. In some instances differences appeared only for the total group when the sexes were combined.

It is of some interest that of the 23 significant findings for the Residential population, 12 favored the Father drawing and 11 the Man. Of the nine significant findings for the Day population, all favored the Man drawing. We might speculate regarding this variation by School on the basis of the psycho-dynamics which may be assumed. However, discussion of such factors is reserved for the following chapter, where analysis of the human figure drawings is made on the basis of personality. The intention here is to accent the fact that although the intelligence quotients for the Man and Father drawings were comparable, there were qualitative differences. These differences are of importance when considering the mental processes and variations in intellectual functioning, which are associated with deafness.

IMPLICATIONS FOR EDUCATION, LEARNING AND ADJUSTMENT

It is more than four decades since Pintner published his first studies of the mental ability of deaf children. Much has been accomplished since the impetus of his pioneering work and only by comparing our present state of knowledge with that of the past can we achieve the perspective needed for creative effort in the future. Furthermore, only through such appraisal can accomplishments be seen in the light of present practices, in the light of present educational methods.

When one views the work covering several decades and sees the various emphases which have been given, a major change in focus appears. The perspective, the frame of reference has shifted from primary consideration of how deafness and mental retardation are related, to the manner in which deafness influences intellectual development and mental processes. That such influence is present is recognized and the fundamental question is, what is the nature of this relationship and what are the implications for educational training, learning and adjustment.

In recent years, perhaps largely since the work of Goldstein,[25] there has been a tendency to view intelligence in terms of a continuum of concrete-abstract. This emphasis has been productive and clarifying in many ways. However, as the work of Guilford[29] illustrates, if only this frame of reference is utilized, there is a danger of unduly restricting the concept of human intelligence. There are types and degrees of concreteness, and types and degrees of abstraction. This is of paramount importance when considering the effects of a sensory deprivation such as deafness.

The factor theory of intelligence and the factor analysis technique can be used to clarify the impositions and implications of deafness in relation to intelligence. This theory holds that there are unique mental abilities and that an individual might be high on certain of these and low on others. Guilford classifies factors of intelligence into five types of mental operations: cognition, memory, convergent thinking, divergent thinking, and evaluation. These may be defined briefly as follows:

> *Cognition*—ability to recognize and to see relationships
> *Memory*—ability to retain and recall

Convergent thinking—ability to see the best and logical order in a given sequence; to see relationships of given information

Divergent thinking—ability to elaborate from given information; trial and error thinking, originality and variety in associations

Evaluation—judgment of goodness, adequacy, suitability and adaptation of the given and familiar to new and unusual purposes.

In terms of these mental operations, what is the effect of early life deafness on intellect? If we assume that each of these consists of both verbal and nonverbal functions, then all five mental operations would be influenced to some degree by language limitation. But what about generalized involvement; does deafness have an equal effect on each of these mental processes? Using nonverbal criteria, such as the Kohs Block Test, it appears that deafness does not influence cognition. We have seen that memory is affected selectively, causing some memory functions to rise and others to fall. Convergent thinking also may be affected only selectively. Guilford places the mental ability measured by the Picture Arrangement Test under this category. Inasmuch as the deaf are not inferior on this test we cannot assume a generalized effect on convergent thinking.

Divergent thinking and evaluation ability both appear to be affected by deafness. These mental functions entail use of experience more broadly, with fluidity, flexibility, and generalizing ability playing a significant role. This does not infer that these two operations are identical. They are grouped here for purposes of convenience in relating these operations to the effects of deafness. The Progressive Matrices Test entails divergent thinking. Common tests of intelligence do not include many measures of evaluation ability. It is difficult to conclude whether those deaf from early life are inferior in general on divergent thinking and evaluation ability, or whether deafness also affects these abilities selectively, only in certain respects. As more specialized nonverbal tests become available, research in this connection will be accomplished more readily.

To think of the mental functions of the deaf only in terms of an abstract-concrete continuum is an obstacle to recognizing the complexity of human intellect. While it is apparent that deafness influences intelligence, a generalized effect is not suggested. The presumption is that those aspects of intelligence, those mental operations which are not affected adversely should be capitalized through training and education. It has long been the practice in guidance to assist the individual in ascertaining those areas in which he has major aptitude. Such assistance seems essential for the deaf if they are to actualize their potentials. Although much knowledge is lacking, there is ample evidence to provide a basic foundation for such guidance programs.

There is another possibility which offers even greater challenge. Present findings disclose that deafness affects specific mental operations more than others. Those requiring verbal-symbolic facility are affected and continued effort to overcome this type of limitation is indicated; this is discussed further in Part Three. However, there are nonverbal aspects in all mental operations. Guilford[29] states that "understanding the behavior of others and of ourselves is largely nonverbal in character." Likewise, many problems of the divergent thinking type, and many judgmental problems are nonverbal. There is clear indication that specific training in these functions should be given to those having deafness from early life. Various activities might be devised, even for the young deaf child, which would give him practice and training on those aspects of intelligence which seem to be most vulnerable to deafness. It can no longer be assumed that the "structure of intellect" is determined completely by heredity. This is demonstrated by sensory deprivation because if stimulation and training do not take place, intellect itself is formed differently. The extent to which mental operations are determined by heredity and through training is not known even for the normal. The extent to which the effects of deafness on intellect are irreversible, or can be altered by training procedures specifically designed for the purpose, likewise is not known. The educator, therefore, is confronted with the need to assume that these effects can be alleviated. His task is to devise techniques and methods for the alleviation of these intellectual impositions to the greatest extent possible.

Considerable work and experimentation will be necessary before the most suitable and most effective methods for such training can be evolved. However, categories of activities can be outlined. To start with it must be recognized that certain training procedures now used with deaf children emphasize a type of mental operation in which he needs training the least; this seems most true of "matching" activities and work referred to as "sense training." Such training might be minimized and greater emphasis given to the child's need for training in memory abilities, such as memory for digits, dot patterns, bead patterns, and for word sequences. Correlation statistics indicate that if this type of intellectual behavior could be improved, there would be a concomitant increase in all verbal behavior, especially in reading.

There are other mental operations for which specialized training might be given. These can be illustrated best by referring to the processes involved in various types of mental tests; the mental tests themselves are not used for training. For example, the pictorial analogy test on the Hiskey[37] requires an ability commonly referred to as reasoning by analogy: father is to *home*—as bird is to *nest*. Problems of this type can be devised for the young child and through all age levels to adulthood. Another example is that of being required to deduce a principle. This can be done through the use of numbers, pictures and words. In the number series 8–16–24–32, the principle is to increase by 8 at each interval. The child might be given the numbers 8–32 and be required to deduce the principle and complete the problem. Activities using pictures can be devised which require grouping, sorting, and categorizing. This is the basis of training in conceptualization. These, too, can cover the range from the simple to the complex. Perhaps the most difficult to devise nonverbally are those requiring *if* and *because* mental processes. One type of approach is through the use of pictures in which is presented the problem of, "If a fire starts—what would you do?" The pictures used for the child's response should include a range of possibilities. Many problem situations stressing the relationship between cause and effect could be used. This type of training accents the critical mental operation of evaluation and judgment.

The involvements of deafness are not limited to the intellectual; other aspects are considered in the following chapters. It is unlikely, however, that there are more important consequences than those noted on the structure of the intellect. These are the bases of learning and adjustment. They provide the foundation for remedial education and training. The educator has the challenging responsibility of determining the extent to which these influences can be altered.

REFERENCES

1. Amoss, H.: Ontario School Ability Examination. Toronto, Ryerson Press, 1936.
2. Arieti, S.: Interpretation of Schizophrenia. New York, Robert Brunner, 1955.
3. Arthur, G.: A Point Scale of Performance Tests. Chicago, C. H. Stoelting, 1943.
4. _____: A Point Scale of Performance Tests, Revised Form II, New York, Psychol. Corp., 1947.
5. Baldwin, B. T.: The physical growth of children from birth to maturity. Iowa City, Studies in Child Welfare, #1, 1921.
6. Benda, C. E.: Developmental Disorders of Mentation and Cerebral Palsies. New York, Grune and Stratton, 1952.
7. Bender, L.: Psychopathology of Children with Organic Brain Disorders. Springfield, C. C. Thomas, 1956.
8. Benton, A. L.: A visual retention test for clinical use. Arch. Neurol. and Psychiatry, 54, 212, 1945.
9. Binet, A. and Simon, Th.: The Intelligence of the Feeble-Minded. Baltimore, Wilkins and Wilkins, 1916.
10. Birch, J. R. and Birch, J. W.: The Leiter International Performance Scale as an aid in the psychological study of deaf children. Am. Ann. Deaf, 96, 502, 1951.
11. Blair, F.: A study of the visual memory of deaf and hearing children. Am. Ann. Deaf, 102, 254, 1957.
12. Bowlby, J.: Maternal Care and Mental Health. New York, Columbia University Press, 1952.
13. Brain, R.: The Nature of Experience. London, Oxford University Press, 1959.
14. Brown, A. W., Stein, S. P. and Rohrer, P. L.: The Chicago Non-Verbal Examination, Manual of Directions. New York, Psych. Corp., 1947.
15. Cassirer, E.: The Philosophy of Symbolic Form, Vol. I, II, and III. New Haven, Yale University Press, 1953.
16. Cobb, S.: Foundations of Neuropsychiatry. Baltimore, Wilkins and Wilkins, 1958.
17. Costello, M. R.: A study of speechreading as a developing language process in deaf and in hard of hearing children. Evanston, Northwestern University, Unpublished Doctoral Dissertation, 1957.
18. Doll, E. A., Phelps, W. and Melcher, R.: Mental Deficiency Due to Birth Injuries. New York, Macmillan, 1932.
19. Drever, J. and Collins, M.: Performance Tests of Intelligence. London, Oliver and Boyd, 1936.
19a. Farrant, R.: A factor analytical study of the intellectual abilities of deaf and hard of hearing children compared with normal hearing children. Unpublished doctoral dissertation, Northwestern Univ., 1960.
20. Fiedler, M. F.: Good and poor learners in an oral school for the deaf. Exceptional Children, 23, 291, 1957.
21. Fisher, S. and Cleveland, S. E.: Body Image and Personality. Princeton, D. Van Nostrand, 1958.
22. Freud, S.: Collected Papers. London, Hogarth Press, 1950.
23. Frisina, D. R.: A psychological study of the mentally retarded deaf child. Evanston, Northwestern University, Unpublished Doctoral Dissertation, 1955.

24. Fuller, C.: A study of the growth and organization of certain mental abilities in young deaf children. Evanston, Northwestern University, Unpublished Doctoral Dissertation, 1959.

25. Goldstein, K.: Language and Language Disturbances. New York, Grune and Stratton, 1948.

26. _____ and Scheerer, M.: Abstract and concrete behavior. Psychol. Monog., #53, 1941.

27. Goodenough, F.: Measurement of Intelligence by Drawings. New York, World Book, 1926.

28. Graham, F. K. and Kendell, B. S.: Performance on brain damaged cases on a Memory-for-Designs Test. J. Abnormal Soc. Psychol., 41, 303, 1946.

29. Guilford, J. P.: Three faces of intellect. Am. Psychologist, 14, 469, 1959.

30. Hall, C. S. and Lindzey, G.: Theories of Personality. New York, John Wiley and Sons, 1957.

31. Halstead, W.: Brain and Intelligence; A Study of the Frontal Lobes. Chicago, University of Chicago Press, 1947.

32. Hayes, S. P.: Measuring the intelligence of the blind, in Zahl, P. A. (ed.) Blindness. Princeton, Princeton University Press, 1950.

33. Hebb, D. and Penfield, W.: Human Behavior after extensive bilateral removal from the frontal lobes. Arch. Neurol. and Psychiat., 44, 421, 1940.

34. Heider, F. and Heider, G. M.: Studies in the psychology of the deaf. Psychol. Monog. #242, 1941.

35. Henmon, V. and Nelson, M.: Henmon-Nelson tests of Mental ability. Teacher's Manual. New York, Houghton-Mifflin, 1932.

36. Hiskey, M.: A study of the intelligence of the deaf and hearing. Am. Ann. Deaf, 101, 329, 1956.

37. _____: Nebraska Test of Learning Aptitude for Young Deaf Children. Lincoln, University of Nebraska, 1955.

38. Hovland, C. I.: Human learning and retention, in Stevens, S. S. (ed.) Handbook of Experimental Psychology. New York, John Wiley and Sons, 1951.

39. Jersild, A. T.: Emotional Development, in Carmichael, L. (ed.) Manual of Child Psychology. New York, John Wiley and Sons, 1946.

40. Jones, H. E.: Motor performance and growth. Berkeley, University of California Press, 1949.

41. Kanner, L.: Child Psychiatry. Springfield, C. C. Thomas, 1957.

42. Kirk, S. and Perry, J.: A comparative study of the Ontario and Nebraska Tests for the deaf. Am. Ann. Deaf, 93, 315, 1948.

43. Knox, H. A.: A scale based on the work at Ellis Island for estimating mental defect. J. Am. Med. Assoc., 62, 741, 1914.

44. Kohs, S. C.: The Block Designs Test. Chicago, C. H. Stoelting, 1923.

45. Langer, S. K.: Philosophy in a New Key. Cambridge, Harvard University Press, 1957.

46. Lavos, G.: The Chicago Non-Verbal Examination: A study in retest characteristics. Am. Ann. Deaf, 95, 379, 1950.

47. Leiter, R. G.: The Leiter International Performance Scale. Santa Barbara, State College Press, 1940.

48. Long, L. and Welch, L.: Factors affecting efficiency of inductive reasoning. J. Exper. Ed., 10, 252, 1942.

49. McAndrews, H.: Rigidity and isolation; a study of the deaf and the blind. J. Abnormal. and Social Psychol., 43, 476, 1948.

50. McFie, J.: Cerebral dominance in cases of reading disability. J. Neurol. and Psychiat., 15, 194, 1952.

51. MacKane, K.: A comparison of the intelligence of deaf and hearing children. New York, Bureau of Pub., Columbia University, T. C., Contrib. to Ed., #585, 1933.

52. MacPherson, J. and Lane, H.: A comparison of deaf and hearing on the Hiskey Test and on performance scales. Am. Ann. Deaf, 93, 178, 1948.

53. Machover, K.: Personality Projection in the Drawing of the Human Figure. Springfield, C. C. Thomas, 1949.

54. Macmillan, D. P. and Brunner, F. G.: Children attending the Public Day Schools for the Deaf in Chicago. Chicago Public Schools, 1906.

55. Masland, R., Sarason, S. and Gladwin, T.: Mental Subnormality. New York, Basic Books, 1958.

56. Meredith, H. V.: The rhythm of physical growth. Iowa City, Studies in Child Welfare, #1, 1921.

57. Milner, B.: Intellectual function of the temporal lobes. Psychol. Bull., 51, 42, 1954.

58. Morrison, W.: The Ontario School Ability Examination. Am. Ann. Deaf, 85, 184, 1940.

59. Morsh, J. E.: Motor performance of the deaf. Comp. Psychol. Monog., #66, 1936.

60. Murphy, K. P.: Tests of abilities and attainments, in Ewing, A. (ed.) Educational Guidance and the Deaf Child. Washington, D. C., The Volta Bureau, 1957.

61. Myklebust, H. R.: The Psychological effects of deafness. In press, Am. Ann. Deaf, 1960.

62. _____: Towards a new understanding of the deaf child. Am. Ann. Deaf, 98, 496, 1953.

63. _____ and Burchard, E. M. L. A study of the effects of congenital and adventitious deafness on the intelligence, personality, and social maturity of school children. J. Ed. Psychol., 34, 321, 1945.

63a. Neyhus, A.: The personality of socially well-adjusted adult deaf as revealed by projective tests. Unpublished doctoral dissertation, Northwestern Univ., 1962.

64. Nielsen, J.: Memory and Amnesia. Los Angeles, San Lucas Press, 1958.

65. Oléron, P.: Conceptual thinking of the deaf. Am. Ann. Deaf, 98, 304, 1953.

66. _____: Recherches sur le Développement Mental des Sourds-Muets. Paris Centre National de la Recherche Scientifique, 1957.

67. Penfield, W. and Roberts, L.: Speech and Brain Mechanisms. Princeton, Princeton University Press, 1959.

68. Peterson, E. G. and Williams, J. M.: Intelligence of deaf children as measured by drawings. Am. Ann. Deaf, 75, 273, 1930.

69. Piaget, J.: The Psychology of Intelligence. New York, Harcourt, Brace, 1950.

70. Pintner, R.: The Pintner Nonlanguage Mental Test. New York, Columbia University, Bureau of Publications, 1929.

71. _____, Eisenson, J. and Stanton, M.: The Psychology of the Physically Handicapped. New York, F. S. Crofts, 1946.

72. _____ and Paterson, D. G.: A Scale of Performance Tests. New York, Appleton-Century-Crofts, 1923.

73. _____ and Reamer, J. F.: A mental and educational survey of schools for the deaf. Am. Ann. Deaf, 65, 451, 1920.

74. _____ and _____: Learning tests with deaf children. Psychol. Monog. #20, 1916.

75. Porteus, S. D.: The Porteus Maze Test and Intelligence. Palo Alto, Pacific Books, 1950.

76. Rapaport, D. Emotions and Memory. New York, International Universities Press, 1950.

77. _____: Manual of Diagnostic Psychological Testing. New York, Josiah Macy Foundation, 1944.

78. Raven, J. D.: Guide to Using the Progressive Matrices. London, H. K. Lewis, 1938.

79. Reamer, J. F.: Mental and educational measurements of the deaf. Psychol. Monog. #29, 1921.

80. Reitan, R.: Certain differential effects of left and right cerebral lesions in human adults. J. Comp. and Physiol. Psychol., 48, 474, 1955.

81. Schick, H. F.: A performance test for deaf children of school age. Volta Review, 34, 657, 1934.

82. Schilder, P.: Mind: Perception and Thought in their Constructive Aspects. New York, Columbia University Press, 1942.

83. Shirley, M. and Goodenough, F. A survey of intelligence of deaf children in Minnesota schools. Am. Ann. Deaf, 77, 238, 1932.

84. Soddy, K. (ed.): Mental Health and Infant Development, Vol. I and II. New York, Basic Books, 1956.

85. Spitz, R.: Infantile depression and the general adaptation syndrome, in Hoch, P. and Zubin, J. (ed.) Depression. New York, Grune and Stratton, 1954.

86. Springer, N.: A comparative study of the intelligence of a group of deaf and hearing children. Am. Ann. Deaf, 83, 138, 1938.

87. Strauss, A. and Lehtinen, L.: Psychopathology and Education of the Brain-injured Child. New York, Grune and Stratton, 1947.

88. Streng, A. and Kirk, S. A.: The social competence of deaf and hard of hearing children in a Public Day School. Am. Ann. Deaf, 83, 244, 1938.

89. Templin, M. C.: The Development of Reasoning in Children with Normal and Defective Hearing. Minneapolis, University of Minn. Press, 1950.

90. Terman, L. M. and Merrill, M.: Measuring Intelligence. New York, Houghton Mifflin, 1937.

91. Teuber, H.: Physiological Psychology. Ann. Rev. Psychol., 6, 267, 1955.

92. Thurstone, L. I. and Thurstone, T. G.: SRA Primary Mental Abilities. Chicago, Science Research Associates, 1948.

93. Treacy, L.: A study of social maturity in relation to factors of intelligence in acoustically handicapped children. Evanston, Northwestern University, Unpublished Thesis, 1952.

94. Tuddenham, R. D. and Snyder, M. M.: Physical growth of California boys and girls from birth to eighteen years. Berkeley, University of California Press, 1954.

95. Van der Lugt, M.: Psychomotor Test Series for Children. New York, New York University Press, 1948.

96. Vigotsky, L. S.: Thought and speech. Psychiatry, 2, 29, 1939.

97. Walker, H. M. and Lev, J.: Statistical Inference. New York, Henry Holt, 1953.

98. Wechsler, D.: The Measurement of Adult Intelligence. Baltimore, Williams and Wilkins, 1944.

99. _____: Wechsler Adult Intelligence Scale, New York, Psychol. Corp., 1955.

100. _____: Wechsler Intelligence Scale for Children. New York, Psychol. Corp., 1949.

101. Witkin, H. A. et al.: Personality through Perception. New York, Harper and Brothers, 1954.

102. Whorf, B. J.: Language, Thought and Reality. New York, John Wiley and Sons, 1956.

103. Wright, R.: The abstract reasoning of deaf college students. Evanston, Northwestern University, Unpublished Doctoral Dissertation, 1955.

104. Zeckel, A. and Van der Kolk, J. J.: A comparative intelligence test of groups of children born deaf and of good hearing by means of the Porteus Maze Test. Am. Ann. Deaf, 84, 114, 1939.

Suggestions for Further Study

Anastasi, A.: Psychological Testing. New York, Macmillan, 1954.

Bridgman, O.: The estimation of mental ability in deaf children. Am. Ann. Deaf, 84, 337, 1939.

Brown, A.: The correlation of non-language tests with each other, with school achievement and with teachers' judgments of the intelligence of children in a school for the deaf. J. Appl. Psychol., 14, 371, 1930.

Capwell, D.: The performance of the deaf on the Grace Arthur Test. J. Consult, Psychol., 9, 91, 1945.

Cronbach, L.: Essentials of Psychological Testing, 2nd. ed. New York, Harper, 1960.

Doctor, P.: On teaching the abstract to the deaf. Volta Review, 52, 547, 1950.

Graham, E. and Shapiro, E.: Use of the performance scale of the Wechsler Intelligence Scale for Children with the deaf child. J. Consult. Psychol., 17, 396, 1953.

Guilford, J. P.: Psychometric Methods. New York, McGraw Hill, 1936.

MacKane, K.: A Comparison of the Intelligence of Deaf and Hearing Children. New York, Columbia University Press, T. C. Cont. to Ed., #585, 1933.

Max, L.: Experimental study of the motor theory of consciousness. J. Comp. Psychol., 24, 301, 1937.

Oléron, P.: A study of the intelligence of the deaf. Am. Ann. Deaf, 95, 179, 1950.

Watson, R. I.: Psychology of the Child. New York, John Wiley and Sons, 1959.

Chapter VI

PERSONALITY DEVELOPMENT AND EMOTIONAL ADJUSTMENT

FROM LITERATURE AND FOLKLORE we learn that assumptions have been made for centuries regarding relationships between physical and emotional factors. During the period of the Graeco-Roman Empire, physique was of primary importance. There was little tolerance for physical defects and the supposition grew that when there was a crippled body there was a crippled mind. This feeling of association between physical handicaps and abnormality of the mind has pertained also to those who have sensory deficiencies. The deaf and the blind frequently are cast in a stereotype by novelists who describe them as secretive, suspicious, cruel, and unfriendly. Brunschwig[5] surveyed such references in literature.

The feelings and attitudes of the public toward those who are different from the majority group is an area for investigation in and of itself. In this regard often it is beneficial to think of the hearing impaired as a minority group. They are subject to biases and prejudices because they are different from the usual, the typical, and the familiar. They may be refused employment or rental of living quarters because they are deaf. Such attitudes and generalizations are inaccurate, harmful, and degrading. While a relationship between deafness and personality adjustment might exist, only objective study can adequately describe such a phenomenon. Moreover, only after such definition and objectification can effective programs be evolved for those maladjustments which are indicated. Study of the influences of sensory deprivation on personality has significance in the understanding of all people. Knowledge regarding the relevance of deafness to psychopathology can contribute to our understanding of hysteria, hallucinations, psychogenic deafness, anxiety neurosis, and schizophrenia.

Study of deafness in relation to personality raises many questions concerning critical aspects of human behavior. Individuals deaf from early life are confronted with one of the most difficult problems encountered by Man, that of acquiring the language of their culture without being able to hear it. What is the effect of inability to communicate on personality development? This consideration is pertinent to personality theory because it indicates the need for knowledge concerning the influence of language on ego development and on the general structure of personality.

However, in the psychology of deafness the problem is not limited to the effect of limitation in language. The deaf baby does not hear the "baby talk," the "cooing" of his mother; he does not hear himself, or others, laugh or cry. He does not hear the inflectional and intonational meanings which often convey more significance than the words themselves; the word *mother* might be spoken several times, each time conveying a different meaning depending on *how* it is spoken. Presumably it is through intonation and innuendo that biases and prejudices usually are passed from father to son. While scientific evidence is lacking, experienced educators of the deaf have observed that people deaf from early life often do not acquire the same biases and feelings of taboo that characterize the normal population. Perhaps they do not acquire these feelings in the same way because they do not hear the innuendos and other unverbalized meanings which are so much a part of daily conversation. Then, too, what is the emotional significance of not hearing the myriads of nonvocal sounds which we call noise? Does not hearing a dog bark stimulate or reduce feelings of fear? Such questions are significant to social psychology and the psychology of personality as well as to the psychology of deafness.

These questions lead us to consider a basic aspect of personality development, identification, which has received attention from psychologists and psychiatrists interested in psychopathology. *Identification* refers to the unconscious development of feelings and attitudes similar to those of the peers, especially of the same sex group. Personality disorders might arise if females *identify* with males, and vice versa. There are many other factors involved in identification, including attitudes toward one's family, community, state, nation, the world, and mankind. As Myklebust[29] and Mowrer[28] have emphasized, identification seems fundamentally related to language acquisition itself. More broadly, audition must play a significant role in the total development of feelings of identification. Conversely, we may hypothesize that it is more difficult to develop such feelings when the many sounds which enhance interpersonal relationships are not heard. When identification is restricted it is reflected especially in ego development, but also in other ways, as shown by the work of Bowlby,[4] Spitz,[43] Goldfarb,[13] and Ribble,[40] who have emphasized the importance of early infancy in personality development and structure. They have stressed that preverbal experience is consequential to later emotional well being. They have revealed that isolation, lack of stimulation and lack of interaction between the infant and his parents might have a disintegrative effect on the emotional growth of the child. The implications are striking for the child having deafness from early infancy. As Pellet[34] has stated, this child has a long preverbal period. While he learns to use gesture, he is largely nonverbal for a period of a few years. Yet he must identify, he must learn to conform, to dress, to feed himself, and to maintain adequate emotional relationships with his environment. Homeostatic equilibrium must be established and preserved. Although he is deprived of an important avenue through which to learn about society's demands and expectations, he must make an adjustment between his environmental circumstances and his inner needs.

Conceivably there is no more important factor than *isolation* in the emotional adjustment of the hearing impaired. By this we refer to the isolation resulting from a hearing loss; the antennae-like distance sense is impaired. There are many ramifications psychologically. An example is the way in which it deprives the individual of the monitoring function of hearing, of the innumerable ways in which audition automatically supplies information concerning the status and fluctuations of the environment. Audition not only provides information about external happenings, it provides a means for monitoring our thoughts and feelings. Hebb[21] has stressed the importance of this function through experiments with artificial sensory deprivation. When the normal individual is isolated, when he is deprived of sensory stimulation and removed from other people, he becomes disturbed and hallucinated. He no longer has the means whereby he can monitor his own feelings and ideas. Apparently a fundamental criterion for maintaining emotional stability is being able more or less continuously to compare one's thinking and feelings with others. This type of monitoring seems essential to maintain a firm hold on reality so as not to escape into autistic behavior. When deafness is present, especially when it is sustained in early life, the monitoring of one's feelings, attitudes, and ideas is more difficult. The individual naturally is more isolated with the implication that he must be more detached and autistic. Most persons having deafness, even when the extent is moderate, must achieve monitoring and realistic contact by other means, notably through vision and taction. From the study of the hard of hearing reported below it seems that the use of hearing aids lessens but does not eliminate this problem. Evidently a moderate hearing loss sustained in adulthood results in a degree of isolation from the majority group. If this is true, then the imposition on monitoring processes might be a factor of substantial consequence in the personality dynamics of those having impairment of hearing.

Deafness can result in isolation in various ways. Intimate contact with families of deaf children discloses that it is extremely difficult to keep the hearing impaired child informed of daily occurrences and circumstances. To explain such happenings, incidental as they may be, is in itself demanding of patience and maturity on the part of parents. Often because of the limitations in the ability to communicate, such explanations cannot be given. This, too, in the final analysis, is a problem resulting from an inability to monitor one's world through hearing. There is a deficiency of total experience which forms the basis of feelings, attitudes, and personality per se.

These considerations, practical and theoretical, serve as a frame of reference in this chapter. It has been hypothesized that a relationship exists between deafness, personality development, and emotional adjustment. There is an assumption that deafness alters experience, that it causes an imposition on monitoring, and that it forces detachment and isolation. Furthermore, language is viewed as a significant factor in the development of personal-social contacts and interaction. Language is assumed to be the primary means whereby experience is internalized, crystallized, and structured. Hence, when language is limited there might be a reciprocal restriction in ability to integrate experience; the personality might be less structured, more immature, less subtle, and more sensorimotor in character. These are fundamental problems to be investigated by the student of the psychology of deafness.

In the study of the psychological consequence of deafness perhaps the two most critical variables are the age of onset and the degree of the impairment. Unfortunately research evidence is meagre relative to the specific influence of these factors. Most investigations of the impact of deafness on personality have pertained to children with profound deafness from early life. Variations of involvement can be expected according to at least four levels of hearing loss. These may be described as:

I. *A loss of 30 to 45 db:* This is a moderate loss affecting mainly the scanning and background functions of hearing. It is also the point at which conversation becomes difficult without amplification. Psychologically, however, it is the impaired awareness and the environmental detachment which are of most importance. At this level the restriction imposed on communication can be alleviated by getting closer to the speaker and by the use of amplification. Thus, it is not socialization, but basic awareness and monitoring that suffer most.

II. *A loss of 45 to 65 db:* With this degree of hearing loss, social intercourse is clearly affected, and the background-foreground use of audition is essentially precluded. Because the scanning function of hearing is largely eliminated, the individual responds only in a foreground manner; whenever he hears, he scans, thus treating all sound as it first reaches his threshold as a sound requiring direct attention. The use of amplification makes conversation readily possible, but because he must give all sound equal attention, conversation is essentially limited to one person, or to a small group. The individual experiences considerable detachment and seeks social relationships with others having a similar degree of deafness.

III. *A loss of 65 to 80 db:* The use of amplification, while effective for maintaining social inter-relationships, is less satisfactory than for those in Group II. Both personal-social and general environmental contact is difficult. There is need for considerable reliance on other systems for monitoring, particularly on vision and taction. Feelings of identification are impeded and personal-social relationships are most satisfying when they are with others having deafness, usually to a similar extent.

IV. *A loss of 80 to 100 db:* This is a profound hearing loss. The use of amplification is effective mainly in maintaining intelligible speech and focusing attention to loud environmental sounds. The use of vision and taction is mandatory in maintaining homeostatic equilibrium. Personal-social interaction with the normally hearing is arduous. Most social relationships are with others having profound deafness.

This classification is given as an indication of the importance of the degree of hearing loss psychologically. However, behavioral reaction to deafness, like all human behavior is complex. *Other factors must be considered*, particularly the *age of onset*. For example, if the degree of involvement were at the level of category IV and were sustained in infancy, the impact on all aspects of behavior can be assumed to be greater than if this extent of hearing loss were to occur in adulthood. Before discussing research evidence, a classification is given which has been found useful in noting the possible effects of deafness according to the age of onset. In the use of this classification, *other factors must be considered*, particularly the *degree of the involvement*.

I. *Prenatal or before 2 years:* This group has the greatest effect on ability to communicate, with implications for impact on personality and emotional adjustment. Basic psychological processes, such as identification, are disturbed. When the deafness is profound, isolation is more apparent than in any other group. Reliance on vision and taction may be marked. Specialized educational training is necessary.

II. *From 2 to 6 years:* There is evidence that if a child hears normally for the first two years of his life, he not only has some benefit verbally, but the psychological effects of his hearing loss may be lessened. This is true particularly the later the onset occurs before 5 to 6 years of age. After 5 years there is a noticeable benefit verbally, with concomitant advantage to personality development and structure. It is with those where onset occurs after 5 years that the classification of *deafened* is most useful, but this implies a profound degree of hearing loss.

III. *School years:* Language function is well retained for inner language purposes, and in other ways. The greatest effect is on personal and school adjustment; often special education is necessary. Friendships and identification with the majority group are difficult to maintain, but ego development and general emotional growth are less affected than for groups I and II. Individuals in this group who sustain profound deafness often become leaders in the deaf community.

IV. *Early adulthood:* The age range for this group is from 18 to approximately 30 years. Except for those deafened by diseases such as meningitis, the degree of deafness often is moderate with otosclerosis being a common etiology. Basic personality patterns are not altered although undesirable traits may be accentuated. Disturbance of social relationships including marital plans, educational programs, and vocational choice often is severe. Attitudes and patterns of behavior may be characteristic. Choice of friends and social contacts may shift to others having impaired hearing.

V. *Early to late adulthood:* This group includes those from 30 to 60 years. Etiologies include otosclerosis, progressive nerve involvement, endolymphatic hydrops, acoustic trauma, and other diseases. Marital adjustment may be affected but a more common problem is occupational status; complete shift of career often follows the onset of the hearing loss. Change of friends and social group also occurs frequently, with the possibility of characteristic attitudes developing on the basis of the sensory deprivation.

VI. *Later life:* In this group we classify the aged with presbycusic hearing loss. The basic effect of the deafness is viewed more in terms of increased withdrawal and isolation, increased insecurity and emotional stress rather than as an effect on personality per se. This is the age group that is threatened with mandatory retirement, with lack of employment, and the need for assistance with a gradually developing problem in self care. In our society they often feel useless and unwanted. The hearing loss can be a significant factor in this matrix of factors, precipitating anxiety and depressive episodes. Usually the isolating effect of the inability to maintain contact auditorially can be readily recognized.

These categories and the classifications according to the degree of the deafness are given to emphasize that these factors are fundamental to considerations of the emotional impact of impaired hearing. As the data given below indicate, the greater the extent of the impairment and the earlier the onset, the more a characteristic personality pattern seems to emerge. Also, because a given culture has patterns, such as typical ages for marriage and for beginning an occupation, a hearing loss has critical implications for each group. These are of importance when analyzing the significance of deafness on personal-social adjustment.

STUDIES OF PERSONALITY

Study of the emotional adjustment of children deaf from early life presents difficult scientific problems. Although children are suspected of having deafness earlier than in former years, the average age at which they are seen for diagnosis is approximately two years. The sensory deprivation has been present for some time before the child is seen for study. A more difficult problem is the inadequacy of the techniques for studying personality development in young nonverbal children. Tests for the evaluation of emotional factors, including projective techniques, are notoriously dependent on verbal facility. The two most useful procedures for young children deaf from the preverbal age are free play and drawing tests. Unfortunately objective studies of this age group are limited. Investigations of those having onset of deafness in early life have been made, but only after they have achieved some degree of verbal facility. The question of procedures is less critical when the deafness is moderate or if the onset is after language has been acquired, but to explore the relative effects of deafness, it is necessary to study all age levels, including the presbycusic.

As in the area of intelligence, early work on emotional factors in relation to deafness was initiated by Pintner.[38] Studies under his direction included both children and adults. With Brunschwig[5] he devised special tests of personality for use with the deaf. These were questionnaires using simple language in an attempt to overcome the verbal limitations involved. These tests were standardized on control groups of hearing children. He compared deaf groups on the basis of the teaching methods used, the presence or absence of other deaf persons in the home, the age of onset, and other variables. Pintner emphasized the similarities of personality adjustment in deaf and hearing children, although he found differences in favor of the hearing. Deaf children from homes where there were other deaf persons, such as deaf parents, were found to be better adjusted than other deaf children. This is an interesting finding and warrants further investigation. In a study of fears, there was only slight difference from the normal, but the fears of deaf children tended to be more unrealistic. Furthermore, deaf children chose immediate satisfactions rather than greater rewards which were delayed. From this he concluded that deafness resulted in emotional immaturity.

Springer[45] and Springer and Roslow[46] used the Brown Personality Inventory to study the emotional stability of deaf children. The groups were matched in intelligence and socio-economic status. They found psychoneurotic tendencies to be much higher in the hearing impaired. Springer[44] also used the Haggerty-Wickman-Olson Behavior Rating Schedules[33] in a study of 377 deaf children compared to 415 hearing children. The deaf had more problem tendencies.

Using the same technique Myklebust and Burchard[31] studied 187 children in a Residential School. The findings confirmed the work of Springer in that the deaf presented a higher incidence of behavior problems. No differences were found between the congenital and acquired groups, or between those in residence at the school more than four years or less than four years.

Gregory[16] and Nafin[32] studied the effect of deafness on social grouping and relationships. Gregory concluded that deaf children formed less adequate social relationships as compared to the hearing. Nafin reported that the limitation in language caused inferior social grouping in the preadolescent age, but thereafter there was no difference. However, he emphasized that deaf children sought other deaf children as playmates.

Pellet[34] made an interesting investigation of persons with early life deafness. He classified their thinking processes and compared them with the hearing according to the work of Piaget.[35, 36] He found that the deaf were more aggressive and competitive, that a leader of the deaf depended more on admiration than on organization and direction of activities. He also found them more immature emotionally and related this to the limitation of language. The results presented below tend to confirm these observations.

Lyon[25] studied the emotional maturity of deaf youth. His population included 87 males and females, with an average age of 19 years who were in attendance at a Residential School. He used the Thurstone Personality Schedule and found that compared to the norms there appeared to be twice as many deaf who were poorly adjusted.

Only a few studies have been made of hearing impaired adults. Pintner, together with Fusfeld and Brunschwig,[39] used the Bernreuter Personality Inventory in a study of deaf college students and other adults. They found the deaf slightly more neurotic, more introverted, and less dominant than the hearing. Welles[49] also used the Bernreuter Test in investigating the emotional adjustment of hard of hearing persons enrolled in various Hearing Societies; he included a control group of adults with normal hearing. He reported that the hard of hearing were more introverted and had more problems of the neurotic type.

Heider and Heider[23] used a questionnaire to study the social and emotional adjustment of the adult deaf. The individual was asked to write about his early life experiences with hearing children, what he missed by being deaf, and what his social relationships were after leaving school. They found that some withdrew from contacts with hearing people and concluded that this might be a realistic adjustment for some deaf persons. Others tried to force their way socially and attempted to educate the hearing regarding the problems resulting from deafness.

These early studies are in agreement that deafness causes disturbance of emotional growth, instability, and maladjustment. However, the nature of these involvements is not clarified, which presumably can be explained by the techniques used. Except for a few inventories, such as the Minnesota Multiphasic Personality Inventory,[19] this type of test does not specify areas of personality disorder or other factors diagnostically. Rather, the findings are largely in terms of more or less disturbance as compared to the average. Another limitation of these procedures is that they require verbal facility, limiting their use and validity when applied to most individuals who have deafness from early life. On the other hand to overlook these results would be unfortunate because more recent work using other techniques is not in disagreement with the trends indicated by these investigators. Moreover, other methods for the study of personality also have limitations, particularly when used with deaf people.

Projective tests of personality now are in common use and increasingly this method is being applied to the hearing impaired. McAndrew[26] used the Rorschach in a study comparing the deaf and the hearing. His sample consisted of 25 children in a Residential School and concluded that the deaf were more rigid in behavior. Levine[24] also used the Rorschach with a group of 31 deaf children. She reported that the deaf were inferior in conceptual thinking, had limited interests, and were emotionally immature compared to the hearing.

While the Rorschach Test[40a] is useful in work with the deaf, this test too is highly dependent on verbal facility. It can be used only after adequate language has been acquired. As shown by Neyhus[32a] language facility was related to performance on the Rorschach and the Rotter Incomplete Sentences Test[40b], the better the language, the more normal the personality pattern. Clearly this relationship must be considered when tests of this type are used with deaf persons. Moreover, deaf persons often give substantially fewer responses than the hearing. This was not found by Levine but hers was a small sample where selective factors could have been operative. Clinically, one of the problems in using the Rorschach even with the average deaf adult is that it is difficult to secure enough responses to assure validity and reliability. Furthermore, it is apparent that a deaf person frequently is forced to use the words he knows rather than words which actually describe what he sees. It seems, therefore, that while the Rorschach is useful in the study of the effects of deafness on personality and in clinical work with the hearing impaired, other techniques must be found. This is particularly true for young deaf children and for those whose language facility is poor irrespective of age.

Bindon[3] suggests an interesting possibility. Together with the Rorschach she used the Make A Picture Story Test[42] which is not dependent on linguistic ability. The subject makes a picture by placing human figure "cut-outs" on various backgrounds. In other words, the individual makes a story by choosing and arranging human figures on cards which provide a background; hence, he makes a picture story. Scoring is objective. Bindon used the MAPS as one of the tests in a study of personality characteristics of rubella deaf children compared to children having deafness with other etiologies. She found no differences between these groups, but the Rorschach indicated greater rigidity while the MAPS showed schizophrenic signs. This later indication is interesting in view of the data discussed below.

Another projective test which has possibilities for use with young deaf children is the Szondi.[8] The task is to choose pictures which are liked the most and liked the least. Verbal facility plays a markedly less critical role both in the MAPS and the Szondi tests than in most other projective techniques. We are now experimentally evaluating these various procedures in an attempt to ascertain their usefulness in the scientific appraisal of the effects of hearing loss on emotional growth and adjustment.

EMOTIONAL ADJUSTMENT OF DEAF AND HARD OF HEARING ADULTS

Previous work suggests a relationship between deafness and personality factors. However, this has not been extensively explored. Many assumptions have been made by the layman and even by the more sophisticated. Psychologists and psychiatrists often have assumed that those who have deafness are suspicious and develop paranoid trends. Is this true, or is it only an assumption? Educators have stated that those who were deaf from early infancy have better emotional adjustment because of their lack of awareness of what it means to hear. Another opinion is that it is those who have become hard of hearing who have the greatest emotional disturbance because they are in an ambiguous position of being neither deaf nor normally hearing. To investigate these observations and to explore the emotional effect of deafness in other ways, we inaugurated a study of adults. The population consisted of two groups; one was hard of hearing, with onset of hearing loss in adulthood, while the other was deaf, with onset in early life.

The Hard of Hearing

The hard of hearing were in attendance at a Hearing Society where they were in speechreading classes and participating in other activities. In this group, which included essentially all who were enrolled at the Society, there were 44 males and 83 females; there were approximately twice as many women as men. From this sample it seems that women more often than men avail themselves of the services of a Hearing Society. The mean age of the males was 39.37 years, and for the women 49.66 years; the mean age for the total group was 44.98. On the average the females were ten years older than the males. The males had a mean db hearing loss of 68, while for the females it was 66. As a group, they had the moderate degree of deafness which characterizes the adult hard of hearing. The mean age of onset for the males was 18.75 years, and for the females 24.12 years. These data are summarized in Table 28.

Data were secured regarding the educational and marital status of the subjects. These are given in Table 29. The sexes were comparable; the differences were not significant except that more women had been widowed. This can be attributed to the higher mean age for the females and to their longer life span. One of the most provocative findings from this comparison is the high incidence of unmarried persons in both sex groups. This conforms to the expectations on the basis of the age of onset categories suggested on page 120, inasmuch as this group falls into category IV, onset in early adulthood. This is the critical age for marriage, and these data indicate that this onset impedes personal-social affiliations and restricts possibilities of marriage.

An attempt was made to analyze the dependency status of those who were unmarried, and the extent to which the total group was self-supporting. The findings are shown in Table 30. The Chi-Square test of significance revealed no differences between the males and females on either of these comparisons. This is interesting because it was hypothesized that fewer men would be living with their parents and that more men would be self-supporting; these differences did not occur. In this group of hard of hearing persons the ratio of women who were self-supporting was equal to that of the men; the actual ratio for those who were independent was 75 per cent for the men and 62.5 per cent for the women. In the absence of a control group, comparison with the normal could not be made, but there was an indication that the hard of hearing male was less self-supporting than the average. This was suggested also by the comparison of living arrangements. Of the unmarried males 60 per cent were living with their parents, while only 33 per cent of the unmarried women had this arrangement. This difference might be partially explained by the younger mean age for the males,

TABLE 28. The mean age, decibel hearing loss and age of onset for the hard of hearing

	Males N-44		Females N-83		Total N-127	
	Mean	SD	Mean	SD	Mean	SD
Age	39.37	15.86	49.66	15.38	44.98	15.83
Age of onset	18.75	13.73	24.12	15.58	22.21	15.03
Hearing loss	68		66		67	

TABLE 29. Educational and marital status for the hard of hearing group

	Educational Attainment					Marital Status			
	Men		Women			Men		Women	
	N	%	N	%		N	%	N	%
Grammar school	13	32	17	21	Single	25	57	39	47
High school	14	31	31	37	Married	15	34	18	22
College	10	22	25	30	Divorced	1	2	4	5
No report	7	15	10	12	Widowed	3	7	21	25
Total	44	100	83	100	Separated	0	0	1	1
					Total	44	100	83	100

TABLE 30. Comparison of living arrangements and self-support status for the hard of hearing

Residing with	Men	Women	Self-support	Men	Women
Parents	15	13	Yes	33	53
Relatives	3	7	No	7	24
Others	7	16	No report	4	6
Total	25	39	Total	44	83

but there was a tendency for the males to be less independent than the females.

An extensive questionnaire was used to study the estimated benefits of speechreading and the use of wearable hearing aids. This procedure required the subjects to indicate the benefit or the lack of benefit on a rating scale. The primary findings are given in Table 31. Statistical analysis revealed no difference in regard

TABLE 31.   Comparison of hard of hearing men and women on the benefits of a hearing aid and of speechreading

Hearing aid satisfactory			Benefits from speechreading		
	Men	Women		Men	Women
Yes	13	33	Good	11	20
No	22	41	Average	12	47
No report	9	9	Poor	19	12
			No report	2	4
Total	44	83	Total	44	83

to the satisfactoriness of a hearing aid; males and females found them equally satisfactory or unsatisfactory. In each group 50 per cent found hearing aids unsatisfactory. The significance of this result is not clear; however, we must assume that many who wore hearing aids and found them useful did *not* find them sufficiently beneficial so that they considered them satisfactory. There must be various reasons for this feeling. It may reflect difficulties in adjusting to the hearing loss as well as to the wearing of a hearing aid. Perhaps it reflects a deeper problem. The hard of hearing adult with late onset of deafness presumably judges the effectiveness of a hearing aid on the basis of its providing hearing as he had before he sustained the impairment; his frame of reference is normal auditory function. These results corroborate the impression that although hearing aids are highly beneficial they do not provide normal auditory capacities. In terms of the total psychological significance of audition, as suggested in Chapter IV, a hearing aid provides mainly foreground hearing. Much of the scanning, altering, antennae-like function of hearing remains significantly impaired. From this point of view this expression of unsatisfactoriness of a hearing aid might be entirely realistic and not a manifestation of emotional disturbance.

In contrast to the findings for the use of hearing aids, there was a significant difference between the sexes as to the extent that speechreading was found to be beneficial; females reported receiving much greater benefit. Approximately 50 per cent of the males reported average or good results, whereas 80 per cent of the females reported such benefits. Clearly, as far as this sample is concerned, there was a sex difference relative to the subjective appraisal of speechreading as an effective compensation for hearing loss. It is interesting that this difference was found also when objective data were obtained. In a study of hard of hearing children Costello[6] found females superior to males in speechreading; the same trend appeared for deaf children but the differences were nonsignificant. Furthermore, in Part Three there is evidence that deaf females are superior to males in various aspects of language behavior. In other words, the results of this comparison of hard of hearing adults are corroborated by other findings. Ostensibly there is a sex difference in speechreading ability favoring females, as there is in other language functions. This sex difference, therefore, cannot be attributed only to a selective effect of deafness on the sexes, or to a greater maladjustment in the males. On the other hand, only further study can clarify this complex problem. Some of the data given below do suggest that deafness has greater impact on males with a concomitant greater emotional involvement. Perhaps these hard of hearing males were realistic in estimating that speechreading was a less satisfactory compensation for them, but also seem to be more emotionally disturbed than the females.

To secure information on the individual's attitude toward his disability the subjects were asked to rate the extent to which deafness was a handicap. A four point rating scale was used including no handicap, slight, considerable and serious. The distribution for this comparison is given in Table 32. Chi Square analysis of the

TABLE 32. Comparison on the basis of ratings of the extent to which deafness was considered a handicap

Rating	Men	Women
No handicap	2	10
Slight	15	40
Considerable	16	21
Serious	10	8
No report	1	4
Total	44	83

weighted scores disclosed a significant difference, the males rating their hearing loss as being a greater handicap. At least subjectively these males found their impairment to present more severe problems. The objective test findings given in Table 36 corroborate these estimates; the males were found to have more emotional maladjustment. Also as noted above, apparently fewer males seek assistance with their problem, and they derive less benefit from rehabilitative procedures such as speechreading. Socio-cultural circumstances make a hearing loss more debilitating for males or they develop feelings of greater loss from their sensory deprivation.

TINNITUS AND VERTIGO: Psychiatrists, psychologists, otologists, and other professional workers have been interested in the problems of head noises and dizziness associated with impaired hearing. Information was gathered on the incidence of these conditions in this population, and the results are shown in Table 33. There

TABLE 33. The incidence of head noises and dizziness in hard of hearing adults

	Head noises		Dizziness	
	Men	Women	Men	Women
Yes	23	50	7	26
No	21	33	37	52
No report	0	0	0	5
Total	44	83	44	83

was no difference between the groups for either head noises or dizziness; men and women reported these problems with equal frequency. It is noteworthy that approximately 50 per cent of the males, and a higher ratio of females, reported head noises. Only 15 per cent of the men and 30 per cent of the women reported dizziness. Relatively the more frequent condition seems to be head noises. It has been authenticated clinically that tinnitus, in particular, can noticeably complicate the adjustment of the hearing impaired. Tinnitus and dizziness are complex problems medically and psychologically. The data for the deaf given below show that for this group both conditions are related to emotional stability. This analysis was not done for the hard of hearing but further study is indicated psychiatrically, psychologically, and otologically.

Another type of information was obtained regarding personality and adjustment. Each person wrote an autobiographical account about *What my Hearing Loss Means to Me*. To give more structure to the task the subject was given six sheets of paper and each page was given a title:

1. My experiences with my family when I first realized I was losing my hearing.

2. My experiences with my friends when my hearing began to fail.

3. My experience with my employer and other working associates since my hearing loss occurred.

4. How my hearing loss changed my life.

5. How I feel about my hearing loss.

6. How do you think your experiences and what you have learned can be of help to others who are hard of hearing?

Allport[1] has indicated the usefulness of personal documents in the study of personality. However, such material does not lend itself to statistical analyses; only general trends are given.

This autobiographical study showed that even moderate hearing loss sustained in adulthood had many and diverse implications for daily living. Life became more stressful in various ways. Most of the hard of hearing found their families helpful and sympathetic, but emphasized that it required considerable patience on the part of the family members. Throughout the discussion of family relationships was the indication of greater necessity for dependence, including need for assistance with messages, as well as in seeking employment and in maintaining friends. One of the striking revelations was that very few held the same friendships they had prior to the onset of deafness. The social isolation resulting from impaired hearing was markedly apparent. Some found their loss of old friends one of the greatest hardships associated with deafness and because of this experience many were despondent and cynical regarding "the hearing." It was this circumstance that frequently led them to seek associations and services for the hard of hearing. *Very few maintained primary identification with the normally hearing.* Almost all found it necessary to develop a basic identification with others who had impaired hearing. This highlights the feelings of isolation which occurred, with the need to shift social contacts, friendships, and affiliations. Apparently, even when deafness is sustained in adulthood, and when verbal facility remains at a high level, it is difficult to maintain normal social relationships with the majority group. This was also demonstrated by many references to "those who are hard of hearing" and to "the hearing." With virtually no exceptions this group thought of themselves as being different from the hearing. There was repeated reference to "us," with the clear connotation that when hearing is impaired it is not typical to be included with the hearing, that isolation is inherent with the need to make adjustments accordingly. Inasmuch as this group found it necessary to identify with others who had deafness, it seems wise to secure information concerning the extent to which a child with profound deafness from early life also needs such identification.

Under the item "My experience with my employer and other working associates," the most frequently encountered circumstance was the need to change occupations, and in many instances their hobbies. Usually occupations were sought that did not necessitate good hearing; research analyst, accountant, technician, and jeweler are examples. The need for hobbies, "to keep your mind busy," was mentioned. Hobbies suggested included photography, books, horticulture, and museum visits. It was interesting how the hobbies and occupations chosen were those that directly accented the use of vision. They also reflected a type of withdrawal, perhaps realistic, in that companions and group participation were essentially unnecessary. Except for certain contacts with others who were hard of hearing, the adjustment most frequently seemed to be a type of "going it alone." Most considered their employers and co-workers fair, but, as with their families, mentioned the need for all to have patience, as there was inconvenience and increased tension in most working relationships.

In connection with the way in which the hearing loss had "changed my life," statements ranged from little to "It changed everything." Frequently the effect on the career was mentioned as the primary indication of change. Similarly in "How I feel about my hearing loss," the most often mentioned worry was in connection with obtaining and holding employment. Good acceptance was shown by many, and a certain resignation was obvious in expressions such as "things could be worse." Under suggestions for others having impaired hearing, there was a strong feeling that it was necessary to take advantage of speechreading instruction and the use of hearing aids. Also, directly and indirectly, there was the suggestion that it was necessary to seek and develop friendships with others who had deafness. Further discussion of this study is given below in comparison with those who had profound deafness from early life.

The Deaf

To study the relationship between impaired hearing and emotional adjustment more fully the hard of hearing and deaf were compared. The hard of hearing group had a moderate degree of hearing loss with onset in adulthood. The deaf group had profound hearing loss with onset in infancy. This group of adults was in attendance at a College for the Deaf. Their grammar and high school education had been obtained in Day and Residential Schools throughout the United States. Admission to the college is by entrance examination. This group was a highly selected population of deaf people relative to both intellectual capacity and educational attainment. The college curriculum consists of five years rather than the usual four; preparatory, freshman, sophomore, junior, and senior classes.

There was considerable difference in age between the deaf and hard of hearing groups. The age and educational levels for the hard of hearing were given in Tables 28 and 29. The chronological age levels, the extent of hearing loss and the median age of onset for the deaf are shown in Table 34. In this group 26 per

TABLE 34. The mean chronological age in years, the classification of hearing loss, and the median age of onset for the deaf group

	C.A.	Hearing loss	Median age of onset
Males	21.56	Profound	1.6 years
Females	21.46	Profound	1.8 years

cent of the females and approximately 20 per cent of the males reported that they were born deaf. The extent of deafness was profound and comparable to the populations in schools for the deaf for whom data were presented in Table 7.

The primary measure of personality in this study of both the deaf and hard of hearing was the Minnesota Multiphasic Personality Inventory (MMPI).[19] This test has been used widely and studies have been made indicating its validity.[12] Hanes[17] has shown that a third grade level of reading ability is required. On the basis of the educational attainment of the hard of hearing group this was assumed to be no limitation for these subjects. Moreover, from Fusfeld's[10] studies, it seems unlikely that this group of deaf college students was significantly handicapped by the language entailed, also indicated by the various statistical analyses discussed below. However, the MMPI was selected with the knowledge that it required a minimal level of reading ability. As mentioned previously, this is true also of most other commonly used tests of personality. Our discussion of results includes the possibility that verbal facility is one of the variables in this study.

The MMPI test consists of ten scales and a separate score is derived for each. These scales are Social Introversion, Hypochondriasis, Depression, Hysteria, Psychopathic Deviate, Interest, Paranoia, Psychasthenia, Schizophrenia, and Hypomania. Only a brief definition of these conditions based on the manual can be given here. *Social Introversion* is a measure of attitudes toward social participation. High scores indicate a desire to withdraw and to be seclusive, whereas low scores are associated with a desire to be an active participant socially. *Hypochondriasis* indicates abnormal worry, apprehension and concern about bodily functions, and possible physical illness. It was assumed that those with physical defects might be unduly concerned about physical factors. The meaning of *Depression* is rather self-evident. It is an inability to feel normally optimistic about oneself and the future. Poor morale, a feeling of uselessness, and much concern with death are characteristic of depressives. It was hypothesized that deafness might contribute to feelings of depression. *Hysteria* as used in this test means the extent to which one converts emotional conflicts into physical symptoms. The hysteric may complain of physical disorders for which no organic basis can be found. Many with psychogenic deafness have "conversion hysteria." High scores on the three scales of Hypochondriasis, Depression, and Hysteria frequently occur together and make up the characteristic profile of the individual who is referred to as neurotic.

Psychopathic Deviate is the condition wherein the person

cannot develop normal feelings regarding what is expected of him so he disregards the social mores. He cannot profit from his experiences and often repeats anti-social acts; he can be viewed as being unable to acquire a normally functioning conscience. Like most who are abnormal, he may be dangerous to himself and to others. This scale was considered relevant as an indication of the extent to which sensory deprivation influenced ability to conform; an inference was that it would provide evidence concerning the normal development of conscience.

The *Interest Scale* is a measure of how much a man or woman is interested in the activities of others of the same sex. High scores for men indicate more than average interest in the activities of women, and high scores for women indicate a more than average interest in the activities of men. Terman[48] has shown the relationship between masculinity-femininity and psychosexual development. Apparently normal development of masculinity and femininity feelings derives largely from appropriate identification with the same sexed parent in early life. This frame of reference was included in this study, and it was hypothesized that this Scale might indicate the effect of deafness on the development of normal feelings of masculinity and femininity.

Paranoia is a type of psychosis and is viewed as being a subcategory of schizophrenia. An individual having this mental illness is characterized by suspiciousness and delusions of persecution. Often such persons feel that others want to take advantage of them. Lay opinion, and even some professional opinion, has assumed that those with impaired hearing become paranoid in their behavior. It was thought that this Scale might provide significant information as to the validity of these opinions.

Psychasthenia is the condition wherein the individual engages in phobic, ritualistic, and compulsive behavior. This might include simple activities such as excessive handwashing and fear of touching doorknobs because of apprehension of being contaminated. Obsessive thinking and ideas are characteristic. Individuals who score above average on this Scale often have high scores on Hypochondriasis, Depression, and Hysteria; Psychasthenia usually is viewed as characteristic of neurosis. However, high scores also may be associated with psychosis. Here we assumed that it might indicate whether deafness contributed to uncontrolled thinking and other types of obsessive, compulsive behavior.

Schizophrenia is the most common and debilitating of the psychoses. It is a disease of early childhood with onset being common before 25 years of age. This condition is characterized by an inability to understand and to accept reality as evidenced by detachment, feelings of isolation, bizarre thinking and behavior. Rather than accepting life and the world realistically, the individual establishes an inner world of his own. The schizophrenic who is seriously ill behaves essentially on the basis of this inner world alone, without regard for external circumstances. Obviously such behavior might be entirely irrational and abnormal. In this study we were interested in the possibility that deafness might cause greater detachment and feelings of isolation. The findings presented in Table 36 indicate a critical relationship between deafness and the scores on this Scale; this is one of the most revealing outcomes of the study.

Hypomania is another Scale which measures psychotic trends. The term refers to a "lesser state of mania," characterized by the person's wanting to do too much. He engages in an abnormal number of activities and is in need of undue stimulation and excitement. Reasonable goals and objectives cannot be established. This type of mentally ill person might conform to the lay stereotype of the "insane." It was hypothesized that this Scale might give an indication of the extent to which deafness influences reason and emotional control in planning and setting of objectives; the need for undue stimulation and self-instigated emotional states such as extreme excitement. High scores on Hypomania, Paranoia, and Schizophrenia are indicative of psychoses, as contrasted with high scores on Hypochondriasis, Depression, and Hysteria which indicate neuroses.

Raw scores for each of these ten Scales are derived first; then T scores are computed. These T scores are standard scores for normal adults; the mean has been adjusted to a score of 50 and the standard deviation to a score of 10. Therefore the average score on each Scale is 50 with an SD of 10. The authors of the MMPI have taken precautions to assure validity by providing for "true," "false," and "can't say" responses. If an individual cannot state that an item is true or false, he can respond by checking the "question" category. However, if the "question" replies exceed a T score of 70 his scores are assumed to be invalid. None of the deaf and only three of the hard of hearing, all females, had too high question scores. Because the manual states that the actual effect of these scores statistically is to move them toward the mean, they were not eliminated.

Two other validating types of scores are used. One of these is the L score, which yields a measure of the extent to which a person makes deliberate attempts to put himself in a good light; he "fakes" responses which might make him seem to have an unusually good personality adjustment. Only two of the deaf, both males, and one of the hard of hearing, a female, had unduly high L scores. Because of the few cases involved, these were not excluded from the statistical treatment.

The third validating procedure, the F score, can be viewed as the opposite of an L score. The subject, perhaps unconsciously, responds in a manner which puts him in an unusually bad light. His total scores show that he might have replied indiscriminately and inconsistently. This can occur because the individual cannot read well enough to respond in a reliable and definitive manner. A high F score can occur also because of unusually frank and honest replies. For a number of reasons 23 per cent of the deaf males and 27 per cent of the deaf females had F scores above the critical T score of 70. In the hard of hearing population 16 per cent of the males and 10 per cent of the females had such scores. Because of this high incidence of F scores in both groups statistical analyses were made two ways, with the high F scores included and with the high F scores excluded. The findings of a high incidence of F scores in itself may be of significance. Why did a substantial number of individuals with deafness respond in such a way that they seemed to have unusually "bad" adjustment instead of unusually "good" adjustment? Inasmuch as this trend was true for both the deaf and hard of hearing it seems unlikely that it was due to poor ability to read or comprehend the meaning of the items. On the basis of the total findings, as discussed below, it seems more logical to infer that more unfavorable adjustment scores as compared to the normal existed in the population of hearing impaired people. Thereby, a greater incidence of high F scores occurred. This agrees with the findings that when the F scores were eliminated, the basic finding of more maladjustment in the hearing impaired was not altered. Analysis of K score did not disclose deviation from the normal.

The validity of certain items on the MMPI must be questioned when this test is used with the hearing impaired because they refer specifically to hearing, speech, or balance; normal function is assumed. It is interesting that both the deaf and hard of hearing responded to these items without difficulty. This was manifested by their not leaving these items blank or by their giving "can't say" responses. Nevertheless we hypothesized that these items might influence the validity of the test scores. Therefore ten items for the deaf and eight for the hard of hearing were judged as "loaded." Statistical analysis of the total findings was made with these items included and with them excluded. The differences which occurred are discussed below. The items judged as "loaded" for the deaf are 5, 25, 119, 134, 180, 185, 192, 281, 332, and 341. With the exception of 134 and 180, the same items were judged "loaded" for the hard of hearing. The responses of both the deaf and hard of hearing to these items are given in Table 35.

These responses are of considerable interest. They indicate the validity and significance of the total findings. Empirically they conform to expectations when deafness is present, and strongly suggest that neither group had difficulty in comprehending the items of this test. In terms of the psychology of deafness one is intrigued by the fact that approximately 50 per cent of the deaf stated they were easily awakened by noise, while only about 10 per cent of the hard of hearing gave this response. Why did so many of the deaf respond in this manner? Perhaps this is quite natural for a deaf person. In Chapter IV it was suggested that when hearing is impaired other sensory channels must be used for scanning contact with the environment. When he is not using vision, such as when in darkness or when asleep, the deaf person is dependent on tactual-kinesthetic-vibratory sensations. He is aware of loud noises through feeling, and he has learned to rely on vibratory sensations to alert him concerning the stability of his environment. Furthermore, he has learned that his safety often depends on such sensations so he is easily alerted by them. From

TABLE 35. The per cent of the deaf and hard of hearing giving each of the responses on the MMPI items which assume normal speech, hearing, or balance

| Item | Deaf | | | | | | Hard of Hearing | | | | | |
| | Males | | | Females | | | Males | | | Females | | |
	T	F	CS*	T	F	CS	T	F	CS	T	F	CS
5. I am easily awakened by noise	45	55	0	47	53	0	6	90	4	24	71	5
25. I would like to be a singer	16	84	0	24	74	1	43	55	2	19	79	2
119. My speech is the same as always	48	48	2	39	53	8	61	36	3	67	29	4
134. At times my thoughts have raced ahead faster than I could speak them	81	19	0	88	12	0	68	29	3	67	32	1
180. I find it hard to make talk when I meet new people	53	47	0	57	41	2	45	55	0	48	52	0
185. My hearing is apparently as good as most people	2	94	4	3	93	4	10	87	3	5	95	0
192. I have no difficulty in keeping my balance in walking	63	37	0	62	38	0	68	29	3	81	19	0
281. I do not often notice my ears ringing or buzzing	63	36	1	60	40	0	42	55	3	43	54	2
332. Sometimes my voice leaves me or changes even though I have no cold	37	55	8	37	57	6	26	71	3	19	79	2
341. At times I hear so well it bothers me	9	85	6	14	76	10	6	94	0	8	87	5

* T = True; F = False; CS = Can't Say.

their responses it can be inferred that the deaf, both males and females, and to the same extent, found the vibratory sensations associated with loud noises disturbing to sleep. Pertinent to this finding, we have often been asked by deaf persons why they were so readily startled by sounds which they *felt* when hearing people present paid no attention to these sounds. The explanation seems to be that the deaf person must monitor his world differently. *He must be alert to signals which the hearing person has learned it is safe to ignore.* This presumably explains why the deaf are more readily alerted by feeling sound than those without auditory impairment are by hearing it. These results for item 5 emphasize the critical importance of cautious interpretations of test results for the handicapped. We cannot infer that the deaf who stated that they were easily awakened by loud sounds were necessarily maladjusted, although this would seem the indication according to the norms. On the contrary it seems that these deaf individuals were responding realistically. This problem of interpretation of results is considered more extensively in relation to the more inclusive findings given below.

The other items judged as "loaded," 119, 134, 180, 185, and 332, also pertain to speaking and hearing. Both the hard of hearing and the deaf reported that their speech was "the same as always." The deaf more than the hard of hearing expressed difficulty with their thoughts racing ahead of their ability to speak. This might be expected when speech is labored. The groups were equal in finding it difficult to "make talk" when they met new people, which may depend on whether the new people also have impaired hearing. Likewise, the groups were equal concerning the "voice changing or leaving me." Very few in either group reported hearing so well that it was disturbing, or hearing as well as most people. These items conform closely to what would be expected from a realistic person having impaired hearing. This indicates that the items were comprehended and responded to appropriately by both groups. It is obvious, however, that these items had meanings for the hearing impaired which were different from the original intent, and therefore require special interpretation.

THE PERSONALITY TEST RESULTS

The findings for the deaf and the hard of hearing on the Minnesota Multiphasic Personality Test with the "loaded" items included are presented in Table 36.

Statistical analyses showed that the deaf males were significantly different from the normal on all ten scales. Except for Social Introversion, this difference was in the direction of greater maladjustment. Taking these results literally, this group of deaf college men was more emotionally disturbed and immature than the average male. This was true for all of the psychological conditions measured, with the possible exception of Social Introversion. The two most deviate scores were on the Scales of Schizophrenia and Hypomania.

TABLE 36. The mean scores for deaf and hard of hearing adults on the MMPI

| | Deaf | | | | Hard of Hearing | | | |
| | Males | | Females | | Males | | Females | |
Scale	Mean	SD	Mean	SD	Mean	SD	Mean	SD
Social Introversion	24.94	7.56	29.33	8.46	28.48	8.78	31.11	7.43
Hypochondriasis	55.17	9.62	51.81	7.93	58.94	10.65	54.08	10.27
Depression	55.66	11.16	51.83	9.90	63.68	14.40	55.84	9.58
Hysteria	55.17	8.80	51.44	8.49	56.94	9.37	54.71	10.28
Psychopathic Deviate	57.82	10.86	53.20	10.19	56.84	12.04	50.43	10.73
Interest	59.06	8.55	55.99	9.37	61.35	12.09	54.65	12.50
Paranoia	59.16	12.73	61.54	13.40	54.68	10.90	53.13	10.79
Psychasthenia	60.88	11.07	56.88	9.64	59.10	10.80	52.56	9.25
Schizophrenia	70.12	15.03	66.08	12.14	64.19	16.27	54.51	11.32
Hypomania	66.44	11.21	66.03	11.77	57.23	13.28	50.11	12.65
	N-104		N-90		N-31		N-63	

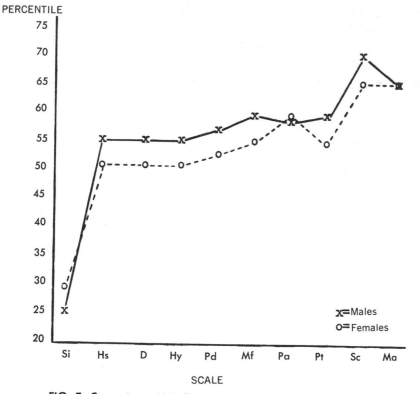

FIG. 7. Comparison of MMPI scores for deaf males and females.

The deaf females showed less deviation; no differences from the normal were found on the Scales of Hypochondriasis, Depression, and Hysteria. However, significant differences in the direction of maladjustment appeared on the remaining Scales. As with the males, the most deviate scores were on Schizophrenia and hypomania. A graphic comparison of the results for the deaf males and females is shown in Figure 7.

The hard of hearing males were found to be more emotionally maladjusted on all of the Scales as compared to the normal with the exception of Paronoia. Interestingly this group too scored most deviate on the Schizophrenia Scale and their second highest score was on Depression. There was a marked similarity of scores for the deaf and hard of hearing males. Nevertheless the opinion that the hard of hearing are suspicious was not confirmed. It is the Paranoia Scale which measures heightened suspicion, yet this is the one Scale on which these males did not differ significantly from the normal.

The hard of hearing females, like the deaf females, showed less emotional maladjustment than their male counterparts. They deviated significantly from the normal on Depression, Hypochon-

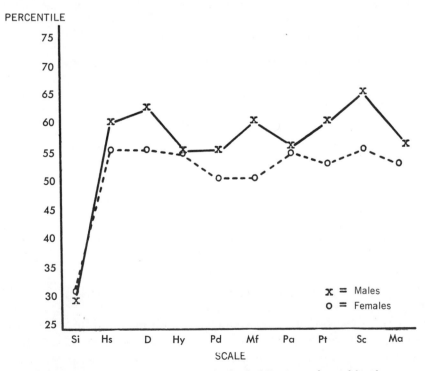

FIG. 8. Comparison of MMPI scores for hard of hearing males and females.

driasis, Hysteria, Interest, and Schizophrenia. They did not differ from the normal on Psychopathic Deviate, Paranoia, Psychasthenia and Hypomania. The results for the hard of hearing are shown graphically in Figure 8.

From this comparison of the hearing impaired with the normal both the deaf and hard of hearing had greater emotional problems. Moreover, these problems were greater in males as compared to females. The hard of hearing females showed the least maladjustment. It is noteworthy that for the deaf, males and females, the high scores were on Scales which indicate psychotic rather than neurotic involvements. This was true to some degree also for the hard of hearing males but not for the females. The hard of hearing as a group showed more depression than the deaf. These findings suggest that deafness affects personality selectively on the basis of sex, age of onset, and degree of hearing loss.

Comparison by Sex

Significant differences were found between deaf males and females on all of the Scales except Social Introversion, Paranoia, and Hypomania; on the remaining seven Scales the males showed the greater maladjustment. Inasmuch as these subjects were comparable in intelligence, age of onset, degree of hearing loss, site of the lesion, educational attainment, and socio-economic status, we cannot assume that deafness influences personality factors equally in men and women. Reasons for this variation are obscure. It seems unlikely that it can be explained wholly by the differing roles of the sexes in society, although this factor may be relevant.

The same sex difference was found for the hard of hearing as shown in Figure 9. Although the number of hard of hearing males was limited, the similarity between the deaf and hard of hearing males was striking. Significant variation was present on all but three Scales, Social Introversion, Hysteria and Paranoia; on the remaining seven Scales the hard of hearing males showed greater emotional disturbance than the normal. There was no sex difference on Paranoia for either the deaf or hard of hearing. Although variables such as age of onset, age, and socio-economic factors were less controlled in the hard of hearing, it is unlikely that such variation within the group explains the greater maladjustment of the hard of hearing male. As for the deaf, this variation of per-

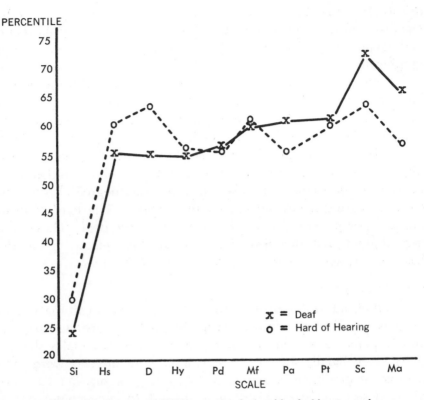

FIG. 9. Comparison of MMPI scores for deaf and hard of hearing males.

sonality involvements on the basis of sex is not readily explicable.

The Interest Scale on the MMPI measures feelings of masculinity and femininity. High scores for males indicate femininity whereas high scores for females indicate masculinity as compared to the average. Both the deaf and hard of hearing, males and females, deviated from the normal on the Interest Scale. The mean scores were highly similar for the deaf and hard of hearing males, and for the deaf and hard of hearing females. (See Figures 9 and 10.) This suggests that deafness, irrespective of degree and other factors, feminizes the male and masculinizes the female. The analysis of interest patterns, discussed in Chapter XIII, shows a comparable trend. The deaf males manifested interest in occupations which for the average are associated with less masculinity, while the deaf females expressed interest in areas related to more masculinity. These findings disclose an intricate relationship between

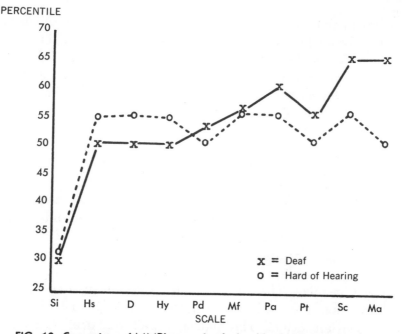

PERCENTILE

FIG. 10. Comparison of MMPI scores for deaf and hard of hearing females.

deafness and psychosexual adjustment but because extensive data are lacking, inferences can be made only with caution. For the deaf, who sustained deafness in infancy, it may be that the masculinity-femininity involvement can be attributed to impositions on identification; it is assumed that audition greatly enhances this process. For the hard of hearing, who sustained deafness in adulthood, this interpretation seems less adequate. On the other hand it cannot be denied that a hearing loss, regardless of age of onset, has importance in terms of self-concepts, in ego functioning, and in psychosexual relationships.

Results with "Loaded" Items Eliminated

Reference to the MMPI Manual[18] showed that the items judged to be "loaded" were distributed among the ten Scales, with some represented on as many as three Scales and some only on one. The net effect of eliminating these items was to reduce the raw score and cause the individual to score lower on the T scale; it reduced the maladjustment score. As might be expected the changes in the scores were slight; the deaf were not significantly different from the normal on Hypochondriasis but on the remaining nine Scales the differences remained significant. Likewise, a single change occurred for the deaf females; the deviation on Psychopathic Deviate was no longer significant. There were no changes in the scores for the hard of hearing males. A single change was observed for the hard of hearing females in that they no longer deviated significantly on Schizophrenia.

Elimination of the "loaded" items resulted in some changes in the differences by sex. For the deaf there was no difference between the males and females on Schizophrenia and Interest Scales. For the hard of hearing there was no sex difference on Hypochondriasis. With these items excluded the deaf males continued to show greater maladjustment than the hard of hearing males on the scales for Hypochondriasis, Depression, Paranoia, and Hypomania. The deaf females showed greater emotional problems than the hard of hearing females on all but the Psychopathic Deviate Scale. This indicates that the deaf and hard of hearing males were more similar than the deaf and hard of hearing females. Also the deaf females in comparison to the hard of hearing females were much more emotionally disturbed.

Results with High F Scores Eliminated

The F score indicates the extent to which an individual tends to give responses which might cause him to earn a maladjustment score which is not valid because he "makes himself worse than he really is." Because a number of the deaf and hard of hearing had unduly high F scores, the data were reanalyzed with these cases eliminated. No changes occurred for the deaf males; all of the mean scores remained significantly different as compared to the normal. One change occurred for the deaf females in that they were not different from the normal on Psychopathic Deviate; the other Scales on which deviations were found on the original analysis remained the same. Two changes were found for the hard of hearing males; their scores on Psychopathic Deviate and Hypomania did not show differences from the normal. The other differences remained unchanged. The greatest variation was noted for the hard of hearing females. Four Scales on which significant differences were found in the original analysis dropped to nonsignificance; these were on Hypochondriasis, Hysteria, Interest, and Schizophrenia. Hence, when the F scores were eliminated, the only significant deviation remaining for hard of hearing females was on Depression.

No change occurred in the comparison between deaf males and females, whereas comparison by sex for the hard of hearing showed two changes; differences were not found for Hypochondriasis and Hypomania. Otherwise the significant differences found in the original analysis were unchanged.

The high F score cases exerted an influence on the trends mainly for the hard of hearing, and in this group, mainly for the females. In the deaf group only one change was noted and this too was for the females. It cannot be presumed that the high F scores caused the basic trends indicated by the original analysis. On the other hand if the data were more valid with the F scores eliminated, then the female hard of hearing deviated from the normal in their emotional adjustment only in that they were more depressed. The deaf, males and females, and the hard of hearing males showed considerable deviation from the normal whether or not the high F score cases were excluded.

Comparison with Other Studies

Some investigators have questioned the norms for the MMPI. For example, Gilliland and Colgin[12] and Goodstein[15] showed that university students scored above the norms as given in the manual for the MMPI. Because these studies were pertinent to our findings for the deaf, statistical comparisons were made with the data of these investigators. Inasmuch as our deaf sample was composed of college students it was thought that they should be compared with other college students. The Schizophrenia Scale was chosen for this detailed analysis because it was on this category that the deaf were most deviate. Through the courtesy of Gilliland and Colgin the actual test responses for their subjects were made available to us and an item by item comparison was made between the deaf and hearing college students. The Chi-Square technique was used. This statistical analysis showed that the deaf gave deviate responses, as compared to the hearing, on 63 per cent of the items on the Schizophrenia Scale. They gave *unexpected* responses much more frequently than did the hearing college students, despite the fact that Gilliland and Colgin's sample scored above the means for the standardization group. Furthermore, the high mean score for the deaf on Schizophrenia cannot be attributed to their giving unusual responses to a few items. They gave deviate responses on many more items than the average hearing college student. We concluded that the indications of greater maladjustment of the deaf could not be explained by the findings that university students score above the norms for the average population.

Critical Scores

The authors of the MMPI suggest that a T score of 70 is critical in terms of maladjustment. They also state that a score of 70 on one of the Scales is of importance but does not necessarily indicate abnormality. On the other hand, people who score above 70 on two or more of the Scales usually are found to be clearly abnormal.[18] Gilliland and Colgin[12] computed the number of subjects in their population who scored above a T score of 70 on one or more of the ten Scales. They found that 39 per cent had such scores on one of the Scales, 14 per cent on two, and 7 per cent on three. They concluded that this was an unusually high incidence of scores indicating maladjustment. For comparison we computed the incidence of critically high T scores for the deaf and hard of hearing. These data are presented in Table 37.

TABLE 37.   The per cent of T scores above 70 on one, two, three, and four of the Scales on the MMPI

	Deaf		Hard of hearing	
	Males	Females	Males	Females
Above on one	70	61	68	32
Above on two	50	23	42	16
Above on three	29	20	29	13
Above on four	18	9	19	5

The number of deaf and hard of hearing having such scores far exceeded that found by Gilliland and Colgin. When two or more critically high T scores are taken as an indication of significant emotional disturbance we find that one-half of the deaf males fell into this classification. Slightly less than one-half of the hard of hearing males, approximately one-fourth of the deaf females, and one-fifth of the hard of hearing females had scores which usually indicate clearly abnormal behavior.

Tabulation also was made of the number of critically high T scores for each Scale, with the exception of Social Introversion. These figures are given in Table 38. The total number in this

TABLE 38. The number of T scores above 70 on nine of the MMPI Scales

	Deaf		Hard of hearing	
	Males	Females	Males	Females
Hypochondriasis	9	0	5	4
Depression	14	7	12	3
Hysteria	8	1	4	6
Psychopathic Deviate	11	6	5	3
Interest	13	6	6	·8
Paranoia	21	22	5	4
Psychasthenia	22	7	6	2
Schizophrenia	49	32	9	7
Hypomania	42	33	9	6

Table exceeds the actual number of individuals studied because many subjects had T scores above 70 on more than one Scale. The abnormally high scores for the deaf males were concentrated on the Scales of Paranoia, Psychasthenia, Schizophrenia, and Hypomania. For the deaf females the concentration was on Paranoia, Schizophrenia, and Hypomania. The highest incidence for the hard of hearing males was on Depression, Schizophrenia, and Hypomania, while for the hard of hearing females it was on Interest, Schizophrenia, Hysteria and Hypomania. This analysis corroborates the mean score findings presented in Table 36. The hard of hearing females showed least concentration in a given area of maladjustment. For the deaf there was a clear indication of greater deviation on those Scales indicative of psychotic behavior, and a similar trend was present for the hard of hearing males.

Age of Onset

We hypothesized that age of onset might be closely related to the extent of relationship between deafness and personality involvements. The comparison between the deaf and the hard of hearing disclosed that this was true but to a lesser extent than we had anticipated, particularly for the hard of hearing males. It was possible to study the influence of the age of onset more fully by comparing the meningitic and the nonmeningitic deaf. These groups were comparable in intelligence, degree of deafness, and chronological age. They differed significantly in age of onset, as can be seen from the data in Table 39. The mean age of onset for

TABLE 39.   The mean age of onset in years for the meningitic and nonmeningitic deaf

	Males			Females		
	N	Mean	SD	N	Mean	SD
Meningitic	41	6.63	3.56	19	6.03	3.85
Nonmeningitic	63	3.12	4.43	71	2.29	3.60

the meningitic group was approximately six years as compared to two to three years for the nonmeningitic. These data disclose that the meningitic as a group became deaf after five years of age. They had normal auditory experience prior to the onset of deafness, with implications for both personality and language development. The foundations of personality structure are well advanced by five to six years of age. Furthermore, there is considerable evidence which indicates that when deafness is sustained after five years of age, essentially normal language patterns are retained. Although in this study there was no indication that the nonmeningitic group did not comprehend the meaning of the items, it is possible that the meningitic were more subtle in the use of language. Perhaps the most important factor to be considered in the comparison of these groups is that the meningitic had the benefit of the *total impact* of audition for a sufficient period of time so that psychologically these individuals have been found more comparable to the hearing.

When the meningitic and nonmeningitic were compared with the Hathaway and McKinley norms[19] and with the norms provided by Goodstein,[15] significant differences appeared. These differences favored the meningitic; they were less deviate emotionally as compared to the nonmeningitic. For example, the deaf males as a group differed from the normal on all ten of the MMPI Scales, whereas the meningitic males differed only on five Scales: Depression, Paranoia, Psychastenia, Schizophrena, and Hypomania. According to these results the later onset of deafness was advantageous to adjustment. However, it is noteworthy that this later onset did not preclude marked emotional problems. The pattern of deviation was the same for the meningitic and nonmeningitic, with the area of greatest disturbance being on those Scales indicative of psychotic trends.

The meningitic and nonmeningitic also were compared by sex. The female nonmeningitic were significantly more masculine than the female meningitic, further indicating that deafness in early infancy affected identification processes adversely. The male nonmeningitic showed greater emotional disturbance than the male meningitic on the Scales of Psychasthenia and Schizophrenia. This analysis on the basis of age of onset disclosed the trend which we anticipated. The greatest personality deviations were present when hearing was lacking from very early life, as compared to after five years of age.

The high incidence of individuals having meningitic deafness in the population studied was noteworthy in and of itself. The incidence of meningitically deaf has stabilized at approximately 10 per cent in school age groups. In sharp contrast in this sample of deaf college students nearly 40 per cent of the males and 21 per cent of the females gave meningitis as the etiology of their deafness. This is in agreement with the data given in Table 2 suggesting that this etiology is more common in males. In relation to the psychology of deafness this high rate of meningitically deaf in the college population is provocative in many ways. In the first place it corroborates the observation from experience that leaders among the deaf often are *deafened* rather than congenitally deaf. Furthermore, it seems that the deafened have an advantage over the congenitally deaf on the college entrance examinations; they more frequently attain the required level of educational achievement. Presumably if a college program for the deaf is to be comparable with similar programs for the hearing, it is the deafened who are most able to fulfill the standards.

Comparison Between the Well and Poorly Adjusted

Those with MMPI scores showing "good" adjustment were compared with those having scores indicative of "poor" adjustment. Arbitrary statistical limits were established, such as no T score above 70, to permit categorical classification. The "good" and "poor" groups were compared on several factors. The hard of hearing males were not included because the samples derived were too small to warrant statistical treatment. For the deaf the variables were head noises, vertigo, self-estimated degree of deafness, the use of a hearing aid, the age of onset, and a self-estimate of the extent to which deafness was a handicap. For the hard of hearing females the variables were marital status, the age of onset, a self-estimate of degree of hearing loss, the age, the use of a hearing aid, the educational level, and a self-estimate of the extent to which deafness was a handicap.

In all instances, for the deaf and for the hard of hearing, the use of a hearing aid was associated with better adjustment. This cannot be interpreted as being simply a function of the hearing aid itself, although this must be considered, because those wearing aids might have had the least degree of deafness, as well as other advantages. Likewise, both for the deaf and for the hard of hearing, there was a relationship between adjustment and the age of onset; when deafness was not congenital, and when it occured later in life for the hard of hearing females, less emotional involvement was manifested. These results are in agreement with those obtained from the comparison between the meningitic and nonmeningitic. The total evidence in regard to the age of onset suggests that the later deafness is sustained, the less impact it will have on personality factors.

As a part of the study of objective feelings and attitudes, the subjects were asked to make an estimate of the degree of their deafness. The Scale used was moderate, severe, very severe, and total. Statistical weightings were assigned to each rating so that mean scores could be computed. The results showed that in the deaf group the males estimated their loss to be greater than did the females. This was in agreement with other findings indicating that the males who sustained deafness judged their problem to be greater when compared to the females. Interestingly the better adjusted deaf males judged their loss to be more severe than the poorly adjusted. The opposite occurred for the females. In both the deaf and hard of hearing groups the poorly adjusted females judged their loss to be greater than the well adjusted. These findings, as in the case of the total MMPI results, indicate a sex difference in regard to the impact of deafness. When the male was asked to make a judgment concerning his handicap, he manifested that it was a more serious problem, that the loss was of more consequence to him personally than in the case of the females. This trend was more consistent for the hard of hearing than for the deaf males.

As shown in Table 33, no sex differences were found for vertigo and tinnitus in the hard of hearing. The same was true for the deaf. However, the deaf who had no vertigo showed better adjustment than those reporting vertigo. This was true also of tinnitus; those having no "head noises" had significantly less emotional disturbance. These results are noteworthy and reveal the need for more psychological and psychiatric study of persons presenting these problems. Presumably a psychosomatic approach would be most advantageous with an attempt to ascertain whether tinnitus and vertigo usually cause more emotional conflict or whether they follow when more marked emotional problems are present. The findings from the study of interest patterns also are of interest in relation to these factors. (See Chapter XIV.)

In the group of hard of hearing females, those who were married were significantly better adjusted emotionally than those who were single, divorced, or separated. Furthermore, in this group there was a difference on the basis of chronological age. The well adjusted female had a mean age of 51 years while for the poorly adjusted, the mean was 41. Moreover, those with the higher educational attainment had the better adjustment scores. The extent to which deafness was a determining factor in these relationships is not clear because less emotional conflict might be associated with age or educational status whether or not hearing loss is present. These results are included to describe the hard of hearing females and to indicate the need for further study of these factors.

We have noted that the hard of hearing males judged deafness to be a greater handicap than did the hard of hearing females. This finding was reversed for the deaf where it was the males who judged deafness to be the least handicap. When the deaf and hard of hearing were compared, the order of the estimate from the greatest to the least handicap was hard of hearing males, hard of hearing females, deaf females, and deaf males. The deaf males who were most deviate on the MMPI rated themselves as having the least handicap. Apparently this group sustained the greatest impact psychologically from their sensory deprivation and, therefore, had less insight into its consequences.

Other observations from this analysis included the circumstance of a remarkably high number of the deaf estimating that deafness was *no* handicap. This judgment was given by 42 per cent of the males and 40 per cent of the females. For the deaf males who considered it to be a handicap, the mean judgment fell at "slight." For the deaf females who found deafness to be a handicap the mean was between "slight" and "considerable." As mentioned above, in the hard of hearing group it was the males who estimated deafness to be the greatest handicap. The hard of hearing females, like the deaf females, had a mean judgment which fell between "slight" and "considerable." Other comparisons revealed that the poorly adjusted deaf males rated themselves as being more handicapped than the well adjusted, the well adjusted deaf females judged themselves as more handicapped than the "poor," the poorly adjusted hard of hearing females rated themselves as the most handicapped in comparison with the other groups; their mean fell between "considerable" and "serious."

The most extreme category on the scale for estimating the extent to which deafness was a handicap was "serious." This judgment was given by 17 per cent of the males and 18 per cent of the females in the deaf group; there was no difference by sex. We found, therefore, that 42 per cent of the deaf males stated that deafness was *no* handicap and 17 per cent stated it was a "serious" handicap. Of the deaf females 40 per cent judged deafness to be *no* handicap and 18 per cent stated it was a "serious" handicap. Inasmuch as there were no differences by sex the males and females were combined and treated homogenously. This resulted in a total of 80 subjects in the "none" group and 35 in the "serious" group. The mean scores for these groups were compared on nine of the Scales on the MMPI; Social Introversion was not included. The results are shown in Table 40. Six of the nine mean scores were higher for the "none" group but these differences did not reach statistical significance; there was a trend for those who judged deafness to be *no* handicap to be more emotionally deviate. One

TABLE 40.   The MMPI scores for those who reported deafness to be no handicap and a serious handicap

	None		Serious	
	Mean	SD	Mean	SD
Hypochondriasis	49.51	8.16	53.11	8.08
Depression	57.71	8.99	54.00	10.51
Hysteria	52.86	7.82	48.44	8.31
Psychopathic Deviate	53.37	9.33	54.85	8.92
Interest	57.56	8.92	58.31	8.24
Paranoia	60.06	12.24	58.05	12.03
Psychasthenia	57.43	10.28	55.60	9.97
Schizophrenia	64.97	13.24	62.20	13.36
Hypomania	63.86	11.38	59.51	11.15

statistically significant difference did occur from this analysis. Those who estimated deafness to be a "serious" handicap were more hypochondriacal than those in the "none" group, which is interesting inasmuch as it is the Hypochondriasis Scale that measures concern about bodily function. Again there is an indication that the MMPI Test was a valid measure for this group because it is logical that those who thought deafness was a considerable handicap would have more apprehension about bodily function than those who stated that it was no handicap. On the other hand literal interpretation of this result would mean that those who judged deafness to be the greater handicap were the more maladjusted. This inference cannot be made. If deafness *is* a considerable handicap such a response would indicate adjustment, not maladjustment. Hence, the lower score for those in the "none" group might manifest poorer insight and greater emotional problems. This interpretation is consistent with the trend of higher mean scores for this group on six out of nine of the Scales.

Although there were no sex differences in the deaf group in the incidence of "none" and "serious" estimates, comparisons by sex were made and statistically significant differences appeared. The males in the "serious" group scored higher on Hypochondriasis than did the males in the "none" group. This finding is consistent with the results of the total group comparison discussed above. Furthermore, the "none" males scored higher than the "serious" males on Hypomania, indicating that those who stated that deafness was *no* handicap were less reasonable and objective, that they were more in need of activity, undue stimulation, and excitement. Another difference which appeared was that the males in the "none" group scored higher than the females in this group on Hysteria. This too is in agreement with the total MMPI findings indicating that the males had a greater emotional disturbance. In general this analysis based on judgments of the extent to which deafness was a handicap disclosed that those who estimated that it was *no* handicap had more emotional problems.

A Study of Socially Well Adjusted Adults

Previously we indicated the meagreness of information concerning adults profoundly deaf from early life. Securing evidence is an arduous task because adults are less available for scientific study than children. Neyhus[32a] has made both the most intensive and extensive study to date of the emotional adjustment of the adult deaf. His primary objective was to broadly define the mental and personality characteristics of those making a successful everyday life adjustment. His criteria for successful adjustment included completion of some formal educational curricula, history of continuous employment, normal intelligence, and ability to read and write. The sample consisted of 40 males and 40 females. In addition to tests of mental ability and language, the techniques employed were the Human Figure Drawing Test,[14] The Rorschach Test,[40a] the Make-a-Picture Story Test,[42] and the Rotter Incomplete Sentences Blank.[40b]

Neyhus' conclusions are in agreement with the findings of previous investigators in that deafness from early life has a pervasive effect on the development of personality. The deviant emotional and social behavior reported in studies of deaf children persisted into adulthood, even among those who made a successful societal adjustment. The characteristic pattern was one of being rigid, concrete, and socially and emotionally immature.

Summary and Implications

This study of hearing impaired adults compared those who sustained moderate deafness in adulthood with those who had profound deafness from childhood. The results indicated a relationship between this sensory deprivation and emotional adjustment. The age of onset, the degree of hearing loss, and sex were found to be significant variables affecting this relationship. Those with profound deafness from early life manifested the greatest emotional deviations. Moreover, the males irrespective of the age of onset and the degree of the involvement showed more personality disorder than did the females. While the female having severe impairment from early life presented an adjustment profile which resembled that of the males, the hard of hearing female showed no characteristic adjustment pattern. Despite the fact that the deaf showed greater emotional disorder than the hard of hearing, the deaf seemed largely unaware of deafness as a handicap. In this regard they lacked insight into the significance of hearing. The hard of hearing, who had long experience with normal auditory faculties, estimated deafness to be a greater handicap and showed more depression concerning their disability. The naïveté of the deaf cannot be taken as an indication of better emotional well-being. On the contrary those who stated that deafness was no handicap, those who showed the least understanding of what it means to hear, were the most disturbed emotionally.

As suggested in Chapter IV, it was hypothesized that a sensory deprivation such as deafness might bring about organismic effects. The results of this study support this supposition. A characteristic profile of personality did emerge, albeit this profile was most obvious and consistent for those who sustained marked deafness in childhood. The adjustment pattern was not of the type which is associated with neurosis, but it was similar to the profile found in psychosis. This was consistent from the MMPI results to the subjective judgments which were secured. The pattern was one of lack of apprehension, worry and concern with oneself, and the manifestation of obliviousness in regard to the true circumstances. The most pronounced feature of this profile was the way in which it was peaked on the Schizophrenia Scale. A total of 47 per cent of the males and 35 per cent of the females in the deaf group, and approximately 30 per cent of the males and 10 per cent of the females in the hard of hearing group had T scores above 70 on the Scale. It was also on this Scale that the meningitic group deviated most markedly.

A critical question which arose was the extent to which these findings could be interpreted according to the norms for the hearing. Specifically the question was whether the results indicated true mental illness or whether they might be more adequately explained on other bases. In the discussion of the "loaded" items we noted that in terms of the psychology of deafness, it might be expected that a deaf person would state that he was easily awakened by noise. Perhaps the total profile found for the hearing impaired on the MMPI must be viewed in these terms. From this frame of reference the high mean score on Schizophrenia might be due to the inherent isolation resulting from deafness rather than from true mental disease. This particular Scale is a measure of feelings of detachment, lack of empathy, and inability to understand reality. If one has normal capacities, high scores on this Scale can be interpreted to mean serious emotional disturbance of this type. On the other hand if one has deafness, he actually might be isolated and detached from interpersonal relationships with others, without having mental illness. In fact the Schizophrenic Scale seems to be an effective means for measuring the isolation which ensues from deafness. This is suggested also by the scores on the Scale of Social Introversion. It was the only Scale on which the hearing impaired fell below the norm for the average. Such a result would be expected only if the group were *not* truly schizophrenic. Their low score on Social Introversion means that the hearing impaired were extrovertedly seeking social contacts, not withdrawing from them. The scores for both the deaf and hard of hearing were so low on Social Introversion that we must infer that they were over-compensating in being gregarious. They were *aggressively* socially extroverted. Such behavior would be markedly inconsistent with schizophrenia.

The personality pattern which emerges is a feeling of severe isolation and detachment with aggressive, almost desperate attempts to compensate and thereby maintain interpersonal contacts. The primary conclusion to be drawn from this study, therefore, is that deafness, particularly when profound and from early life, imposes a characteristic restriction on personality but does not cause mental illness. Despite the significance of the impact of deafness on emotional adjustment it is not comparable to conditions such as schizophrenia. What is normal or realistic for a hearing person may not be realistic for an individual who has impaired hearing.

THE EMOTIONAL DEVELOPMENT OF DEAF CHILDREN

Study of adults having impaired hearing has been rewarding from the point of view of acquiring an understanding of the effects of such sensory deprivation. It is essential that we learn of the influences of longstanding profound deafness as well as of the consequences of a moderate hearing loss sustained after maturity has been attained. Various fields of endeavor, however, emphasize the importance of studying growth as an ongoing process. In the psychology of deafness this means there is a need to ascertain the consequences of deafness in the growing child. Through such study we may find ways in which the structure of personality is being altered during the time of its development and growth.

Earlier in this chapter we considered the difficulties in studying the emotional development of deaf children. Most techniques for the study of personality assume normal verbal facility and are not readily applicable to children who have had profound deafness from early life. Nonverbal tests of personality are being developed gradually. One of these, given considerable impetus by the work of Machover,[27] is the Drawing of the Human Figure Test. We prepared a modification of this technique for use in the National Study of the psychology of deafness. Our procedure consisted of having the child draw four human figures, a Man, his Father, his Mother, and Himself. Except for the need to comprehend the simple instructions, this is a nonverbal test. Both in clinical work and in research, we have found that this technique can be used readily with deaf children above seven years of age; it can be administered to most deaf children at six and to some at five. Experience has revealed that other techniques must be developed for the study of emotional factors in preschool deaf children.

No personality test can be expected to cover all aspects of an individual's emotional life. All tests have limitations, but the Drawing of the Human Figure Test, in addition to being essentially nonverbal, has been used widely in psychoneurology, psychiatry, and psychology and has a vast literature which is growing constantly. This test has been used as an indicator of emotional problems as well as in the study of the behavioral concomitants of neurological disturbance.

The concept of body image arose chiefly through neurology. Although it had prior origin, Pick[37] gave impetus to this concept through his work in the early 1900's. He introduced the term *autotopagnosia* to describe the inability to perceive one's body parts; such disorders are commonly recognized in psychoneurology. Head[20] first developed a rather elaborate concept of body imagery. His contribution was followed by the well known work of Schilder,[41] Critchley,[7] and Bender.[1a] Gerstmann's[11] observations have been of outstanding significance because he first noted the relationship between distortions of body image and psychological functions such as the ability to distinguish right from left, to write, and to do arithmetic. His findings have been confirmed by workers in psychoneurology; our studies have shown aspects of the "Gerstmann Syndrome" to be present in children, deaf or hearing, if they are dyslexic. Benton[2] has made extensive analysis of this syndrome.

The Human Figure Drawing Test is useful in the diagnosis of brain disease and in addition it has been beneficial in the evaluation of human behavior. Machover[27] indicated its applicability to the study of emotional adjustment. It has been used more broadly by Witkin[50] in his studies of perception and by Fisher and Cleveland[9] in their investigation of body image in relation to personality. All of this work has relevance to the utilization of the Human Figure Drawing Test in the psychology of deafness. It might serve as a measure of the relationship between impaired hearing and emotional adjustment. Our frame of reference stressed the points of view presented by Tagiuri and Pertullo[47] and by Heider[22] which emphasizes the psychology of interpersonal relationships and person perception. Stated differently, we assumed that the Human Figure Test might indicate the nature of the deaf child's perception of himself, as well as of other persons. We were especially interested in the possible effects of early life deafness on self-perception, person-perception, and identification.

The Human Figure Drawing Test used in this investigation is an adaptation of the Goodenough Test,[14] and the Scales devised by Witkin[50] and by Machover.[27] Many of the items were modified, and others were designed specifically for our purpose. The Scale is presented in Appendix B. After the Test was initially prepared, a pilot study was made analyzing the drawing of 50 hearing and 50 deaf children matched in pairs by age and intelligence. Thereafter it was revised and completed in its present form. The definition of the items and the scoring procedure essentially eliminated subjectiveness in scoring. Through the use of a template, actual measurements were made in most instances. Each drawing was scored by at least two trained workers, and a psychologist trained in projective test techniques checked the scoring of all of the drawings. When a discrepancy occurred, the score given represented a combined judgment.

The Drawing of the Human Figure Test, consisting of a Man, Father, Mother, and Self was administered to 830 children in schools for the deaf; 511 were in Residential Schools, and 319 were in Day Schools. The Draw-a-Man part of the test was given to a control group of 274 hearing children. Thus, the study included comparison with the normal on the drawings of a Man but not on the other three figures. A personality score was not computed; instead, each of the 100 items on the Test was scored separately, and the chi-square technique was used to determine the presence of significant differences. The basic statistical comparisons included Deaf versus Normal, Males versus Females, and Day versus Residential. The comparisons by school included total groups, males versus females, males versus males, and females versus females. The mass of significant differences which occurred could not be presented in the usual tabular form. Rather, a total listing of these findings is presented in the Appendix. A brief discussion of the results for each of the 23 body parts scored is given immediately below, followed by a more general summary of the results.

Results of the Drawing of the Human Figure Test

SIZE: The size of the drawing was studied by noting the number of children who drew figures covering less than $\frac{1}{3}$ of the length of the drawing space and the number who drew figures covering more than $\frac{2}{3}$ of the length of the drawing space. The Deaf drew more large figures than the Normal, while the Residential group drew more large figures than the Day group. However, these trends were not consistent and occurred mainly at the 9 and 11 year age levels. In some instances differences by age, sex, and school were reversed.

POSITION: The position of the drawing was determined by measuring whether it was at an angle toward the right or toward the left. The Residential children drew more figures than the Normal which were at an angle toward the left. No marked trends were found in comparison with the Normal.

PLACEMENT: The placement of the drawing on the paper has been considered of importance in the interpretation of performances on this Test. When the groups were compared statistically, 14 differences occurred on this item. All but two were found at the upper age levels studied; also, all but two of the differences were on point c—the drawing touches or is within ½ inch of the top of the drawing space. The Deaf used such placement more than the Hearing and in the drawing of the Mother, the Day group favored this placement as compared to the Residential. However, there were no outstanding trends for any Deaf group.

PHYSIQUE: There were no statistically significant differences.

VIEW: The view of the drawing was scored on the basis of whether it was in full profile, in full face, or whether it had characteristics of both of these; that is, whether it was partially in profile and partially in full face. A total of 25 differences appeared, most of them at the 9 and 11 year age levels. There was a sex difference in the Normal control group in that the Females drew more full profile drawings than the Males, which must be considered in the interpretation of the findings for the Deaf. Goodenough has shown that the full profile drawing developmentally occurs between 11 and 12 years of age. On this basis some of the differences which appeared can be attributed to variations in intelligence. In the comparison between the Day and Residential groups the most consistent findings were for the mixed view drawings; the differences favored the Day School children. The Residential population drew more figures that were a confusion of full profile and full face drawings. This suggests that a perceptual distortion was present more often in the children attending a Residential School.

TRANSPARENCY: Transparencies were scored through a refinement of the Goodenough scoring procedures with the number of drawings having one or more transparencies being determined. A total of 24 differences appeared with all but six of these falling at the 13 or 15 year age levels. Because the differences clustered at the upper age levels, they cannot be explained on the basis of intellectual factors. The Deaf showed more transparencies than the Normal, the Residential showed more than the Day, and there was a trend for the Deaf males to show more than the Deaf females. These results are curious and intriguing. Perhaps the Deaf were less perceptually aware of the incongruity of a transparency, perhaps they were less autocritical, to use an explanation first suggested by Pintner. But to what shall we ascribe their decreased autocriticism?

Ability to be autocritical seems to assume an objective and mature attitude which can be achieved only through normal ego development. Accordingly the results from this item indicate that the drawings of the Deaf were more naive, less mature, and more primitive perceptually. Although this was true of many of the drawings by the Deaf, it was most characteristic of the figures drawn by the Residential School population.

PORTRAIT: There were no statistically significant differences.

PROPS: One way in which an individual might reveal his attitudes in the drawing of the human figure is through the use of props. He might include such objects as a pipe, tree, chair, cane, or a gun. The specific importance of props in a drawing seems not to have been determined. Ours was an attempt simply to study the frequency of the use of props and to learn something of their nature. Two types of scores were derived. One pertained to the use of props such as mentioned above, while the other was a score on the use of a line or a sidewalk for the figure to "stand on." Including both types of scores, 25 differences were found. Of these, 20 favored the Residential population with only five of the differences occurring below the age level of 13 years. The Residential children clearly used more props of both types than those in the Day School. It is interesting that no differences appeared between the Deaf and the Hearing. In the comparisons between the Deaf, props were used more frequently by the Males than by the Females. Also, the props were used more frequently on the male figures than on the female figures. The Residential males used props in drawing of Father more than in the drawings of Self, or than in the drawings of a Man. Since this trend was not found in the drawings of the Day Males, a marked difference between the Day and Residential Male groups was revealed. This may be explained by differences in the level of identification attained by the two groups. The use of props can be viewed as indicating feelings of warmth and empathy. If this were true, the Residential Males showed such feelings more than the Day Males. That these male groups were perceiving and projecting different feelings regarding their fathers there can be little question. However, the nature of these different feelings is not really apparent and must be studied further.

SEX CHARACTERISTICS: In psychological diagnosis considerable attention has been given to the masculine and feminine traits of the figures drawn; such sex characteristics have proved useful in the study of personality. Previously in this Chapter we have suggested that deafness may influence the development and maintenance of feelings of masculinity and femininity. To explore this possibility further, the sex characteristics present in the drawing were scored in three ways; the drawing was not clearly male or female, or it manifested either masculine or feminine characteristics. No differences between the Deaf and the Normal were found in the drawing of a Man. Comparison of the Deaf groups revealed that more males than females drew figures which were not clearly male or female; these differences occurred mainly at the nine year level. Moreover, the Day Males drew more such figures than the Residential Males. If drawing figures which are not clearly male or female is taken as an indication that identification with the same sexed parent has not developed normally, then this problem of psychosexual maturation was more prevalent in the Day School males. Also, it occurred more frequently in the males than in the females, irrespective of type of school attended.

Evaluation of the results for the masculine characteristics disclosed a number of significant differences which varied by age, sex, and type of school attended. The Deaf population, especially the males, more often than the Normal portrayed a hat; the Residential males included this article more frequently than the Day males. However, the Normal more than the Deaf drew figures which had a masculine neckline with a collar and tie, and the Residential males included this feature to a greater extent than the Day males.

The most noteworthy characteristics seemed to be that the Normal control group drew more male figures who had broad shoulders, had a square stance, and a muscular appearance. This was true for both sexes and was consistent at the 9, 11, 13, and 15 year age levels, which suggests that Normal males and females portrayed male figures with more masculineness in the body build than did either Deaf males or females. This must be viewed as a trend for the Deaf to portray the male figure in a more frail, effeminate manner. Interestingly, although the Residential population exceeded the Day in including articles such as a tie and buttons, the Day exceeded the Residential in the portrayal of a beard or a mustache; at 15 years they also exceeded the Normals in portraying this feature. This may be indicative of differences in perceptual awareness as well as in feelings of identification.

Study of the items used to reveal feminine characteristics also disclosed a number of variations between the groups; however, these items revealed no differences between the Deaf and the Normal. As expected, the females drew more feminine figures with rouged lips, spike heels, and eyelashes. There were substantially fewer differences between the Day and Residential females than between the Day and Residential males when all of the sex characteristics were considered.

In general, with few exceptions the masculinity-femininity evaluation manifested that Deaf children had established basic identifications to a high degree. While there was evidence that this psychosexual aspect of the personality deviated from the Normal in certain respects and varied to some extent on the basis of school environment, no gross abnormalities were revealed. On the other hand the differences which were found must be considered consequential when studying the effects of deafness on personality development.

Mood: Four scores were obtained on Mood—positive, meaning that the drawing definitely reflected happiness and enjoyment; negative, the drawing reflected definite unhappiness, aggressiveness, or hostility; mixed, a drawing that manifested moods in opposition to each other, such as sadness and levity; neutral, a drawing that gave no clue as to mood. This item disclosed one of the most consistent and provocative findings concerning the emotional adjustment of deaf children.

There was a clear and definite trend for the Residential children to draw figures showing positive mood and for the Day School children to draw figures showing negative mood. These differences, which appeared primarily at the 13 and 15 year age levels, cannot be explained simply as difficulties of adjustment at the age of entering school. Furthermore, the Day population drew more negative mood children than the Normal at the 11, 13, and 15 year age levels. Such a difference was not found between the Normal and Residential groups. Another finding denoting a similar pattern was that the Day School children drew more figures which showed a mixture of moods than did either the Normal and Residential subjects; these differences were found principally at the 9 and 11 year age levels. At the

13 year level the Total Deaf sample drew more figures than the Normal showing mixed moods. Consistent with these results was the finding that the Normal drew more neutral mood figures than did the children in the Day Schools.

If we interpret these results as indicating attitudes toward self and toward others, especially the parents, then we must infer that the Day School children were less happy and showed more emotional conflict. Inasmuch as this finding was on the basis of the type of school attended it seems that the Day School environment presented a more stressful situation emotionally.

CLOTHING: The use of clothing in drawing the human figure has been evaluated in various ways. Our approach was to study the completeness and unusualness of the costume, and the filling in of space by cross-hatching. This provided five scores pertaining to clothing. There was a trend for the Normal to draw more figures than the Deaf showing complete costumes without incongruities, but this was not marked and pertained chiefly to the females. Comparisons between the Deaf groups disclosed that the Residential children drew more complete costumes than the Day School population, indicating a higher level of perceptual awareness and identification. This pattern was consistent for the other scores on details of clothing portrayed.

No differences were found on the portrayal of unusual costumes. Consistent with the findings on several other items, the Residential included cross-hatching more than the Day School children. The significance of this result is obscure but it can be attributed to some extent to the more completeness of the costume drawn by this group. In general, it may reflect more feelings of security and greater feelings of identification.

HEAD: Study of the portrayal of various body parts in human figure drawings is one of the most revealing and useful in this method of personality investigation. We included a number of items of this type and devised specific procedures for scoring them. The first of these body parts to be considered is the Head, for which three scores were obtained: head drawn as a circle only, head drawn too small or too large. If the head were portrayed only as a circle, it was viewed as being a more primitive or a more immature drawing, as indicated by Goodenough. This type of drawing of the head was made more often by Residential than by Day School children.

This was true for all four of the figures drawn, but of the 11 differences found, six fell at the age level of 11 years, which suggests that this variation by school group may have been largely on a developmental basis, with the Residential children showing slower maturation. On the other hand, from the results for other body parts as given below, there is a possibility that this difference in body image was not an isolated phenomenon. There is evidence suggesting that the Residential population deviated in the perception of other body parts.

No variations were found on the basis of the head's being drawn proportionately too small, but several differences were disclosed in relation to drawing the head proportionately too large. These did not reveal a trend except that the Deaf males more often than the Deaf females seemed to draw heads that were too large. Most of these variations appeared at the 9 year age level.

Eyes: Goodenough demonstrated that the portrayal of eyes occurs early developmentally. The eyes have been given considerable attention as a feature of the drawing when studied projectively. In our investigation five scores were obtained: eyes present, eyelashes present, eyebrow present, pupils present, and the horizontal measurement of the eye greater than the vertical measurement. No differences were found for the eyes being present. The Deaf and the Normal, males and females, Day and Residential groups portrayed eyes with equal frequency. In the portrayal of eyelashes, the most noteworthy result was that this feature was included more frequently by the Residential children. They showed eyelashes more often than the Normal and the Day School group, and several variations occurred within the Day and Residential School populations. This is an interesting finding, especially in view of the fact that the reverse was found for the eyebrows. On this feature the Day exceeded the Residential group, albeit to a lesser extent. These results are made more complex by the additional fact that the Day School children consistently and clearly drew more pupils than the Residential sample. No pattern emerged in the drawing of eyes so that the horizontal measurement exceeded the vertical, except that the Deaf females more often than the Deaf males portrayed the eyes in this manner.

These results indicate differences in the perception of body parts, in details relating to the eyes, which are highly specific and which vary according to the type of school attended. The most clearly revealed variations are the higher incidence of eyelashes in the Residential population and the more frequent portrayal of pupils by the Day School population.

NOSE: Two scores were obtained on drawings of the nose—nose present and nostrils shown. No differences appeared on the inclusion of the nose in the drawing; all groups portrayed it with equal frequency. However, a curious and intriguing result was obtained on the portrayal of the nostrils. The Residential children clearly included this feature more often than did the Day School group. Moreover, the females in the Residential School portrayed this feature more often than any other group. With one exception, the variations appeared at the seven or nine year age levels. Again we note that the self-perception and the perception of body parts varied on the basis of the type of school attended.

MOUTH: Drawing of the mouth was scored in three ways— mouth present, two lines for the lips, and the lips shown in two dimensions. All groups, Normal and Deaf, drew the mouth with equal frequency. However, there were differences between the groups of Deaf children on the other two features. The trend was for the Males to draw lips with two lines and for the Females to draw them in two dimensions, apparently explicable on the basis of females routinely giving more attention to the lips. It may be of some importance that this sex difference was not found for the Normal. Moreover, at the age level of 13 years, the Day School males gave more attention to the lips than either the Normal or the Residential School males. Consistent with other findings, the Residential population more than the Day at the 15 year age level, drew lips with two lines on the Father figure. For a number of the features there was a trend for the Residential group to portray more details than the Day group, especially on parental figures. While the tendency was not marked, Deaf children, especially those in Day Schools, seemed more perceptually aware of the lips than the Normal. This may be a function of their training in speechreading.

TEETH: Teeth were scored only as being present or not present. Only two differences appeared on this item, both on drawings of the Self and both at the age level of 15 years. The males in Residential Schools exceeded the females, and also the Day males in the portrayal of teeth. This revealed a sex difference in the Residential population which did not appear for the Day Group, with a difference between the males on the basis of the school attended. This is consistent with the finding of the Residential males including more details in their drawings as compared to the other Deaf groups.

HAIR: Two scores were obtained for the drawing of hair—hair present and hair shown in detail. Many differences emerged on this item. A variation occurred by sex in the Normal control group with the Females drawing hair more frequently than the males at the 7 and 9 year age levels. Furthermore, the Deaf males exceeded the Normal males at 7 years of age. Otherwise the trend was for the Deaf females to portray hair more often than the Deaf males, which was in agreement with the results for the normally hearing. The data for the Deaf disclosed that the Day School females consistently drew hair in detail with greater frequency than the Residential School females, and more often than the Normal females at 15 years of age.

Another trend appeared in that the Residential males consistently exceeded the Day males in portraying hair in detail, and in some instances they showed this feature with greater frequency than the normally hearing males. Least attention was given to drawing of the hair by the Day School males and the Residential females. Perhaps the most revealing finding was the greater use of hair detail in the drawings by the Residential males. The total findings for this item indicate differences between the Deaf and the Normal by school, and by sex. Portrayal of hair was related psychodynamically to deafness, especially in the Males.

EARS: We hypothesized that the ear as a body part might have a special meaning for deaf children; this postulation was confirmed. Five scores were derived: ears present, ear shown in detail, horizontal measurement greater than vertical; too large or too small in proportion to the head. Many statistically significant results were obtained and some trends were manifested. A sex difference appeared in the Day School group, with the Males portraying ears much more frequently and in greater detail than the Females; this was not true for the Residential population. As anticipated, ears were drawn more often on male than on female figures. An indication of the psychic significance of the ear to the Deaf was that at the age level of 7 years, they drew more ears than the Normal. Apparently they were perceptually aware of the ear at an earlier period developmentally.

There were other indications that the Deaf were psychically sensitive to this body part. The total hearing impaired, to a greater extent than the Normal, drew the ear in such a manner that the horizontal measurement exceeded the vertical measurement. This variation between the Deaf and the Normal was highly consistent, occurring at the age levels of 7, 11, 13, and 15 years. Furthermore, drawings of the ear by the Deaf consistently were proportionately too large as compared to the Normal. While these trends occurred for the total population of hearing impaired, the differences were greater for the Day School subjects.

These data revealed two major patterns in portrayal of this body part by the Deaf. They drew it so that the horizontal measurement exceeded the vertical, and so that it was proportionately too large in relation to the size of the head. In other-words they portrayed the ear in a "cupped" position as well as being larger in comparison with the Normal. Developmentally, psychodynamically, and in terms of body image these children were more perceptually aware of the ear. This may be explained by the focusing of attention on this body part from early childhood and may not necessarily be detrimental to personality and emotional adjustment. However, such a possibility cannot be overlooked.

ARMS: Detailed study was made of the limbs. Three scores were obtained for drawings of the arms: arms present, proportionately too large, and proportionately too short. No variations were found for "arms present" or for "arms too long." A highly consistent difference did appear for the item "arms obviously too short in relation to the torso." The Deaf more than the Normal drew arms that were disproportionately too short and this finding was generalized, occurring at the 9, 11, 13, and 15 year age level. Perception of the size of this body part, as well as some of the others, seems to be affected by deafness. While no major trends appeared in comparisons between the groups of Deaf children, there were a few specific variations. In the Residential population at the lower age level, the Females drew shorter arms than the Males; at the upper age level the pattern was reversed. This variation by sex was not found for the Day School group.

HANDS: Hands were studied as distinct from arms or fingers. We postulated that hands might be accentuated in the drawings of children with markedly impaired hearing. While differences did not appear between the Deaf and the Normal, interesting dissimilarities were found according to the type of school environment experienced by the child; these variations were present principally at the age level of 11 years. The most consistent finding was that the Residential group portrayed hands as being too large in comparison with the Day School subjects. They also tended to draw hands more often, whereas the Day group in drawings of the Father, tended to conceal the hands. This may reflect more perceptual awareness of the hands, more psychic value of the hands, on the part of the Residential children who used the manual sign language as an important means of communication. There is a possibility also that the Day School group manifested some reticence concerning hands because of their often being restricted in the use of gesture and the sign language. Whatever the reasons, differences in body imagery and in the perception of others again were evident on the basis of the type of school.

FINGERS: In a similar manner as for the hands, we assumed that fingers might have a meaning unique to the Deaf. This hypothesis was verified more conclusively than for the hands. At two age levels, 7 and 13 years, the Deaf drew significantly more fingers than the Normal. Furthermore, comparison by School revealed differences which were in agreement with those found for the hands; the total Residential exceeded the total Day subjects in the portrayal of fingers, while the males in Residential Schools exceeded the males in Day Schools. Details of the fingers were more prevalent in the drawings of Normal children as compared to the Deaf. Thus, those with deafness were developmentally and perceptually more cognizant of fingers, but they portrayed them in less detail than did the Normal.

LEGS: Legs were scored in the same way as the arms—as being present, too long or too short in proportion to the torso. In contrast to the findings for arms, however, there were no differences between the Deaf and the Normal. On the other hand, the deaf groups were dissimilar with a tendency for the Residential children to draw legs too short in comparison to the Day. These variations were constant for the drawing of Mother and Self at the 11 year age level.

In general these results for the limbs suggest that deaf children have a distortion of body image in relation to the arms. As compared to the Normal this distortion does not include the legs, but in comparison to the Day the Residential child is more likely also to perceive the legs as being too short. This must be considered of consequence and as being related to the total alteration of psychological organization found in deaf children.

FEET: Six scores were derived for the drawing of feet—any attempt to show feet, clubbed feet, perspective shown, details portrayed, feet too big, and feet too small. Dissimilarities were found on all items with the exception of "any attempt to show feet"; all groups, Deaf and Normal, made such attempts with equal frequency. Deaf children as a group drew more clubbed feet than the Normal at 7 years of age. Perhaps this indicates that deaf children learn to perceive feet accurately at a developmentally later age than normally hearing children. Otherwise, Day School subjects consistently exceeded the Residential in portraying clubbed feet. This was consistent for all four of the drawings. Curiously they also drew more feet in perspective, but this difference appeared only at the 9 year age level. The occurrence of more clubbed feet in their drawings was chiefly at the 11 and 13 year age levels. It is difficult to reconcile these findings, but aparently while the Day School children achieved more perceptual accuracy of the foot by 9 years, they did not maintain this superior ability as they reached the higher levels of age.

There were other significant and interesting variations. The Residential population exceeded the Normal in the drawing of details of the feet. They also exceeded the Day group on this feature and they exceeded the Day in drawing the feet "too big." In contrast, at 13 years of age in the drawing of the Father, they drew more feet that were too small than did the Day group. We see, therefore, that not only were alterations present in both groups but also that these alterations differed from one group to the other. Both groups differed from the Normal and from each other in certain respects. These findings are congruent with other results of this study which indicate that deafness and the type of school are influential in the perception of self and of other persons.

Summary of Emotional Development in Deaf Children

The drawing of the Human Figure is a widely used projective Test for the study of personality and emotional adjustment. From the results of our investigation we concluded that this Test can be used to study emotional development and other psychodynamic factors in children having profound deafness from early life. It might be a critical tool diagnostically, but its applicability is more inclusive. It can be utilized to appraise the effects of deafness on perceptual organization, body image, self-perception, and on the perception of other persons. This study of the emotional development of deaf children manifested that the sensory deprivation of profound loss of hearing has far-reaching consequences. As these ramifications become clarified, it will be necessary to devise additional methods and approaches to the education and training of deaf children. Conceivably this might result in the deaf child's actualizing his potential to a substantially greater degree than is characteristic for him at this time.

The results from this investigation emphasize that a sensory deprivation, such as profound deafness from infancy, alters the perceptual processes and awareness of the individual. This was indicated by previous study but only in regard to form and figure-ground.[30] The deaf child has characteristic perceptual distortions regarding himself and presumably projects these in his perception of others. His body image includes altered perception of various body parts, entailing the perception of the head, hands, fingers, ears, limbs, lips, hair, feet, and characteristics such as mood, maleness, and transparencies. The specific psychological processes which are operative are not apparent and must await further investigation. The implication of paramount importance is that perceptual behavior is altered, the deaf child's body image is different from the normal; his perception of himself and of others varies characteristically. Furthermore, the nature of his body image varies by sex and on the basis of the type of school which he attends.

It was hypothesized that the deaf child's psychological organization would be different from the Normal, and a rationale for such modification of his psychic structure was discussed in Chapter IV. The point of view expressed was that deprivation of a distance sense causes the organism to *shift,* to integrate experience differently.

Our results indicate some of the ways in which the organism shifts to maintain balance between inner needs and external circumstances. Psychological equilibrium is attained principally through developing greater dependence on residual sensory capacities. While the hierarchy of psychological organization suggested in Figure 5 is not revealed in detail, the premise for this rationale is supported. The deaf child is more psychologically sensitive to specific body parts indicating greater reliance on vision, taction, olfaction, and gustation. Thereby, his experience is constituted differently. Deprivation of hearing results in a modification of figure-ground organismically.

The results of the study also might be viewed in terms of emotional immaturity. The deaf children drew body parts that were proportionately too large, a characteristic of younger children. They showed immaturity also in the use of space, in placement of the figure on the page, and in the use of transparencies. A notable result psychodynamically was the indication that deafness impedes the process of identification, manifested principally by the males. The findings of greater emotional involvement in males corresponds to the results found for the adults and discussed previously in this chapter. Moreover, the indication of immaturity and more emotional problems in deaf children when compared with the normal is in agreement with the results of other investigators.

A prominent aspect of this investigation was comparison on the basis of the type of school attended. A remarkable number of differences were found between the Day and Residential populations, with implications for theory and educational practice. No outstanding advantages emerged for either school. Rather the results indicated advantages and disadvantages for each type of school program. The Day School children showed more emotional stress, conflict, and frustration, both in comparison with the Residential group and with the Normal. Identification was most disturbed in the Day School sample and this may be the primary basis of their less adequate emotional adjustment. The Residential School child usually has association with children like himself and of his own age. Also, most often he has more frequent contact with deaf adults. From the study of the emotional adjustment of hearing impaired adults, we can assume that contact with others having deafness is a fundamental factor in feelings of belonging and of general well-being. The Day School children had more difficulty attaining such feelings of adequacy.

In comparison with the Day, the Residential population had attained a more satisfactory emotional adjustment. However, sex differences must be considered. The greatest variation occurred between the male groups. In comparison to the Day, the Residential children drew more figures that were proportionately too large, more too large heads and hands. They also drew more mixed view figures, more transparencies, eyelashes, nostrils, teeth, hair detail, fingers, and more details of the feet. In addition they more frequently portrayed props, details of clothing, complete costumes, and cross-hatching. A major variation on the basis of School was the substantially greater use of detail in the drawings of the Residential group. The significance of these variations in body image psychodynamically is obscure and interpretation must remain tentative. However, it seems that the Residential child had attained a more successful shift, that he had achieved more adequate "altered" psychological structure and organization, albeit, this organization, in certain respects, may be at a lower level in comparison with the Day School child. The Residential group seemed to be encountering less struggle. In contrast, there was evidence that the Day subjects were making a vehement attempt to behave in ways more comparable to the norm for hearing persons and that they were being successful to a degree. It is noteworthy in this connection that they gave more attention to ears, lips, and pupils of the eye. Furthermore, they portrayed fewer transparencies, mixed view figures, and more accurate perspective in drawing the feet. We might generalize to the extent of suggesting that the Day School children manifested more accuracy of body image, of self-perception, and of person perception in comparison to the Residential. However, this was not achieved without deleterious effects on the personality. In contrast, the Residential group, while showing more stable identification, more adequacy of emotional adjustment, manifested more of the organismic involvements related to profound deafness from early life. Their portrayal of more complete drawings, with greater detail, suggests less feeling of isolation and more of an attitude that when one is deaf he must behave accordingly.

These differences between Day and Residential groups must not be stressed unduly. Neither should the results be construed as being advantageous to either type of school program. For the deaf child, as for any child, the school of choice, the preferred school, is a highly personal matter entailing one's total orientation, convictions, and experience. It is of importance to secure objective evidence relative to the differences in learning and adjustment which might be anticipated from each type of school program. We attempted to add to this body of knowledge. A question which arises from this research is to what extent should a child deaf from early life be expected to attain adjustment which is equivalent to that of the hearing; to what extent should he be encouraged to adjust to a "norm" for the deaf instead of a "norm" for the hearing? Perhaps the most logical frame of reference is that deaf children, as all other children, present wide variations and individual differences. While characteristic shifts in psychological structure and learning processes must be assumed, only through choosing programs according to the individual child's total capacities and needs will he attain the maximum benefits from training. An important implication of these findings is that the effects of deafness are being modified in specific respects according to the type of school attended. While some aspects of the psychology of deafness might be irreversible, it is apparent that through specialized methods, procedures, and school environments, the child can be assisted to actualize his potential more successfully.

The most forthright conclusion from this investigation is that a relationship was found between deafness and personality development. While there was evidence of emotional disturbance, this was not the primary involvement. The predominant indication was that psychological organization and structure are different when deafness is present from infancy. It is these differences which must constitute the fundamental basis for educational planning and for instituting guidance programs designed to alleviate the specialized problems in learning and adjustment.

It has been suggested that Man matures chiefly in three ways, mentally, emotionally, and physically. In Chapter V we considered the relationships between deafness and intellectual functioning. In this chapter our concern has been the way in which impaired hearing influences personality development and emotional adjustment. A relationship was found between deafness and psychodynamic factors in both children and adults which conforms to the conclusions of past investigators. The primary implication is that deafness cannot be viewed as a unitary factor. A sensory deprivation has organismic effects. Although the defect is limited to his ears it is the total person who has deafness. Therefore, the true significance of the deprivation can be realized only when the individual is viewed wholistically. Like other human beings, children and adults who have deafness are striving for adequacy and psychological equilibrium. It is the criterion of relevancy which changes and which remains as a constant challenge for all of us concerned with the auditorially deprived.

REFERENCES

1. Allport, F.: Theories of Perception and a Concept of Structure. New York, John Wiley and Sons, 1955.

1a. Bender, L.: Psychopathology of Children with Organic Brain Disorders. Springfield, C. C. Thomas, 1956.

2. Benton, A. L.: Right-Left Discrimination and Finger Localization. New York, Paul B. Hoeber, 1959.

3. Bindon, M.: Make-a-Picture Story Test findings for rubella deaf children. J. Abnormal and Soc. Psychol., 55, 38, 1957.

4. Bowlby, J.: Maternal Care and Mental Health. New York, Columbia University Press, 1952.

5. Brunschwig, L.: A Study of Some Personality Aspects of Deaf Children. New York, Columbia University, T. C. Contribs. to Ed., #687, 1936.

6. Costello, M. R.: A study of speechreading as a developing language process in deaf and in hard of hearing children. Evanston, Northwestern University, Unpublished Doctoral Dissertation, 1957.

7. Critchley, M.: The Parietal Lobes. London, Edward Arnold, 1953.

8. Deri, S.: Introduction to the Szondi Test. New York, Grune and Stratton, 1949.

9. Fisher, S. and Cleveland, S.: Body Image and Personality. Princeton, D. Van Nostrand, 1958.

10. Fusfeld, I.: Research and testing at Gallaudet College. Am. Ann. Deaf, 85, 170, 1940.

11. Gerstmann, J.: Syndrome of finger agnosia, disorientation for right and left, agraphia and acalculia. Arch. Neurol. and Psychiat., 44, 389, 1940.

12. Gilliland, A. and Colgin, R.: Norms, reliability and forms of the MMPI. J. Consult. Psychol., 15, 435, 1951.

13. Goldfarb, W.: Effects of psychological deprivation in infancy and subsequent stimulation. Am. J. Psychiat., 102, 18, 1945.

14. Goodenough, F.: Measurement of Intelligence by Drawings. Yonkers, World Book, 1926.

15. Goodstein, L.: Regional differences in MMPI responses among male college students. J. Consult. Psychol., 18, 437, 1954.

16. Gregory, I.: A comparison of certain personality traits and interests in deaf and hearing children. Child Develop., 9, 277, 1938.

17. Hanes, B.: Reading ease and MMPI results. J. Consult. Psychol., 9, 83, 1953.

18. Hathaway, S. and McKinley, J.: Minnesota Multiphasic Personality Inventory: Manual. (Revised) New York, Psychol. Corp., 1951.

19. _____: The Minnesota Multiphasic Personality Schedule. Minneapolis, University of Minnesota Press, 1942.

20. Head, H.: Studies in Neurology, Vol. 2. London, Hodder and Stoughton, 1920.

21. Hebb, D. O.: A Textbook of Psychology. Philadelphia, Saunders, 1958.

22. Heider, F.: The Psychology of Interpersonal Relations. New York, John Wiley and Sons, 1958.

23. _____ and Heider, G.: Studies in the psychology of the deaf. Psychol. Monog., #242, 1941.

24. Levine, E.: Youth in a Silent World. New York, New York University Press, 1956.

25. Lyon, V.: The use of vocational and personality tests with the deaf. J. Appl. Psychol., 18, 224, 1934.

26. McAndrew, H.: Rigidity and isolation; a study of the deaf and the blind. J. Abnormal and Social Psychol., 43, 476, 1948.

27. Machover, K.: Personality Projection in the Drawing of the Human Figure. Springfield, C. C. Thomas, 1949.

28. Mowrer, O. H.: Learning Theory and Personality Dynamics. New York, Ronald Press, 1950.

29. Myklebust, H. R.: Babbling and echolalia in language theory. J. Speech and Hearing Disorders, 22, 356, 1957.

30. _____ and Brutten, M.: A study of the visual perception of deaf children. Acta Oto-laryng., Suppl. 105, 1953.

31. _____ and Burchard, E. M. L.: A study of the effects of congenital and adventitious deafness on intelligence, personality, and social maturity of school children. J. Ed. Psychol., 34, 321, 1945.

32. Nafin, P.: Das soziale verhalten taubstummer schulkinder. Konigsberg, Unpublished Thesis, 1933.

32a. Neyhus, A.: The personality of socially well-adjusted adult deaf as revealed by projective tests. Unpublished doctoral dissertation, Northwestern University, 1962.

33. Olson, W. C.: Problem Tendencies in Children. Minneapolis, University of Minn. Press, 1930.

34. Pellet, R.: Des Premieres Perceptions du Concret a la Conception de l'Abstrait. Lyon, Bosc Freres, 1938.

35. Piaget, J.: The Construction of Reality in the Child. New York, Basic Books, 1954.

36. _____: The Origins of Intelligence in Children. New York, International Universities Press, 1952.

37. Pick, A.: Ueber Störungen der Orientierung am eigenen Körper. Berlin, Karger, 1908.

38. Pintner, R.: Eisenson, J. and Stanton, M.: The Psychology of the Physically Handicapped. New York, F. S. Crofts, 1946.

39. Pintner, R., Fusfeld, I. and Brunschwig, L.: Personality tests of deaf adults. J. Genetic Psychol., 51, 305, 1937.

40. Ribble, M.: The Rights of Infants. New York, Columbia University Press, 1943.

40a. Rorschach, R.: Psychodiagnostic. New York: Grune and Stratton, 1942.

40b. Rotter, J. and Rafferty, J. The Rotter Incomplete Sentences Blank manual. New York, Psychol. Corp., 1950.

41. Schilder, P.: Image and Appearance of the Human Body. New York, International Universities Press, 1951.

42. Shneidman, E.: A Manual for the MAPS Test. Proj. Tech. Monog., 1, #2, 1951.

43. Spitz, R.: No and Yes. New York, International Universities Press, 1957.

44. Springer, N.: A comparative study of the behavior traits of deaf and hearing children of New York City. Am. Ann. Deaf, 83, 255, 1938.

45. _____: A comparative study of the psychoneurotic responses of deaf and hearing children. J. Ed. Psychol., 29, 459, 1938.

46. _____ and Roslow, S. A further study of the psychoneurotic responses of deaf and hearing children. J. Ed. Psychol., 29, 590, 1938.

47. Tagiuri, R. and Petrullo, L.: Person Perception and Interpersonal Behavior, Stanford, Stanford University Press, 1958.

48. Terman, L. and Miles, C.: Sex and Personality. New York, McGraw-Hill, 1936.

49. Welles, H.: Measurement of Certain Aspects of Personality Among Hard of Hearing Adults. New York, Columbia University, T. C. Contrib. to Ed., #545, 1932.

50. Witkin, H. A., et al.: Personality Through Perception. New York, Harper and Brothers, 1954.

Suggestions for Further Study

Altable, J.: The Rorschach diagnostic as applied to deaf mutes. Rorschach Research Exchange, 11, 74, 1947.

Barker, R., Wright, B., Meyerson, L. and Gonick, M.: Adjustment to Physical Handicap and Illness. New York, Social Science Research Council, 1953.

Bartlett, F.: Remembering. New York, Macmillan 1932.

Davitz, J. (ed.): The Communication of Emotional Meaning. New York, Mc-Graw Hill Book Co., 1964.

Ewing, A. (ed.): Educational Guidance and the Deaf Child. Washington, D. C., The Volta Bureau, 1957.

Habbe, S.: Personality Adjustment of Adolescent Boys with Impaired Hearing. New York, Columbia University, T. C. Contribs. to Ed., #697, 1936.

Hall, C. S.: Theories of Personality. New York, John Wiley and Sons, 1957.

Hathaway, S. and Meehl, P.: Atlas for the Clinical Use of the MMPI. Minneapolis, University of Minnesota Press, 1951.

Healey, R.: A study of personality differences between hearing and non-hearing girls as determined by the Mosaic Test. Washington, Catholic University, Unpublished M.A. Thesis, 1951.

Kelly, G.: The Psychology of Personal Constructs, Vol. 1 and 2. New York, W. W. Norton, 1955.

Knopp, P.: Emotional aspects of hearing loss. Psychosomatic Med., 10, 203 1948.

Munn, N.: The Evolution and Growth of Human Behavior. Chicago, Houghton Mifflin, 1955.

Murphy, L.: Personality in Young Children, Vol. 1 and 2. New York, Basic Books, 1956.

Myklebust, H.: Psychological and psychiatric implications of deafness. Arch. of Otolaryngology, 78, 790-93, 1963.

Rainer, J., Altshuler, K., Kallman, F., and Deming, W.: Family and Mental Health Problems in a Deaf Population. New York, Columbia University, 1963.

Schaefer, E.: A comparison of personality characteristics of deaf and hearing college students as revealed by a group Rorschach method. Washington, Catholic University, Unpublished M.A. Thesis, 1950.

Schanberger, W.: A study of the personality characteristics of deaf and non-deaf as determined by the Mosaic Test. Washington, Catholic University, Unpublished M.A. Thesis, 1951.

Simon, B. (ed.): Psychology in the Soviet Union. Stanford, Stanford University Press, 1957.

Zechel, A.: Psyche and deafness. Amer. J. Psycho-therapy, 7, 321, 1953.

Chapter VII

DEAFNESS AND MOTOR FUNCTIONING

IN CHAPTER V we noted a relationship between deafness and intellectual abilities, while the influence of deafness on personality was considered in Chapter VI. Here we are concerned with the interaction of hearing loss on the third way in which Man matures, the problem of deafness and motor functioning.

A number of pioneers in psychology studied these aspects of growth and maturation. Outstanding investigations were made by Baldwin,[1] Goddard,[20] Binet and Simon,[5] Doll,[14] Gesell,[18] Thompson,[42] and McGraw.[29] It was physical development and behavior which were studied most extensively by the early students of psychology. This was followed by studies of the relationship between physical and mental growth and included the question of interaction between physique and personality. The work of Sheldon[39] and Jones[25] illustrate the importance of such investigations in human behavior.

Although motor maturation has been studied extensively, virtually no attention has been given to the possible effects of sensory deprivation on such development. Experimental psychology has indicated a relationship between sensory channel and reaction time.[4] In general, the quickest reaction time has been associated with auditory sensation. From this we might infer that those having deafness will have reduced reaction time in situations which require audition. This presumption has relevance to the study of motor capacities in the auditorially handicapped.

The study of the psychology of deafness, however, must be concerned with many other questions regarding the relationship between hearing loss and motor functioning. One of these is the evident association of defects in the inner ear and disturbances of motor function. Although definite experimental evidence is meagre, it has been known for some time that impairment of the semicircular canals results in reduced ability to maintain motor balance and equilibrium.[33] There are other difficult questions. For example, does the lack of auditory experience, resulting in altered perceptual organization, in turn alter the dynamics of motor function? In other words we must consider whether deafness, especially when it is severe and is from early life, causes a change in visuo-motor organization and behavior. Furthermore, is motor-kinesthetic functioning enhanced or reduced? Does deafness with or without semicircular canal dysfunction affect proprioception, somasthesis, and tactual motor performance?

Psychomotor disorders are of many types and derive from many causations. Various systems for classification have been suggested.[11, 13, 27] A broad grouping of motor disabilities is on the basis of whether they are paralytic or nonparalytic. The *paralytic involvements* have received generous attention in the study of the cerebral palsies. This is relevant to the psychology of deafness because a number of individuals, those with spasticity or athetosis, have deafness with motor disorders of the paralytic type. The etiologies commonly associated with deafness and paralytic motor disorders are maternal rubella and Rh blood incompatibility, although other etiologies might be involved.

The *nonparalytic* motor disabilities have been studied less extensively and, hence, are less well understood. These include primarily the ataxias and apraxias. Neurologists have added significantly to the knowledge of these conditions in recent years.[10, 16, 34] The most frequently encountered ataxia is that which results from damage to the cerebellum, referred to as *cerebellar ataxia*, not uncommon in deaf children. Often it is characterized by a staggering, swaying gait. The child gives the appearance of losing his balance. This condition is readily confused with the disturbance of gait and balance following destruction of semicircular canal functioning through diseases such as meningitis. Other characteristics of the cerebellar ataxic are slight chorieform movements in the fingers, awkwardness in manual manipulations, and poor coordination of the tongue. It should be emphasized that ataxia is not a paralytic involvement but is an ability to coordinate motor movements normally. As Cobb[8] states, the motor movements can be made, but they are made in a disorderly manner.

Apraxia is a complex problem and has been defined in various ways. Nielson[34] and Critchley[10] have attached terms which add to the basic concept entailed in apraxic disorders. Nielson uses the term *ideational* with apraxia, while Critchley emphasizes the term *constructional* apraxia; both are useful and add to the understanding of this condition. Hughlings Jackson[41] clarified apraxia in relation to expressive aphasia. Expressive aphsia is a type of apraxia and is one of the best examples of this condition. *Apraxia* is an inability to associate a mental image, or idea, with the motor system involved. Therefore, an expressive aphasic cannot speak, not because he cannot *think* the word, he has the word in mind, but because he cannot *think* the motor plan for saying the word. This condition results from damage to the premotor area in the frontal lobes. Apraxias can affect many types of voluntary actions, such as the ability to protrude the tongue and the ability to button. In addition to expressive aphasia, it might cause another consequential language disorder, *dysgraphia*. This is an inability to write because the individual cannot relate the word he has in mind to the motor system for writing. Perhaps, as in other areas of clinical work, the most commonly observed nonparalytic motor disabilities seen in deaf children are expressive aphasia and dysgraphia. Dysgraphia, even in those having deafness from early life, can be readily diagnosed by the trained clinician. Obviously it is a difficult diagnosis in any child before five or six years of age. Expressive aphasia, on the other hand, is a difficult diagnosis in those having a profound hearing loss from early life, and perhaps can be determined on an inferential basis only.

The language imposition which occurs in conjunction with deafness is discussed in Part Three. Here we emphasize that the nonparalytic motor disorders must be included in the study of motor problems related to deafness, not because these disorders are a concomitant of an inability to hear normally; they occur in the population of hearing impaired people who have neurological involvements in addition to deafness. This is true of both paralytic and nonparalytic motor disabilities.

Another broad classification of psychomotor problems is on the basis of retardation versus disorders, suggested by Gesell.[19] This concept is especially useful in diagnosis and also has implications for training and therapy. Much has been learned about motor retardation through studies of the relationship between motor and mental development. Slowness of motor development, as compared to average and rapid development, has been investigated by Doll,[15] Bayley,[2] Gesell,[19] and Tuddenham.[43] *Motor retardation* implies that the rate of development is below the average. For example, a child might be six years of age but fall at a four year level on norms of motor maturation. This retardation might persist into adulthood so that the individual never attains average motor ability. In motor retardation the basic problem is not incoordination, apraxia, or paralysis. Rather, the individual can perform motor acts but only with ability equivalent to that of a person of a younger age.

In *motor disturbance* the problem is an inability to execute a specific type of motor act because of incoordination, paralysis, ataxia, or apraxia. This distinction is highly revealing in the study of motor functioning, as Heath[23] has indicated in motor study of the mentally deficient. He found that the endogenous and exogenous were significantly different when compared on the basis of retardation versus disorder. Myklebust[33] and Frisina[17] have applied this distinction to deaf children and their results are discussed below. While many exceptions are found, those with endogenous mental deficiency show problems of motor retardation. In contrast, those who have exogenous mental deficiency, or who have psychoneurological learning disorders, have problems of motor disturbance. From work in differential diagnosis and from research, it is evident that motor tests can provide information pertinent to etiology. Use of motor tests from this point of view has implications for the study and classification of children with deafness.

Motor study of those having a sensory deprivation such as deafness entails all of these possibilities, as well as others. Both motor retardation and motor disturbance, like apraxias and ataxias, can be expected to occur in addition to deafness in certain individuals. Other motor problems are commonly associated with impaired hearing. The loss of normal balance capacities is an example. When there are defects in the inner ear, not only the acoustic but also the nonacoustic labyrinth may be damaged. When this occurs, balance is affected. Myklebust has shown that such impairment of balance occurs frequently when the hearing loss is caused by meningitis. When deafness and loss of balance are present simultaneously, it is not uncommon for the loss of balance to be the greater problem immediately following the illness. Often in children the ability to walk is lost and they must learn to walk again. Many gradually acquire good balance, apparently through the compensatory use of vision and kinesthetic cues. It is obvious from contact with those who have no semicircular canal function that they have difficulty in maintaining balance in the dark. Their gait then usually is characterized by swaying, staggering, lunging, and generalized disequilibrium.

Perhaps the most challenging consideration is the possible effect of deafness itself on motor behavior. This problem was suggested above in referring to the association between quickness of motor performance and audition, but considerably more is involved than just the factor of speed. An example is the shuffling gait which has been observed by those who work closely with the deaf.[32] Individuals with high degrees of deafness typically shuffle their feet when they walk and many educators attempt to train deaf children to lift their feet more normally. From observation such efforts seem not to have been successful as whatever causes the shuffling gait is not readily amenable to training. Furthermore, this characteristic gait is not limited to those with dysfunction of the semicircular canals. It can be observed in virtually all children having what is referred to as profound deafness. The variables seem not to be etiology or age of onset but the degree of hearing loss. This may reflect the primary nature of the problem as it indicates that hearing is used to monitor the sound or noise one makes when he walks. Apparently the hearing child learns not to shuffle because he hears and unconsciously reacts to the noise which it causes. When one does not *hear* the shuffling, the total organism is not made sufficiently aware of it; hence, the shuffling gait. This illustrates the subtle shifts which result from sensory deprivation and has implications for the alterations that must be considered when studying the relationships between deafness and motor functioning.

Two of the most common ways of studying motor capacities are the strength or force of the motor act, and the speed with which it is performed.[4, 13] A number of investigators have indicated that speed concepts are difficult for deaf children. Hiskey[24] suggested that speed tests should not be used in measuring their intelligence. Psychologists have referred to the sense of time and temporalness as being mainly dependent on hearing. There is evidence which indicates that motor speed might be reduced by deafness. However, as all such functions are complex, it should not be expected that this relationship is a simple one. Rather, it appears that such interaction depends on the nature of the task, on the motor functions involved, and how they are measured. Some study of hearing impaired children has been made in regard to both speed and strength.

A third way in which it is common to appraise motor function is through the study of handedness or laterality. A number of studies have shown that children having reading, speech, or other types of learning disorders, often have disturbances of laterality.[30] Associated with these difficulties is an above average incidence of left handedness and mixed right and left handedness. There is an indication also that these deviations of laterality are more common in those having early life deafness.

There is considerable evidence from motor and neurological studies that integrity of motor behavior is closely related to integrity of the central nervous system. Therefore, an individual having deafness might have motor disorders chiefly because of inner ear involvement or disturbances of the central nervous system; he might have both of these simultaneously. In such instances he has organic damage causing both impaired hearing and motor disability. However, as indicated by the above discussion, another major consideration is that deafness itself might alter motor functioning. In this case the shifts in motor behavior are secondary to the sensory deprivation. This consideration, this question of relationship, is in nature the same as that encountered in the study of mental functioning and personality. Unfortunately less study has been made of the motor abilities of those with deafness but the evidence available has many implications and indicates the need for further study.

STUDIES OF MOTOR ABILITY

Long[28] made one of the early studies of the motor ability of deaf children. He used five tests from the Stanford Motor Skills Unit as adapted by Seashore,[38] and two additional tests. The seven tests used were: spoolpacking, serial discriminator, pursuit rotor, tapping, motility rotor, dynamometer, and balance-board. Long studied 37 deaf girls and 51 deaf boys, matched with hearing children of the same age, sex, and race. The only significant difference was on the balance-board results, in which the deaf were inferior to the hearing. A similar study was done by Morsh.[31] His subjects included older children and some deaf college students. While slight differences appeared, with the deaf superior on some tests and the hearing on some, the only significant difference again was on balance. Morsh blindfolded the subjects for the balance test and found this to be a greater handicap for the deaf. He was not aware of the fact that some deaf people sustain destruction of the semicircular canals; therefore, he was at a loss to explain the complete lack of balancing ability on the part of some of his subjects.

From these two studies we might conclude that with the exception of balance, there is no difference in motor ability between the deaf and the hearing. Such a conclusion may be warranted for the types of measures used in these studies and Pintner came to this general conclusion. These studies included tests involving both speed and strength. Further studies of motor strength in relation to deafness have not been made but it is conceivable that such study would corroborate the findings of Long and Morsh. On the other hand, more recent studies involving speed of motor function indicate that in both of these early studies the nature of this problem was minimized. This illustrates the need for caution in making inferences and generalizations. Additional findings have corroborated the conclusion that as far as speed of manual dexterity is concerned, the deaf are equal to the hearing. It must be emphasized that the Long and Morsh studies dealt with manual dexterity and the subject performed the tasks in a seated position. Evidence presented below suggests that when more complex motor function is required, the deaf are inferior on speed of performance. As in the case of memory, abstraction, and other psychological processes, the effect of deafness on motor speed might not be on all or none basis. This becomes a critical factor in regard to various aspects of the psychology of deafness.

Motor Speed

In an attempt to analyze further the factor of speed in the manual dexterity of the deaf, a study was done using the Minnesota Spatial Relations Test,[3] short form including Boards A and B. Each board consists of 58 pieces which must be placed in the proper recess. It is a rather difficult formboard type of test which is scored for both time and errors, and is administered individually. The sample included 80 deaf males who were in residence at a public Residential School, ranging in age from 12 to 21 years. The mean chronological age was 15.7 years. The mean scores are given in Table 41. It is interesting that the time scores for these deaf

TABLE 41. Results for deaf boys on the Minnesota Spatial Relations Test

| | | Time | | | Errors | | |
	N	Mean	SD	Percentile	Mean	SD	Percentile
Congenital	41	562.5	132.6	50	31.1	12.0	15
Acquired	31	552.2	113.0	50	27.0	11.0	15
Total Group	80	556.3	122.9	50	30.3	11.5	15

adolescents fell at the 50th percentile for the hearing; they were neither inferior nor superior. In contrast, on errors they fell at the 15th percentile. In eye-hand coordination, on visuo-motor spatial perception, this group was equal to the hearing as far as speed of performance was concerned. This is in agreement with the findings of Long and Morsh. However, although the speed of the motor performance was not inferior, many more errors were made as compared to the hearing. An error consisted of an attempt to insert a block into the wrong recess. Hence, an individual who engaged in manual trial and error, trying the block in the recess to determine whether it fit, made many errors. An individual who engaged in mental trial and error, mentally trying the block in the recess without actual attempts at insertion, made few errors. Apparently the deaf group used primarily a manual trial and error approach and therefore, although completing the task as quickly, committed many more errors.

This study disclosed that equality in speed of performance does not assure equality in the type, or the quality, of the psychological processes entailed. We noted the same problem in Chapter V relative to mental capacity and mental functioning. The error score in this study of visuo-motor perception gave us a measure of quality, a measure not used in the Long and Morsh studies. Again we note that to conclude simply that the deaf and hearing are equal on motor performance leads to overgeneralization. Apparently their

approach psychologically might be different and qualitatively inferior, with more motor thinking, more "acting out" as compared to
"thinking out." This has implications educationally and vocationally.
Of major importance is the possibility that this motor thinking approach, as it is further clarified, might be modified through training.
It seems that efforts in this regard are indicated.

Locomotor Coordination

Interest in motor behavior has grown during the past two
decades. This is manifested through work both in the United States
and in Europe. The contributions of European workers such as Van
der Lugt,[44] Oseretsky,[36] and Da Costa[12] have been especially noteworthy. In this country the work of Gesell[18] and of Seashore[38] has
been prominent. Heath,[22] too, has contributed to the concept of
motor development and motor disorders. He developed the Railwalking Test and studied the motor performance of the endogenous
and exogenous mentally deficient. He found that the endogenous
were superior in motor abilities as compared to the exogenous. This
enlarged the concept of etiology and its importance in diagnosis and
in classification for research. In the area of motor behavior it emphasized the significance of distinguishing between motor retardation
and motor disorder. As indicated above, this concept is essential in
differential diagnosis and adds to the knowledge of human behavior.
It is highly consequential when studying the relationships between
deafness and motor function.

Although Heath defined the Railwalking Test as a measure of
locomotor coordination, it is apparent that various factors are involved in such motor performance. Through a pilot study of blind
children we learned that vision plays a very consequential role.
Blind children have marked limitation in ability to walk a rail, even
when the task is explained in detail. Moreover, from the data in
Table 44, it can be assumed that balance is an important factor.
Those having dysfunction of the semicircular canals have considerable difficulty in performing the task. It can be assumed also that
kinesthetic ability is entailed. Therefore, this test involves more
complexities than a test of manual dexterity alone. Visuomotor
factors, balance, kinesthesis, and total body tonus and integration
play a role; audition itself seems not to be a part of the matrix. This

consideration of what the Railwalking Test measures is relevant to the data given below.

Frisina[17] used the Heath Railwalking Test in his study of mentally retarded deaf children. The results are summarized in Table 42.

TABLE 42.   Results for mentally retarded deaf children on the Heath Railwalking Test

	N	Mean	SD	r with M.A.	r with M.A.*
Males	41	55.55	40.98		
Females	40	43.00	30.84		
Endogenous	21	64.38	41.08	.59 ± .13	.78 ± .09
Exogenous	22	34.14	23.71	.32 ± .19	−.09 ± .22

* C.A. held constant.

The mean C.A. for the males was 13.5 and 13.8 for the females. The mean scores for hearing children, as standardized through one of our studies, was 106.1 for males and 93.0 for females at the 13 year age level. The difference between the deaf mentally retarded and the normally hearing was significant, with the deaf being inferior. Furthermore, there was a significant difference between the endogenous and exogenous, in favor of the endogenous. (The groups were equated by C.A., M.A., and degree of hearing loss.) This finding is in agreement with the results of Heath.

When deafness and mental retardation are present because of hereditary defect instead of from disease or birth trauma, the motor performance is more comparable to the normal. When mental retardation and deafness result from brain damage, from exogenous factors, then motor function is disturbed and is more grossly inferior. This is indicated further by the correlations between motor and mental capacities. The correlation was significant for the endogenous but not for the exogenous. Mental and motor capacities are not associated when motor disabilities of the exogenous type are present. Again, this in good agreement with the findings of Heath for the mentally deficient having normal hearing.

These differences between exogenously and endogenously mentally retarded deaf children have implications for their education and training. It can be presumed that the exogenous group especially might profit from the methods and techniques which have been found beneficial for brain damaged children. Motorically, this group is more like children who have psychoneurological disorders than like other deaf children and thus should profit most from training procedures which combine the psychology of brain damage and the psychology of deafness.

Because locomotor coordination, as measured by the Railwalking Test, has been found useful in studying both children and adults having learning disorders, an extensive study was undertaken in which this test was used. The sample included normal, deaf, mentally retarded, speech handicapped, dyslexic, and emotionally disturbed children. Only the results comparing the deaf with the normal are presented here and these results are given in Table 43.

TABLE 43.   Results comparing the deaf and the hearing by age on the Railwalking Test

	Deaf		Hearing	
Age	N	Mean	N	Mean
7	8	40	72	53
9	10	44	45	77
11	16	63	60	82
13	20	70	51	96
15	21	79	47	118

TABLE 44.   Comparative Railwalking scores by age of onset and etiology

Group	N	Mean C.A.	Mean Score	SD
Acquired	41	11.0	74.5	20.0
Undetermined	48	13.5	68.3	17.7
Congenital	86	11.9	71.6	18.4
Meningitis	23	13.3	30.0	7.4

From this comparison we must conclude that deaf children are inferior to the hearing on locomotor coordination as measured by the Railwalking Test. These findings for both the deaf and the hearing are in agreement with the work of Heath, showing there is progression in ability as age increases. This is shown also by Figure 11. Nevertheless, the level of ability attained by the deaf was below that of the hearing throughout the age range. Heath's study did not go beyond the 14 year level. In the present investigation alternate ages were studied from seven through 15 years. Significant differences between the deaf and the hearing appeared at each of these age levels. This indicates that the deaf are inferior in early life and although they show progressive maturation, do not attain normal ability in locomotor coordination. As shown in Table 44, there were no significant differences between the acquired, con-

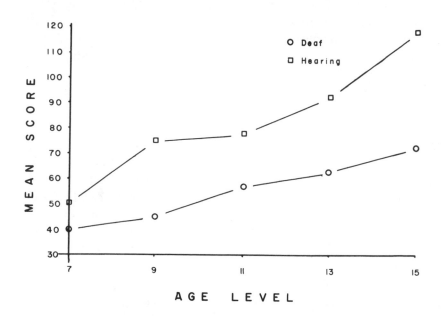

FIG. 11. Comparison of deaf and hearing on Railwalking ability.

genital, and undetermined groups; the meningitic were inferior to all of the others. It appeared that the deaf as a group were inferior to the hearing and that this inferiority could not be explained on the basis of etiology or age of onset alone. While these factors might be influential they do not provide an adequate explanation of the inferiority of the deaf on this type of motor function.

The etiology of meningitis is an exception as it seems to be directly related to motor performance as measured by the Railwalking Test. To further explore this relationship the caloric test was administered to this group by an otolaryngologist. The results were highly positive; it was concluded that all but one child had nonfunction of the semicircular canals. These subjects also were rotated and tested for nystagmic reactions. With one exception they did not have nystagmus after rotation; indefinite rotation did not produce dizziness. The mean I.Q. of this group was 101, the average for the total population studied. There is little question but that the poor locomotor coordination of this group was due to an inability to maintain normal balance as a result of nonfunctioning semi-circular canals. The individual having meningitic deafness is highly characteristic in his locomotor coordination, revealed also by use of the Railwalking Test in diagnostic studies of hearing impaired children and adults. When the test findings indicate nonfunction of the semicircular canals, these indications often are confirmed by medical diagnosis.

Further study was made using the Railwalking Test in order to appraise its reliability as a procedure in the study of the psychology of deafness. We had it administered by a trained educator of the deaf to all of the children above five years of age in a small public Residential School. The results for this school, School Y, were compared with the results from the present study, children in School X. This comparison is shown in Table 45. As can be seen from these results, the mean scores for the two groups are highly similar. From these data we may deduce that the scores from this test are reliable, and substantiates the conclusion that deaf children are inferior to the hearing on this type of function. This conclusion is in disagreement with the broad generalization that the deaf are equal to the hearing in all aspects of motor performance. Railwalking ability requires more inclusive coordination and integration than tests requiring mainly manual dexterity. When this organismic motor behavior is required, the deaf child falls below the norm for the hearing.

TABLE 45. Comparison of two Residential School populations on Railwalking ability

		School X				School Y		
	N	Mean C.A.	Mean Score	SD	N	Mean C.A.	Mean Score	SD
Males	105	13.0	73.8	18.2	40	12.8	72.5	15.4
Females	98	13.0	59.1	14.5	31	12.4	56.8	6.6

The Oseretsky Test of Motor Proficiency

Standardized batteries of tests designed to measure motor maturation have developed slowly in the United States. Perhaps the most extensive test of this type was developed in Russia by Oseretsky.[36] Doll[15] provided a translation and a manual of instructions in English. Sloan[40] and Cassell[7] have published adaptations based on study of the mentally deficient. The Oseretsky Test differs from other motor tests in that it is designed to measure areas, various facets of motor ability. In this way it is comparable to mental tests, such as the Binet, and to the Social Maturity Scale, on which areas of maturation are appraised. The advantage of such a test is immediately evident. The Stanford Motor Skills Tests are principally speed of eye-hand coordination and there are no maturational norms. The Heath Railwalking Test has been standardized on normal children and hence, does provide a guide to maturation, but only for one aspect of motor development, locomotor coordination. Oseretsky apparently used a neurological frame of reference when selecting the aspects of motor ability to be studied. A number of the tests included in his battery are used in neurological evaluation. He selected six areas of motor function: General Static, Dynamic Manual, General Dynamic, Speed, Simultaneous Movement, and Synkinesia. One test of each of these functions is provided; thus, there are six tests at each age level from four through sixteen years. The translation provided by Doll raises questions regarding procedures and scoring. The more inclusive presentation by Oseretsky clarifies many of these ambiguities. There are limitations in the use of this test, however, in that it has not been standardized on American children. While many of the items seem unaffected by cultural factors, in some instances such influences must be assumed.

Before considering results for deaf children on the Oseretsky Test it is advantageous to discuss briefly each of the areas of motor ability included. As indicated previously this test was standardized by age level, hence the scores derived are in terms of *motor ages,* comparable to the mental age used in the measurement of intelligence. Also, comparable to mental tests, a motor age can be obtained for each of the areas measured. These scores can be portrayed in profile form as illustrated in Figure 12.

The motor functions referred to by Oseretsky as *General Static* can be viewed as entailing principally the ability to use and maintain balance; not balance in a narrow sense, but broadly, total balance capacities including the semicircular canals, kinesthesis, and cerebellar controls. It is evident that Oseretsky was aware of the critical role of the cerebellum in maintaining integrity of balance.

The area of *Dynamic Manual* pertains to manual dexterity but not in a static or stationary manner. The individual is required to use his hands while his body is in motion. *General Dynamic* as a category refers to movements of the total body. Generalized integration and coordination of motor activity is emphasized. This is noteworthy inasmuch as motor behavior often is appraised only in terms of one set of functions, such as manual dexterity, without appraising the organism's ability to function as a whole. In our study of the motor capacities of individuals having sensory, language, and other learning disorders, it is appraisal of the organism as a whole that has been most revealing. The area of *Speed* is self explanatory in the sense that it is the rate of motor performance which is being measured. The tests included require complex behavior, not simple repetitive tasks. *Simultaneous Movement* refers to the ability to use one motor component, such as the hands, in an activity while another component, such as the feet, are used in another movement. As an area of motor function, it capitalizes motor control and integration. Neurologically it requires that both hemispheres of the brain be intact and, at least to some extent, that laterality be minimized. *Synkinesia* as a concept in motor behavior has been emphasized by work in cerebral palsy. It refers to involuntary movements in one part of the body while voluntary movements are being made by another part. For example, while voluntarily using the right hand, the left hand might involuntarily be brought into action, a problem often described by the term "overflow."

To ascertain the usefulness of the Oseretsky Test with deaf children we made a pilot study and the findings are presented in Table 46. These results must be viewed as tentative. The sample

TABLE 46. Motor Age scores for deaf children on the Oseretsky Test of Motor Proficiency

	Males N-30		Females N-20		Totals N-50	
	Mean	SD	Mean	SD	Mean	SD
Chronological Age	11.30	1.20	10.11	1.40	11.10	1.30
Motor Age	9.50	1.60	9.50	1.70	9.50	1.70
General Static	8.11	2.90	8.40	2.10	8.70	2.11
Dynamic Manual	10.11	1.70	10.90	2.10	10.10	2.30
General Dynamic	9.80	2.30	9.90	2.40	9.80	2.30
Speed	6.11	1.11	7.10	2.00	7.50	2.00
Simultaneous Movement	8.90	1.70	9.40	1.90	9.00	1.80
Synkinesia	10.40	1.50	10.40	1.11	10.50	1.70

consisted of 30 boys and 20 girls, all in residence at a public Residential School. The age range was from eight through 14 years.
Oseretsky made allowances for sex differences where they were
found so it is possible to make direct comparisons between the
sexes. The scores were markedly similar for both males and females.
Both sexes, and the total group, earned a motor age of 9.50 years;
the mean C.A. was 11.1 years. The hearing impaired children fell
approximately one and one-half years below the norm provided by
Oseretsky for hearing children.

These inclusive motor age scores are useful but the scores for
each of the six areas of motor ability measured are even more revealing. As shown in Figure 12, there is considerable variation from
one area to another. The two areas in which the deaf fall well
within the normal range are Dynamic Manual and Synkinesia. This
finding for manual dexterity is in agreement with other studies that
have found the deaf to be average on manual skills. As far as can
be ascertained, Synkinesia has not been studied previously in deaf
children. As a motor disability it is highly specific to certain types
of neurological disturbances. Inasmuch as it can be assumed that

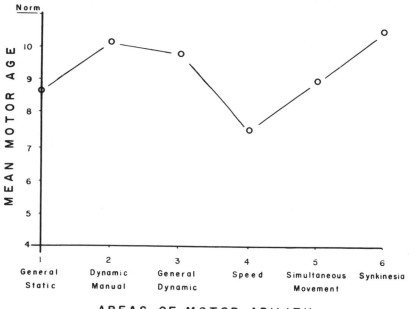

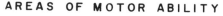

FIG. 12. Motor profile for deaf children on the Oseretsky Test of Motor Proficiency.

most deaf children have peripheral, not central nervous system disorders, it would not be hypothesized that the deaf as a group would show primary inability in this type of motor behavior. This was the finding of this study; the group of children with deafness was not inferior on Synkinesia.

Some motor retardation or disorder was indicated on the remaining four areas of motor ability measured. The results obtained from the highest to the lowest scores were General Dynamic, Simultaneous Movement, General Static, and Speed. When general integration and integrity of motor behavior were involved, there was inferiority. General Dynamic requires total coordination of the type inherent in ability to perform on the Railwalking Test, hence, these performances can be compared. This same type of inferiority seems to prevail in the area of Simultaneous Movement.

The two lowest scores were found on General Static and on Speed, which is in unusually close agreement with clinical experience and research. All studies of the motor ability of the hearing impaired have disclosed inferiority on tests on balance. This is true also in this study and can be attributed largely to dysfunction in the inner ear. The findings on the Speed tests corroborate the impressions of Hiskey[24] and others, who have noted that deaf children have difficulty with speed concepts or actually are inferior in motor speed. Only further study can clarify this complex problem. It is conceivable that they present problems in speed of motor function as the complexity of the task increases. For example, speed tests on the Ozeretsky require more generalized integration than those on the formboards used to secure the data given in Table 41. In any event further study of the relationships between deafness, speed, time, and motor behavior is clearly indicated. The Oseretsky Test seems to offer possibilities in this connection as well as in relation to other aspects of motor performance.

Laterality

Laterality refers to the circumstance of one side of the body being *dominant* as compared to the other. This phenomenon has been referred to by other terms such as handedness and sidedness. Psychologists, neurologists, and educators have been interested in laterality for several decades. The work of Orton[35] was outstanding in noting the relationship between disturbed laterality and learning disorders. He especially stressed the association between confused handedness and disabilities in speaking, reading, and writing. More recently the work of other neurologists, such as Cobb,[9] Neilsen,[34] and Penfield and Roberts[37] has stimulated new attention to this aspect of behavior. Cobb has stated that laterality is unique in Man. He arrived at this conclusion because a dominant cerebral hemisphere cannot be clearly demonstrated in subhuman forms of animal life. This point of view is intriguing and useful, particularly in the study of language development and language pathology.

Laterality is of consequence in the study of motor development and motor behavior. If the development of rightness and leftness is retarded or disturbed in other ways, there is an indication that neurological disorder is present. Laterality does not develop except as the organism can establish cerebral dominance. When disturbances of laterality are present, motor disorders usually are present also. Study of the mentally deficient has disclosed a higher incidence of left handedness as compared to the normal.[30] Approximately 5 per cent of left handedness is found in the general population.[6] Often this has been taken as a criterion and if the incidence of leftness exceeds this estimate, other than normal dextrality is indicated. Because laterality is relevant to motor behavior, this phenomenon was studied in a group of deaf children. This was an attempt to ascertain whether a relationship existed between hearing loss and laterality in children. It was assumed that the same possibilities for deviation were present as in the other areas of the psychology of deafness. Deaf children might have more neurological disorders than the normal, and therefore have more confusions of laterality. Or deafness itself might influence neurological structures as well as the behavioral factors involved in establishing normal laterality and, hence, present a greater problem in this regard as compared to the normal.

The laterality tests used were adapted mainly from the battery suggested by Harris.[21] Hand, leg, and eye dominance were studied. The tests for handedness and leggedness included throwing, grasping, pointing, and kicking. The Key-hole Test was used to study eye dominance. Three trials were given for each test and the subject was scored right or left only when he gave a consistent response for all three trials. The results of this study are presented in Table 47. The children studied were in residence at a Residential School and ranged in age from six through 21 years.

TABLE 47.   Laterality test results for 291 deaf children*

	RH-RL	LH-LL	LH-RL	RH-LL	Indefinite
N	186	21	7	3	2
%	85	10	3	1	1

* RH—right handed   LH—left handed
RL—right legged   LL—left legged

Of the total 85 per cent were both right handed and right legged; 10 per cent were left handed and left legged; 3 per cent had the mixed laterality of being left handed and right legged; 1 per cent had the confusion of being right handed and left legged; and 1 per cent were ambidextrous. Normative studies of leg dominance are not available. Using the estimate of 5 per cent of left handedness being normal, there were twice the average number of left handed children in this population. When those with mixed laterality and ambidextrousness were combined with those who were left sided, there was a total of 15 per cent who had other than right sided laterality. The precise significance of these findings is obscure and interpretation must be made with caution. It seems unlikely, however, that deafness per se is influential in the development of laterality as far as the hand and leg are concerned. A more logical presumption is that the higher incidence of atypical laterality in the deaf can be attributed to a higher incidence of disorders of the central nervous system.

Eye dominance was studied, not as an indication of cerebral dominance, but as an aspect of behavior. Neurologists have shown that when a function has equal representation on both hemispheres, such as in the case of vision, it cannot be used as an indicator of cerebral dominance. On the other hand, eye dominance has been assumed to be related to certain learning disorders, such as inabilities in reading. The findings for eye dominance are given here mainly as an indication of relationship between visual functions and deafness. Eye dominance tests were done on 176 of the subjects who could be classified as having endogenous or exogenous etiology. The results showed that 46 per cent of the endogenous and 42 per cent of the exogenous had left eye dominance. This is a very high incidence of left eyedness. While the significance of this result is not known, some of the implications are considered further under Vision in Chapter XIII.

Motor Maturation

A challenging question in the study of motor maturation is whether profound congenital deafness may be influential. Kendall[26] states that deaf children tend to sit and walk later than the normal. However, he does not provide information relative to the number studied, the actual developmental ages obtained, or whether the factor of intelligence was controlled. Myklebust[32] studied the sitting and walking ages for normal, aphasic, emotionally disturbed, and mentally retarded as compared to those with deafness. The differences between the deaf and hearing were slight and nonsignificant. The deaf were not inferior in this type of motor maturation. Because of the interrelationship between mental age and ages for sitting and walking, it is apparent that intelligence must be controlled when making such comparisons. This was shown by Frisina[17] who found that mentally retarded deaf were significantly inferior to normal deaf children in ages of sitting and walking. Moreover, he found the exogenous more inferior than the endogenous, which is in agreement with various studies of the mentally deficient. Further study of motor behavior is necessary, but present evidence suggests that the sensory deprivation of deafness does not influence psychomotor development such as sitting and walking.

IMPLICATIONS FOR PSYCHOLOGY, EDUCATION AND TRAINING

Studies of the maturation of motor function demonstrate that this is one of the ways in which Man matures. The problem for the psychology of deafness is to ascertain whether such sensory deprivation influences this basic aspect of human behavior. When raising this question, it is of consequence to note that motor function does not directly entail verbal facility. Therefore, the question of relationship between motor functioning and deafness involves the secondary consideration of whether this sensory deprivation has generalized effect on a type of behavior which is nonverbal. As in the study of intellectual functioning and personality adjustment, the

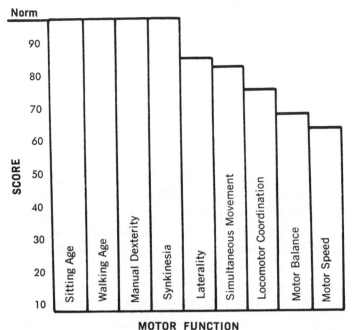

FIG. 13. A graphic illustration of the motor abilities of deaf children.

other primary ways in which Man matures, we find that the question raised is complex and cannot be answered in an all or none manner. This point is emphasized in Figure 13. It shows that the person deaf from early life falls at the normal level in maturation of ability to sit and to walk and that he is not inferior in manual dexterity or synkinesia. However, he falls below the average on laterality, simultaneous movement, locomotor coordination, balance, and motor speed; speed of complex motor acts, not simply acts of manual dexterity.

The obvious implication from this summary of findings for deaf children is that the *strengths* should be capitalized to the greatest extent possible. For example, specifically in regard to motor function, deaf people should be encouraged to compete in activities acquiring manual dexterity inasmuch as they show no inferiority in this ability. A more basic consideration is whether the functions on which they show inferiority are irreversible. Of these functions we might assume that training for laterality and balance would be ineffective and perhaps unwise.

The remaining areas on which inferiority has been indicated are simultaneous movement, locomotor coordination, and motor speed. Could performance in these areas be improved? On the basis of present evidence to assume that it could not, might be a gross error of oversimplification. Stated more positively, an intensive program of remedial physical education seems not only warranted but urgently indicated. In terms of a broad body of knowledge now available, for example, through neurophysiology, such programs could be expected to be most successful if they were inaugurated in early life during the period of the organism's greatest plasticity. Perhaps the primary deficiency of current physical education programs for deaf children is that they are based more or less exclusively on activities which have been successful with hearing children. The program here implied would be based on the specific needs of deaf children, on those aspects of motor behavior which are influenced significantly by hearing loss. Motor speed is an illustration. If deaf children are inferior in speed of complex motor acts, perhaps a series of motor functions progressing from simple manual acts to complex body integrations could be used to improve this aspect of their motor capacities. Many other examples could be given.

More broadly in terms of the psychology of deafness, the area of motor behavior offers an avenue of study with considerable potential. Questions such as whether tactual perception is enhanced by the sensory deprivation of deafness or whether kinesthesis as a perceptual process is impeded, can be expected to reveal significant findings when experimental study is accomplished. Through such study, knowledge will be gained concerning the basic sensory channels for learning when deafness is present, and this knowledge will contribute to the further understanding of all human behavior.

REFERENCES

1. Baldwin, B.: The physical growth of children from birth to maturity. Iowa City, University of Iowa, Studies in Child Welfare, #1, 1921.
2. Bayley, N.: Size and body build of adolescents in relation to rate of skeletal maturing. Child Develop., Monog. #14, 1943.
3. Bennett, G. and Cruikshank, R.: A Summary of Manual and Mechanical Ability Tests. New York, Psychol. Corp., 1942.
4. Bills, A.: Studying motor functions and efficiency, in Andrews, T. G. Methods of Psychology. New York, John Wiley and Sons, 1948.

5. Binet, A. and Simon, Th.: The Intelligence of the Feebleminded. Baltimore, Williams and Wilkins, 1916.
6. Blau, A.: The master hand. Am. Orthopsychiatric Assoc., Research Monog., #5, 1946.
7. Cassell, R.: The Vineland adaptation of the Oseretsky Tests. Vineland, The Training School, Monog. Suppl. #1, 1950.
8. Cobb, S.: Borderlands of Psychiatry. Cambridge, Harvard University Press, 1948.
9. _____: Foundations of Neuropsychiatry. Baltimore, Williams and Wilkins, 1958.
10. Critchley, M.: The Parietal Lobes. Baltimore, Williams and Wilkins, 1953.
11. Crothers, B. and Paine, R.: The Natural History of Cerebral Palsy. Cambridge, Harvard University Press, 1959.
12. Da Costa, M.: Testes de Oseretsky; sua adaptacao em lingua porteguesa. Crianca Portuguesa, 2, 193, 1943.
13. De Jong, R.: The Neurological Examination. New York, Paul B. Hoeber, 1950.
14. Doll, E. A.: The Measurement of Social Competence. Minneapolis, Ed. Test Bureau, 1953.
15. _____: The Oseretsky Tests of Motor Proficiency. Minneapolis, Ed. Test Bureau, 1946.
16. Dow, R. and Moruzzi, G.: The Physiology and Pathology of the Cerebellum. Minneapolis, University of Minnesota Press, 1958.
17. Frisina, D. R.: A psychological study of the mentally retarded child. Evanston, Northwestern University, Unpublished Doctoral Dissertation, 1955.
18. Gesell, A.: Infancy and Human Growth. New York, Macmillan, 1928.
19. _____ and Amatruda, C. Developmental Diagnosis. New York, Paul B. Hoeber, 1947.
20. Goddard, H.: Feeble-Mindedness: Its Causes and Consequences. New York, Macmillan, 1914.
21. Harris, A.: Harris Tests of Lateral Dominance. New York, Psychol. Corp., 1947.
22. Heath, S.: A mental pattern found in motor deviates. J. Abnorm. and Soc. Psychol., 41, 223, 1946.
23. _____: Railwalking performance as related to mental age and etiological type among the mentally retarded. Am. J. Psychol., 55, 240, 1942.
24. Hiskey, M.: Nebraska Test of Learning Aptitude for Young Deaf Children. Lincoln, University of Nebraska, 1955.
25. Jones, H. E.: Motor Performance and Growth. Berkeley, University of California Press, 1949.
26. Kendall, D.: Mental development of young children, in Ewing, A. Educational Guidance and the Deaf Child. Washington, The Volta Bureau, 1957.
27. Lamm, S.: Pediatric Neurology. New York, Lansberger Medical Books, 1959.
28. Long, J.: Motor Abilities of Deaf Children. New York, Columbia University, T. C. Contrib. to Ed., #514, 1932.
29. McGraw, M.: Maturation of behavior, in Carmichael, L. (ed.) Manual of Child Psychology. New York, John Wiley and Sons, 1946.
30. Morley, E.: The Development and Disorders of Speech in Childhood. Edinburgh, Livingstone, 1957.
31. Morsh, J.: Motor performance of the deaf. Com. Psychol. Monog., #66, 1936.
32. Myklebust, H.: Auditory Disorders in Children. New York, Grune and Stratton, 1954.

33. _____: Significance of etiology in motor performance of deaf children with special reference to meningitis. Am. J. Psychol. 59, 249, 1946.

34. Nielsen, J. M.: Agnosia, Apraxia, and Aphasia. New York, Paul B. Hoeber, 1946.

35. Orton, S.: Reading, Writing and Speech Problems in Children. New York, W. W. Norton, 1937.

36. Oseretsky, N. I.: Psychomotorik: Methoden zur untersuchung der motoric. Beih. Zeitschrift Angewandte Psychol., 17, 162, 1931.

37. Penfield, W. and Roberts, L.: Speech and Brain Mechanisms. Princeton, Princeton University Press, 1959.

38. Seashore, R. H.: Stanford motor skills unit. Psychol. Monog., #78, 1928.

39. Sheldon, W., Stevens, S. S. and Tucker, W.: The Varieties of Human Physique. New York, Harper, 1940.

40. Sloan, W.: The Lincoln-Oseretsky Motor Development Scale. Genetic Psychol. Monog., 51, 183, 1955.

41. Taylor, J. (ed.): Selected Writings of Hughlings Jackson, Vol. 1 and 2. New York, Basic Books, 1958.

42. Thompson, H.: Physical growth, in Carmichael, L., Manual of Child Psychology. New York, John Wiley and Sons, 1946.

43. Tuddenham, R. and Snyder, M.: Physical growth of California boys and girls from birth to eighteen years. Berkeley, University of California Press, 1954.

44. Van der Lugt, M.: Psychomotor Test Series for Children. New York, New York University Press, 1948.

Suggestions for Further Study

Bayley, N.: The development of motor abilities during the first three years. Soc. Research Child Develop., #1, 1935.

Espenschade, A.: Motor performance in adolescence. Monog. Soc. Research Child Develop., 5, #1, 1940.

Gesell, A. et al.: The First Five Years of Life. New York, Harper, 1940.

Heath, S.: Clinical significance of motor defect with military implications. Am. J. Psychol., 57, 482, 1944.

Krogman, W.: A handbook of the measurement and interpretation of height and weight in the growing child. Monog. Soc. Research Child Develop., #13, 1950.

Lassner, R.: Annotated bibliography on the Oseretsky Tests of Motor Proficiency. J. Consult, Psychol., 12, 37, 1948.

Murphy, M.: The relationship between intelligence and the age of walking in normal and feeble-minded children. Psychol. Clinic, 22, 187, 1933.

Oseretsky, N. and Payova, E.: Die psychomotorik poliomyelitischer kinder. Beih. Zeitschrift Kinderforsch., 44, 253, 1935.

Seashore, H.: The development of a beam walking test and its use in measuring development of balance in children. Am. Assoc. for Health, Phys. Ed. and Recreation, Research Quarterly, 18, 246, 1947.

Sloan, W.: Motor proficiency and intelligence. Am. J. Mental Deficiency, 55, 394, 1951.

Chapter VIII

DEAFNESS AND SOCIAL MATURITY

In the preceding chapters attention has been given to the effect of deafness on the primary ways in which Man matures. It was found that this sensory deprivation influenced each of these to some degree. In other words, it was concluded that deafness has a modifying effect on intellectual processes, on personality, and on motor functions.

There is another way in which fundamental relationships between behavior and handicapping conditions might be studied. While each of the primary ways in which Man matures requires specialized study, evaluation of the total, of the composite, in terms of effectiveness of interaction with the environment is revealing clinically and scientifically. This concept raises the challenging question of why there might be differences between a person's potential and his adjustment, between innate capacities and productivity. Doll[6] has demonstrated the significance of these questions in the study of human behavior through his development of the concept of social maturity. He has shown that capacities and attainments are not necessarily correlated; furthermore, that it is how a person *uses* what he has, not *what* he has, which is the criterion of value, the criterion used by society. Doll recognized that it was necessary to have a measure of the effectiveness of an individual's interaction with his society, a measure of the extent to which he attains the specific social competences expected from the society in which he lives. He termed this broad aspect of human behavior *social maturity* and devised the Social Maturity Scale to measure it.[6]

Social maturity as an aspect of human behavior refers to the attainment of independence. All maturation and growth assumes progression toward a fully developed organism. Stated differently, the goal of maturation is adulthood; adulthood physically, emotionally, mentally, or adulthood as a socially competent individual. From the point of view of social competence this means that maturation is the process through which one achieves independent behavior, especially as it relates to the acquiring of ability to care for oneself. All growth and maturation lead toward this goal.

Varying degrees of maturity relative to independence of behavior can be seen in divergent forms of life. For example, in some insect life there is no growth so far as independence is concerned. At the time of birth the young are entirely self-sufficient and the parents give no attention or care to their offspring. This circumstance also has been observed and reported by ichthyologists. In contrast, the human infant at birth is almost wholly dependent; he must have appropriate assistance and care from his parents if he is to survive. This *dependence* of the human infant persists for a long period of time. According to Doll the human being has parental dependency of some nature and to some extent until he attains the age of 25 years. This is the equivalent of about one-third of the life span. Cultural factors are assumed to play a part in such dependency so it must be emphasized that this criterion is based on studies in the United States.

It is evident from work in psychology and anthropology that the human being has greater dependency at the time of birth than all other forms of life. From this has grown the concept that there is an inverse ratio between the degree of dependency at birth and the level of behavior achieved at adulthood. In other words, the greater the dependence at birth, the higher the level of behavior attained by the organism at full maturity. Very simple forms of life have little or no dependency at birth and do not reach high levels of social or intellectual competency. The human organism, which is highly dependent at birth, achieves a complex level of behavior, entailing such unique characteristics as language and ability to engage in abstraction.

The human being also can be compared to other forms of life on the basis of instinct versus learning. This concept is consequential in many respects. In general, it appears that the lower the form of life, the more instinct rather than learning determines the level of behavior that will be attained. Using these concepts of dependence at the time of birth as well as instinct versus learning, psychologists, anthropologists and geneticists can study the young organism and predict the level of attainment expected for a given form of life at adulthood. The study of Man's achievement of maturity, of adulthood, has occupied a major role in the study of all human behavior. The exact terminal point of his dependence on his parents, if such a point is ascertainable, varies according to the definition used and from one culture to another. There seems to be little disagreement, however, that irrespective of definition or culture his dependence persists until after puberty and adolescence. This is reflected by all societies through religious rites, indicating that the age of self responsibility has been attained, through the age at which franchise is granted, or in many other ways.

Because Man has a long period of dependency before achieving adulthood, because he has the longest period known for learning, many conflicting opinions have been given as to how he best can attain the maturity expected of an adult. His long period for growing does present many and often serious vulnerabilities. There is ample opportunity for him to develop a type of behavior which society does not condone. If his behavior is fixed largely by instinct, such vulnerabilities and problems would be less; he also would be less human. Our primary concern here is with social maturity, with that aspect of Man's maturity which directly indicates the extent to which he has attained independence from parental assistance and can effectively manage himself according to the demands of the culture in which he lives.

Doll has defined *social maturity as the ability to care for oneself and to assist with the care of others.* Specifically, this indicates that in early life the main task is to achieve the level of *self-help,* of being able to care for one's toilet needs and to feed and dress oneself. The norms of the Social Maturity Scale indicate that this type of independence is achieved during the first seven to eight years of life. The second major goal of the child on the way to adulthood is to achieve the level of *self-direction.* This level of behavior is indicated on the Social Maturity Scale by items such as "going out on his own." Self-direction as an aspect of maturation begins around eight years for the average child; it increases in complexity and grows until approximately 18 years. At this age the individual has attained adulthood as far as self-help and self-direction are concerned. But, according to Doll's definition and according to the expectations of our society, the individual has not yet attained full maturity. He must achieve the level of being able to assist with the *care of others*. In so doing he must learn to provide for the future, to anticipate hardships due to illness, accidents, or even wars and disturbances of nature; he must learn to contribute to the general welfare of society. This level of social maturity is expected to begin at 18 years of age and to achieve full maturity some time after 25 years of age. It is from this point of reference that we consider the question of whether deafness influences the development of social maturity. Does deafness affect the growth of independent behavior? If so, is the greatest effect at the level of self-help, self-direction, or at the level of being able to assist with the care of others? It must be stressed that in measuring social competence, we are not considering mental brightness, integrity of sensory capacities or motor abilities, or the adequacy of emotional adjustment. Rather, we are measuring the person's total attainment in terms of social performance; what he does with his capacities, his ability to care for himself and to assist with the care of others. This is a question of considerable consequence in the psychology and education of those with profound deafness.

In the development of the Social Maturity Scale, Doll divided social maturity into six areas. These areas are comparable to the various factors of intelligence measured by standard tests of mental ability. They also can be compared to the facets of motor ability measured by the Oseretsky Test of Motor Proficiency. No major attribute of human behavior can be simplified to the extent of being studied through only one of its characteristics. Through analysis and experimentation Doll arrived at the following six major attributes of social competence: Self-help, Self-direction, Communication, Locomotion, Socialization, Occupation. From the point of view of the psychology of sensory deprivation or of other handicaps, the problem is to ascertain specifically what effect the disability may have on each area of social maturity. As in all major aspects of behavior, when it is measured according to the various types of functions involved, an individual may fall at the average level or above on certain categories and below on others. Because of the marked imposition of deafness on communication, it can be presumed that this area would be most affected by this sensory deprivation if it is sustained in early life. In comparison, it would be expected that the crippled would fall lowest in the area of Locomotion but that their disability might also be revealed on Self-help because this area of function assumes certain motor skills. Other examples could be given, such as the difficulties experienced by the mentally deficient and the psychotic in attaining Self-direction.

These examples serve to highlight the ways in which handicaps impose limitations on the attainment of social maturity. It is difficult to conceive of maximum independent behavior in an individual who must be helped with dressing or feeding, who cannot assume responsibility for himself in terms of self-direction, locomotion, socialization, and occupation, or *if he has serious limitations in ability to communicate.* In the psychology of deafness we must determine the extent to which the handicap causes increased dependence on others. By implication another need is to study the means by which such dependency may be alleviated. Practically there is no more fundamental question for the psychology of the handicapped. *One of the most significant aspects of any handicap is the extent to which it causes greater dependency on others.* Perhaps this is the inherent meaning of a handicap. If a deviation does not cause increased dependency, there is reason to assume that it should not be defined as a handicap. Furthermore, foremost in the concept of a handicap is the presumption that some of the increased dependency will remain irrespective of best efforts to alleviate it. Hence it is not anticipated that the involvements of any significant handicap can be completely overcome.

It is essential for the educator, psychologist, and rehabilitation worker to recognize the limits beyond which efforts toward alleviation are unrealistic and should be replaced by efforts which encourage acceptance. However, such a judgment can be valid only when the nature of the dependency is understood. Only then can educational methods, vocational training, and other procedures be developed to assist the individual with overcoming the basic involvements of his handicap. Moreover, only then can the psychologist and psychiatrist be in a position to assist the person with the difficult problem of acceptance of those aspects which cannot be alleviated. Obviously the balance between acceptance and alleviation must be realistic and as much as possible be based on scientific verification. Unfortunately, knowledge concerning the social maturity of those with deafness is meagre; such study is still in its infancy. Nevertheless, from the data discussed below, there are indications that those whose deafness dates from early life attain the first two levels of social competence, self-help and self-direction, but they have difficulty in attaining the third, ability to assist with the care of others.

The only standardized developmental scale available for the measurement of social competence is the Vineland Social Maturity Scale. It is a psychometric instrument and must be used as rigorously as any psychological test or other technique of this type. Accurate and valid results assume training in administration and interpertation; as an instrument it apears deceptively simple and often has been used erroneously. Because it is a standardized scale of development, it is scored in the same manner as mental tests; both social ages and social quotients are derived. The quotients are computed in the same way as is done in measuring intelligence; hence, the average social quotient is 100.

STUDIES OF SOCIAL MATURITY

Bradway[4] first investigated the social maturity of deaf children. Her study included 92 children in a public Residential School with an age range of five to 20 years. She found a mean social quotient of 80.70 and concluded that deaf children fall 20 percent below the average for hearing children. As in the normal standardization group, no sex differences were found.

Streng and Kirk[10] studied the social maturity of deaf children in a Day School. Their sample consisted of 97 children from six to 18 years of age. The mean social quotient which they reported was 96.2. However, they used double scoring so these results are not directly comparable to those of Bradway. It seems unlikely that this difference in scoring completely explains the higher mean quotient for their group. A significant trend was indicated by this study inasmuch as these investigators noted a slight decrease in social maturity scores with increase in life age. This has noteworthy implications as indicated by the data presented in Figure 14.

Avery[2] investigated the social competence of 50 preschool deaf children and reported that they fell at the average level. Analysis of the scale as indicated above reveals that this could occur only if the subjects as a group scored above average on areas of social maturity other than communication. This is highly unlikely as such trends have not been revealed by other studies. Rather, subsequent study of preschool deaf children has revealed below average scores also for this age group, although at this age the scores are higher than those found at later ages. Presumably Avery's findings can be explained by the double scoring technique which she used.

Myklebust and Burchard[8] studied 194 children in a public Residential School. This group ranged from seven to 19 years in age and was of average intelligence. The mean social quotient for the congenitally deaf was 85.0 and for the acquired, 82.4; there was no difference between these groups. They concluded that deaf children fall from 15 to 20 per cent below the average for hearing children. These results confirmed those of Bradway. No sex differences appeared. Furthermore, when those in residence at the school more than four years were compared to those in residence less than four years, no significant differences were found. These investigators concluded that the Residential School neither advanced nor retarded the social maturity of deaf children. Subsequent study has revealed a more complex relationship between growth of social maturity, deafness, and school residence.

.More recently Treacy[12] investigated the social maturity of deaf and hard of hearing children and its relationship to factors of intelligence. This study is helpful in clarifying various aspects of the relationship between deafness and growth of independent behavior. The group studied was in attendance at a large Day School. The school consisted of two departments, one for the deaf and one for the hard of hearing. The child's classification was determined by educational criteria, essentially by the extent to which he had acquired language. Those in the deaf department had profound deafness and could not acquire language normally. Those classified as hard of hearing had considerable residual hearing, responded well to the use of amplification, and had less handicap in language. A number of the hard of hearing had only moderate losses of hearing. The mean C.A. for the deaf group was nine years and five months; for the hard of hearing, ten years and two months. This difference was not significant. The mean social quotients are summarized in Table 48. The hard of hearing fell well within the average range, while the deaf fell at the lower limits of normal. The difference in favor of the hard of hearing was statistically significant.

TABLE 48. Comparison of mean social quotients for deaf and hard of hearing children

	N	Mean	SD
Deaf	50	90.03	9.6
Hard of hearing	44	97.51	11.2

These results are in agreement with those of previous investigators who found a relationship between the development of social maturity and deafness. However, the degree of inferiority for the deaf is less than reported by Bradway and by Myklebust and Burchard. This may be explained by the fact that Treacy's sample was from a Day School. Perhaps through community living as compared to Residential School experience, the deaf child achieves a higher level of social competence. Also there is a possibility that selective factors were operative, causing the more mentally and socially mature child to attend the Day School. However, in view of the data considered in Chapter V, this seems unlikely. Comparatively, it is interesting that the hard of hearing children studied fell at the average level in social maturity. Treacy attributed this to their obviously greater facility in language but generalizations must be made with caution because of the small sample involved.

An important contribution of Treacy's study is that she correlated the social maturity scores with chronological age and with factors of intelligence as measured by the Primary Mental Abilities Test.[11] These correlations are given in Table 49. The correlation between general intelligence and social maturity was highly significant for the deaf but not for the hard of hearing.

These data are provocative in other respects. For the deaf statistically significant correlations were obtained between social maturity scores and scores on Verbal, Number, Reasoning, and Perception. For the hard of hearing significant correlations with

TABLE 49.   Correlations between social maturity and factors of intelligence
for deaf and hard of hearing children

| | Deaf | | | Hard of hearing | | |
	N	r	S.E.	N	r	S.E.
P.M.A. IQ	30	.48	.14	36	.11	.16
Verbal	31	.36	.15	36	.24	.15
Space	37	.26	.15	36	−.10	.16
Number	31	.50	.13	35	.38	.14
Reasoning	25	.49	.15	28	.38	.16
Perception	22	.56	.14	22	−.19	.21
C.A.	50	−.36	.12	44	.40	.12

social maturity appeared on the factors of Number and Reasoning;
these results substantiate the discussion in Chapter V regarding
intelligence. Each factor of intelligence, with the exception of
Space, is of importance to the deaf child in attaining social maturity, whereas, for the hard of hearing only two factors were
found to be related to the achievement of social competence. The
highest correlation between social maturity and intellectual factors
for the deaf was on Perception. In the Primary Mental Abilities
Test, Perception consists of visual-perceptual speed. The implication is that when deafness is profound and dates from early life,
it is the visual perceptual processes which must assume a leading
role in the development of independent behavior. These findings
accent the hypothesis that when a sensory deprivation such as
deafness occurs, other capacities take on a more critical role. The
individual is forced to rely heavily on psychological functions
which for the normal serve only as reserve or operate only in a
minor way.

There was another finding of importance in this study. For
the hard of hearing there was a significant positive correlation
between social competence scores and chronological age. As the
hard of hearing child became older, he increased in social competence. This is the expected findings inasmuch as the child becomes more independent as he grows older. In marked contrast,
while there was a significant relationship between social maturity
and chronological age for the deaf, it was negative; that is, in the
opposite direction. As the deaf child became older, he became
less socially competent. Apparently as he grows older it is increasingly difficult for him to show equivalent growth in social maturity.
Instead of achieving independence at a constant rate, he attains

less of the average normal gain each year. Therefore, a negative correlation exists between his life age and scores in socal maturity. This finding has a number of implications which are discussed further below in relation to other relevant data.

SOCIAL MATURITY, LEARNING, AND ADJUSTMENT

To investigate the relationships between social maturity and other aspects of development in deaf children, we studied 150 children in a public Residential School. There were 77 males and 73 females ranging in age from 10 to 21 years. The data collected included scores in social maturity, educational achievement, intelligence, personality adjustment, vocational training, and ratings of behavior. As a group, these children were of average intelligence as measured by the performance section of the Wechsler-Bellevue Scale[13] and the Grace Arthur Performance Test.[1] The social maturity scores are presented in Table 50. Also in this table is given the mean social quotient for a group of preschool deaf children as found in a study by Myklebust.[7]

TABLE 50. Social quotients for deaf children from preschool to 21 years of age

Age group	N	Mean	SD
Preschool	79	91.8	19.3
10–12.9	27	92.5	12.5
13–14.9	32	92.7	11.5
15–16.9	41	82.2	10.0
17–18.9	35	80.4	12.2
19–20.9	15	76.2	9.8

The mean social quotient for the sample of 150 children was 85.8 with a standard deviation of 12.1. This is remarkably similar to that reported by Bradway[4] and Myklebust and Burchard,[8] suggesting that at least as far as Residential School children are concerned, there is an inferiority in social maturity in general to the extent of approximately 15 per cent. There is, however, a more intricate finding from this study which demands attention. The social quotient for the preschool group and for the other age groups up to 15 years was slightly over 90. For the age groups from 15 to 21 years there was a gradual decline in the social quotient; at 15 years it was 82.2; at 17 it was 80.4; and at 19 it was 76.2. For the three age groups below 15 years the average social quotient was 92.3, while for the three age groups above 15 years of age, the average social quotient was 79.9. These differences are statistically significant.

From these results it seems that children deaf from early life are inferior in social maturity to the extent of approximately 10 per cent, up to the age of 15 years. From our discussion earlier in this chapter, we can conclude that prior to 15 years the primary task confronting the child in social maturity is the attainment of ability in Self-help, with beginnings of achievement in Self-direction. The implication is that deaf children are not inferior in achieving Self-help, but as higher levels of social competence become necessary because of increased age, they find attainment more difficult, indicated particularly by the gradual decline in scores after 15 years of age. The inferiority for these age groups is greater, reaching a degree of 15 to 20 per cent at the age of 21 years, the age usually taken as the beginning of adulthood. This is shown graphically in Figure 14.

To analyze further this gradual decline at the upper age levels it is helpful to refer again to the concept of social maturity as measured by the Social Maturity Scale. Until 15 to 18 years of age social maturity entails mainly achieving competence in Self-help and Self-direction, basically learning to care for oneself and attaining the level of responsibility required for Self-direction.

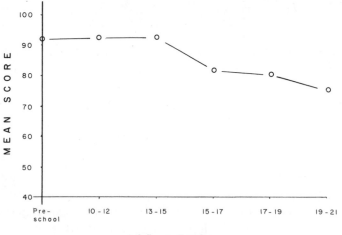

FIG. 14. Graphic illustration of social maturity quotients for a group of deaf children.

Gradually after 18 years, social maturity entails assisting in the care of others, providing for the future, and assuming responsibilities for the general welfare. This is adulthood, the age at which one is expected to have energies and capacities over and above those required to care for oneself. Our study, like those of Streng and Kirk and of Treacy, suggests that it is this level of social maturity which is difficult to achieve when profound deafness is present from early life. These results have important practical implications for psychology, education, and rehabilitation.

Comparison by Etiology

The possible influence of etiology was investigated, and the results are presented in Table 51. There were no differences on the basis of etiology, which is in agreement with the previous findings of Myklebust and Burchard. When deafness occurs in early life, it is the fact of deafness rather than the factor of etiology which is of prime importance in achieving social maturity.

TABLE 51. **Mean social quotients for the etiological groups**

Group	N	Mean	SD
Endogenous	78	85.9	13.0
Exogenous	72	85.6	11.0
Undetermined	33	87.7	10.0

Sex and Age of Onset

Study of the influence of sex and age of onset has been made by various workers.[6, 8, 10] These factors were investigated also in the present study. In agreement with previous studies, sex differences did not appear. Presumably age of onset is a significant variable in the achievement of social maturity by deaf persons. This presumption seems especially warranted if the deafness occurs after five years of age. In the present investigation only 10 children fell into this category so statistical analysis was not made. Further study of the deafened as well as of other groups varying in age of onset is indicated.

Correlation with Other Factors

It has been suggested that the Social Maturity Scale measures the degree of independence of self-sufficiency. It is interesting to note the extent to which this measure correlates with other indications of competence, learning ability and adjustment. The correlation coefficients for the social maturity quotients and other test scores for 150 deaf children are given in Table 52.

TABLE 52. Correlation between social maturity scores and other measures

Brown Personality Inventory	Haggerty Olson Wickman Schedule A	Haggerty Olson Wickman Schedule B	Mental Age	Educational Age	Grades in Vocational Training
−.13 ± .05	−.37 ± .05	−.63 ± .03	.55 ± .04	.70 ± .03	.28 ± .05

The Brown Personality Inventory[5] and the Haggerty-Olson-Wickman Schedules[9] are measures of personal adjustment. High scores indicate more adjustment problem tendencies, hence the negative correlations. The correlation between social maturity and Schedule B is especially significant. This schedule rates the child on subjective aspects of personality, such as easily fatigued, talkativeness, and courageousness. These findings suggest that the more socially mature child also is the more emotionally stable and mature.

The correlations between intelligence and educational achievement scores and social maturity also are significant. The relationship with intelligence is comparable to that found by Treacy. Again, it is apparent that there is a relationship between intelligence and social maturity in deaf children. These results also indicate that a close relationship exists between social maturity and educational attainment. This is not surprising when it is recalled that Communication as an area is represented on the Social Maturity Scale. For this as well as for other reasons, it is apparent that higher educational achievement might be reflected in higher social competence. Likewise, if the social competence level can be increased, educational attainment also may be raised.

Double Scoring

Doll provided a method of double scoring which has usefulness in the study of handicapped individuals. This procedure consists first of selecting those items on the Social Maturity Scale which are failed as a direct result of the handicapping condition. These items are "double scored" plus. For example, item 79 "makes telephone calls," is always failed when significant deafness is present. When double scoring is used, such an item in the case of those having deafness, would be scored plus. The purpose of this precedure is to note the specific effects of the handicap on social maturity. Through such analysis much can be learned about the areas of social competence which are directly influenced by the handicap and thus provide a basis for education, therapy, and rehabilitation.

Unfortunately, this procedure has led to unrealistic appraisal of the handicap in certain instances. Scoring the items plus does *not* change the individual. It merely indicates the primary influence of his disability. Only persons with training and experience can select those items which are related directly to a given handicap. As Bradway[4] has indicated, only item 79 is failed by *all* deaf people. The other most frequently failed items are those in the area of Communication. Therefore, double scoring for the deaf usually is limited to these items. When this is done, the social quotient for deaf children below the age of 15 years approximates the normal. In other words, the inferiority in social maturity manifested by children having deafness from early life is essentially due to the limitation of language before the age of 15 years. After 15 years an *overflow effect* becomes obvious. When double scoring is used for this age group, the quotient is raised only 5 to 7 points on the average. Moreover, the overflow effect becomes greater as age increases. The importance of this procedure and concept can be seen especially when it is recognized that the average normal individual is fully matured in communication by 18 years of age, the age at which standardization of the Social Scale revealed no further growth in Communication. Nevertheless, it is precisely after this age level that the deaf show greatest effect of their sensory deprivation. Therefore, *double scoring, as the individual reaches adulthood, does not raise his score.*

In terms of the development of programs to alleviate the effects of deafness on social maturity, interesting inferences can be drawn. There is an inherent aspect of the handicap, revealed by the double scoring procedures, which is irreversible. This is illustrated by the item, "makes telephone calls." While not being able to make telephone calls does affect one's social competence, *making him more dependent,* it is an inevitable result of the disability and must be *accepted* by the person concerned. On the other hand, it is the only item on the Scale which is failed by *all* deaf people. Presumably *some* persons with deafness achieve the degree of social competence indicated by all of the other items. While other factors, such as age of onset, must be considered, this implies that much of the overflow effect is overcome by at least some of the deaf. The greatest possibility for alleviation of the inferiority in social maturity is specifically in regard to the functions which are affected not directly but indirectly.

The use of the double scoring technique is advantageous in clarifying the relationships between social maturity and deafness. Frequently, it provides an objective basis for guidance, counseling, and rehabilitation programs.

Comparison with Other Handicapped Groups

Handicaps are not readily defined. Often there is discussion of what constitutes a handicap. Perhaps there is no more realistic or thought provoking definition than one which is based on the extent to which the handicap increases dependency on others. Only when a definition of this type is used is it possible to make comparisons between types of handicaps. Such analyses have both practical and theoretical significance.

In the field of sensory deprivation, comparison often is made between the deaf and the blind and these considerations have been helpful in understanding the problems of both groups. The question as to which is the greater handicap frequently arises. In terms of dependency, in terms of social maturity, the differences are immediately apparent because the blind show substantially greater dependency than the deaf. This was first shown by the work of Bradway[3] when she found that the average social quotient for blind children was 63 as compared to 80 for the deaf.

Myklebust[7] has compared the social maturity levels of preschool deaf children with those of the aphasic, emotionally disturbed, and the mentally deficient. These results are given in Table 53. This analysis revealed significant differences between the deaf and the other three groups, the deaf being superior. Deafness from early life increases dependency but handicaps due to central nervous system damage or to marked emotional disturbance might cause greater inferiority in self-sufficiency.

TABLE 53. The mean social quotients for groups of handicapped children

	Deaf	Aphasic	Psychic Deaf	Mentally Deficient
N	79	58	27	29
Mean	91.84	74.21	78.26	56.86
SD	19.36	19.01	25.88	22.87

IMPLICATIONS FOR TRAINING AND ADJUSTMENT

The research findings pertaining to the social maturity of persons deaf from early life indicate an inferiority compared to the normal. This is not unexpected in view of the findings for mental functioning, personality adjustment, and motor performance. Actually, social maturity is a composite of all of these facets of the person and also a combination of various others, such as his abilities in perception. The conclusion that those with profound deafness from early life have increased dependency is confirmed by the experience of educators as well as research workers who recognize that this sensory deprivation is of considerable consequence in the total behavior of the individual.

A basic question confronting all who work with the hearing impaired is the extent to which this greater dependency, this greater need for assistance, can be alleviated. It is not assumed that all dependence can, or should be, overcome. Interdependence is a phenomenon of modern life which is remarkably characteristic. Independent behavior to any complete degree is impossible and perhaps should be viewed as undesirable. Thus, acceptance of dependency is inevitable in all walks of life. From this frame of reference the problem confronting deaf people falls on a continuum; everyone is faced with the need to accept dependency and their problem is only one of being greater than that encountered by most people. This point of view is useful as far as it goes; often it is advantageous when working with the hearing impaired.

To view the problem of the deaf only in terms of a continuum, eventually leads to oversimplification. Moreover, it does not provide a specific basis for planning programs to alleviate the inferiority in social competence. Training programs must draw upon the psychology of normal persons, but the critical factors inherent in the success of these programs is the extent to which they are focused on the specifics of the psychology of deafness. Although much knowledge of the psychology of deafness still is lacking, we can presume that basic factors such as altered perceptual processes, altered memory, and disturbances of ego development are involved. If these basic influences of deafness can be overcome to some degree, there is reason to believe that the level of social maturity will be raised. It is apparent that if the language limitation can be reduced, this, too, will result in an increase in social maturity.

There are other more direct approaches to the alleviation of this problem in social maturity which might be attempted. Unlike the hearing child, the deaf child needs consistent training in social maturity over a long period of time. He is in need of emphasis on all aspects of social maturity, but especially in Self-direction, Socialization, and Occupation. We may assume that such a program warrants inclusion as a regular part of the educational curriculum with a detailed program of instruction in attainment of social maturity being developed for all age levels.

In this connection we developed a pilot study in a public Residential School. A part of the school population, representing certain classes and cottages, was selected as an experimental group, while another segment of the population served as a control group. The teachers and housemothers of the experimental group were given instruction regarding the more difficult aspects of social maturity confronting deaf children. They also were given assistance in inaugurating a program to help these children to overcome these problems. In a period of six months, the period of time covered by the pilot study, the experimental group showed noticeable gains over the control group.

This program of training in social competence stressed the non-verbal aspects. At the lower age levels this included Self-help functions of eating, dressing, bathing, telling time, and use of money. At the upper age levels, where the problem is more difficult, the training stressed the selection and purchase of clothing accessories, assuming responsibility for "routine chores," making arrangements for and traveling alone, recognition and care of health needs, and the assumption of group responsibility. A detailed program for the development of social maturity in deaf persons remains to be developed. This discussion is given mainly to indicate that there is evidence that such a program is needed and that a direct approach to such training is beneficial. It is not hypothesized that the inferiority in social maturity can be completely alleviated. To do so would be to overcome all the increased dependency due to deafness. Then, according to the definition used here, there would be no reason to include this group in the category of the handicapped. It *is* hypothesized that the inferiority in social maturity can be alleviated by programs which are directed specifically at this problem. It seems especially urgent in this connection that studies be made of deaf adults, perhaps through departments of rehabilitation. There is no information concerning the plateau, the level at which the social maturity of the average deaf adult stabilizes. From Table 50 we note that at 19 to 21 years of age, the social quotient is 76.2. Even if we assume that it does not fall below this level at 25, 30, 35 years and above, the degree of dependence represented by a score of 76.2 presents a number of risks for satisfactory, self-sufficient adjustment. Experientially and logically we can expect that the average social quotient of the deaf adult can be raised to 80 or 85 through the efforts of intensive training. Such results would be highly efficacious and rewarding to the persons involved.

REFERENCES

1. Arthur, G.: A Point Scale of Performance Tests. Chicago, C. H. Stoelting, 1943.
2. Avery, C.: Social competence of preschool acoustically handicapped children. J. Except. Children, 15, 71, 1948.
3. Bradway, K.: Social competence of exceptional children. J. Except. Children, 4, 1, 1937.
4. _____: The social competence of deaf children. Am. Ann. Deaf, 82, 122, 1937.
5. Brown, A., Morrison, J. and Couch, G.: Influence of affectional family relationships on character development. J. Abnorm. Soc. Psychol., 42, 422, 1947.
6. Doll, E. A.: The Measurement of Social Competence. Minneapolis, Ed. Test Bureau, 1953.
7. Myklebust, H. R.: Auditory Disorders in Children. New York, Grune and Stratton, 1954.
8. _____ and Burchard, E.: A study of the effects of congenital and adventitious deafness on the intelligence, personality and social maturity of school children. J. Ed. Psychol., 36, 321, 1945.

 9. Olson, W.: Problem Tendencies in Children. Minneapolis, University of Minnesota Press, 1930.
10. Streng, A. and Kirk, S.: The social competence of deaf and hard of hearing children in a public day school. Am. Ann. Deaf, 83, 244, 1938.
11. Thurstone, L. and Thurstone, G.: SRA Primary Mental Abilities. Chicago, Science Research Associates, 1948.
12. Treacy, L.: A study of social maturity in relation to factors of intelligence in acoustically handicapped children. Evanston, Northwestern University, Unpublished M.A. Thesis, 1955.
13. Wechsler, D.: The Measurement of Adult Intelligence. Baltimore, Williams and Wilkins, 1944.

Suggestions for Further Study

Bradway, K.: Social competence of grade school children. J. Except. Education, 6, 326, 1938.

Doll, E. A.: The social basis of mental diagnosis. J. Applied Psychol., 24, 160, 1940.

Kelly, E.: A program to develop social maturity in the orthopedic child. J. Except. Children, 8, 75, 1941.

Lurie, L., Rosenthal, F. and Outcalt, L.: Diagnostic and prognostic significance of the difference between the intelligence quotient and the social quotient. Am. J. Orthopsychiatry, 12, 104, 1942.

Madden, R.: The School Status of the Hard of Hearing Child. New York, Columbia University, T.C. Contrib. to Ed., #499, 1931.

Maxfield, K. and Fjeld, H.: The social maturity of the visually handicapped preschool child. Child Develop., 13, 1, 1942.

Paterson, C.: The Vineland Social Maturity Scale and some of its correlates. J. Genetic Psychol., 62, 275, 1943.

Watson, R.: The Clinical Method in Psychology. New York, Harper, 1951.

Part Three
Language—Speech, Speechreading, Reading and Writing

Chapter IX

LANGUAGE AND LANGUAGE DEVELOPMENT

LANGUAGE AS A PHENOMENON has intrigued scholars for centuries. How and why Man first developed, and now acquires, language has concerned the philosopher, the linguist, the anthropologist, the psychologist, the semanticist, the neurologist, and the psychiatrist. Many theories have been expounded regarding the origin and nature of this phenomenon which Langer[17] has described as "without a doubt, the most momentous and at the same time the most mysterious product of the human mind." Langer's categorization of language as used by Man and by lower animals has been widely accepted. One of the most complete analyses of the nature of symbolism and language was made by Cassirer.[6] He included discussion of the origin of symbolic behavior and the nature of language with illustrations from language disorders.

Early studies of language were made by Müller,[23] Whitney,[35] and Clodd[8]; the classification system suggested by Clodd is given below. Wells,[34] Ceram,[7] and Friedrich[10] have emphasized the importance of phylogenetic aspects and have presented illuminating discussions on the development of reading and writing. Korzybski[16] and Hayakawa[13] have stressed the point of view and the findings in general semantics. Whorf[36] highlighted the importance of language in relation to thought processes and to the growth of the mind, emphasizing that language has a fundamental influence on thought itself. The understanding of the psychology of language development has been greatly enhanced by the work of Piaget,[28] Vigotsky,[33]

McCarthy,[19] Templin,[32] and Mowrer.[21] The significance of communication theory has been manifested by Miller.[20] In relation to children, work in the field of linguistics, which has contributed greatly to the knowledge of language as a process, has been led by Leopold.[18]

LEVELS OF EXPERIENCE

Although much has been learned about language behavior, there is little uniformity in the points of view and theories regarding its nature and development. Study of those having communicative disorders has been revealing in this connection, especially of those having deafness from the preverbal age. From such study we have learned that experience constitutes the basis of all behavior, including language behavior. Language is the instrument, the tool, the means whereby experience is symbolized and communicated. If experience itself is altered, if it is constituted differently, then meaning is changed.

That this question has both philosophical and scientific importance has been indicated eloquently by Brain.[4] While experience cannot be fully described, it is beneficial to view it in terms of levels or hierarchies. Thus we can compare the experience of Man with that of other forms of life. Furthermore, we can compare the experience of the sensorially deprived with that of the normally hearing. The hierarchies of experience might be categorized logically into the levels of Sensation, Perception, Imagery, Symbolization, and Conceptualization as shown schematically in Figure 15. This classification emphasizes that if the level of sensation is impaired, as in the case of deafness, then all of the categories above this level will be altered to some degree. On the other hand, the level of symbolization may be impaired, as in the case of dyslexia, without affecting the levels below symbolization. However, it must not be assumed that these levels are dichotomous; rather, they are overlapping developmental stages. Furthermore, all levels are operative simultaneously in the normal, mature human being.

This frame of reference and theoretical construct is useful in the study of language, language pathology, and the psychology of sensory deprivation. Progress has been made in the development of objective tests to measure the function represented by each of these

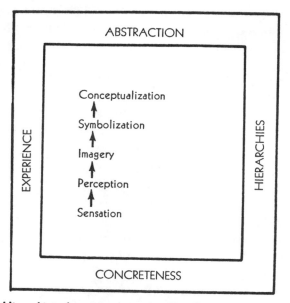

FIG. 15. Hierarchies of experience ranging from the concrete to the abstract.

levels. Such tests are essential for adequate differential diagnosis and when more refined techniques are available, they will provide a means whereby the nature of intellect can be more fully understood. Moreover, they will make it possible to establish an objective basis for differential language therapy and educational training. For the greatest benefit an individual having major impairment at the level of perception requires different training and therapy than one whose major deficit is at the level of symbolization. To alleviate the involvement, remedial training must be focused on the specific level or levels of experience which are affected.

Sensation

Sensation refers to the nervous system activity resulting from the activation of a given sense organ; it is present in all forms of animal life and may occur without perception. For example, an individual may hear a sound but be unable to attach significance to what he hears. Such sensation without perception often indicates the presence of an agnosia. Interestingly, the level of sensation might be impeded by both organic and psychologic conditions. Deafness and blindness are common examples of organic involvement while psychogenic deafness and psychogenic blindness are examples of nonorganic conditions affecting this level of experience.

Perception

Perception has been defined in various ways. Allport[1] has provided a critical review of the primary schools of thought and has contributed to the understanding of this basic psychological process. Strauss[30] in his work with children having neurological deficits defined perception as attaching meaning to sensation. Cantril[5] has emphasized the ways in which culture and socialization are related to one's perceptions. The roles of self-perception and person-perception have been investigated by Tagiuri and Petrullo[31] and Heider.[14] There is general agreement that at the level of sensation there is no integration; perception marks the beginning of integration. At this level according to the total capacities and needs of the organism, sensory stimuli become meaningful. Depending on the level of the specie, the organism learns to interpret sensation and to engage in anticipatory behavior. Contrary to the position of Bartley,[3] many authorities view this process as being nonsymbolic and as being possible only when the stimulus is present. Therefore, it is commonly assumed that no generalizing or categorizing occurs at this level. Perception is viewed as being primitive and present in all forms of animal life, human and subhuman.

Imagery

Imagery has in the past played a significant role in psychology but, with the exception of workers such as Russell[29] and Mowrer,[22] this phenomenon has not been emphasized in recent years. In contrast neurologists, as represented by the work of Penfield,[27] Nielsen,[24] and Brain,[4] have given considerable attention to imagery as a specific attribute of the mental life of humans. Study of the psychology of deafness is difficult without including the concept of imagery. Although philosophers have stressed that there is no thought without words, it is apparent that children deaf from birth engage in thought before they have acquired verbal language. Thus the question arises: By what means do they think? They might think in "gestures" which have become symbolic and take the place of words. This explanation, however, seems inadequate because frequently they have few conventionalized gestures of this type. Another possibility is that they are primarily dependent on imagery. It should not be assumed that words and images necessarily represent dichotomous levels; words, too, might serve as images. Nevertheless, imagery differs from verbal symbols in that it is more pictographic and ideographic. Instead of using a word to represent the object, an aspect of the object itself is recalled and used for the thought process; what it looks like, what it sounds like, and how it feels constitute the image. Such a process may be nonverbal but it is representational; the image represents the object. This is the primary demarcation between perception and imagery. Phylogenetically Man apparently used imagery before he acquired language. Likewise ontogenetically, the infant seems to have images before he acquires verbal facility.

Although it has not been studied extensively, there is evidence on the nature of imagery also from the area of psychopathology, stressed by Brain as important in understanding the nature of experience. When the human being is primitivized by mental illness, he often engages in hallucination. Further evidence of this type derives from the study of dreams. The process of dreaming seems limited essentially to the level of imagery.

As illustrated in Figure 15, imagery, as compared to verbal symbols, is viewed as being more concrete. Although imagery is an essential aspect of human behavior, Man attains a higher level of symbolic representation. The extent to which lower animals engage in imagery has not been ascertained. The work of Yerkes[37] indicates that imagery is present in the chimpanzee. Perhaps as we go down the phylogenetic scale we might find that there is a point at which imagery is not present. It is advantageous scientifically to consider the level of imagery as an overlapping area between human and subhuman behavior. From this frame of reference, all forms of animal life experience sensation and perception, whereas only the higher forms, human and subhuman, engage in imagery with Man alone attaining the level of symbolization and conceptualization.

Verbal Symbolic Behavior

Verbal symbolic behavior is unique in Man. This position has been emphasized by Langer.[17] Cobb[9] also has stressed this point of view by indicating that only Man has the neurological structures which make language acquisition possible. Language is an arbitrary symbol system used to represent objects, ideas, and feelings. This level of behavior is characterized by its not being dependent on the experience itself; symbolization makes re-experiencing possible without the occurrence, circumstance, or stimuli being present. To symbolize is to be able to internalize experientially and to communicate with others. Imagery, too, makes representation and mental manipulation possible. However, in comparison with the symbol it is not so far removed from the actual experience. Symbolic behavior is more flexible, subtle, and abstract. According to Langer, when the experience must be present, as when an animal signals danger, the behavior is at the level of "signification." Lower animals signify but do not symbolize.

Man uses both verbal and nonverbal symbols. Mythology, art, religion, and music are replete with illustrations of nonverbal symbols. While Man's use of nonverbal symbols is intriguing and is of importance in the psychology of deafness, it is with his verbal functioning that we are primarily concerned. It is principally through words that we manipulate experience and are able to communicate with others.

Conceptualization

Conceptualization is the process through which experiences can be classified and categorized according to certain principles or common elements. This is the highest level of behavior yet attained and, as with symbolization, is unique in Man. Concept formation has been studied in various ways, but perhaps the most definite work has been done in relation to schizophrenia and brain disease. The contributions of Vigotsky,[33] Hanfmann and Kasanin,[12] Arieti,[2] Oléron,[26] and Goldstein[11] are notable.

Study of conceptualization raises the complex question of whether this level of behavior is directly dependent on language, as suggested by the schema in Figure 15. Heider and Heider[15] and Oléron[25] have shown that deaf children conceptualize effectively even though verbal language is limited. This was shown also by results given in Chapter V. Nonverbal conceptualization may be possible through the categorization of images, but that normal levels of abstraction are attained thereby seems unlikely. While conceptualization seems not to be limited to verbal symbolic function, it is highly dependent on it.

Deafness and Experience

Study of the psychology of deafness does not indicate that sensory deprivation alters the hierarchy of experience as discussed here. The deaf child receives sensation, perceives, and he develops imagery, symbolization, and concepts. However, when auditory sensations are lacking or present only to a minimal degree, the nature of his perceptions, imagery, symbols, and concepts is altered. The levels of symbolization and conceptualization are most affected; development of certain types of abstract behavior is impeded. Presumably the individual with profound deafness from early life is highly dependent on imagery, especially visual imagery, which may be a predominant factor in the restriction imposed on his psychological development as well as in the concreteness which results. Language is a critical factor in the attainment of the higher levels of experience. When the relationship between deafness and each of these levels of experience is further clarified, new approaches to the learning and adjustment problems can be devised.

LANGUAGE DEVELOPMENT

Much can be gained by viewing the problem of language development phylogenetically. It is apparent that the first verbal system acquired by Man was auditory. He did not first learn to read or to write but rather to comprehend another's vocal utterance and to speak. There is evidence that many centuries of evolution were required after he was able to speak before he acquired the ability to read and to write. Furthermore, as Clodd,[8] Wells,[34] and Friedrich[10] have emphasized, the manner in which Western Man evolved reading and writing was different from that of Oriental Man. This difference in the language of the "West" as compared to the "East" continues to the present day.

This phylogenetic pattern of auditory language developing first, before the visual, also is seen ontogenetically. The infant does not first learn to read; he learns to comprehend and to use the spoken word. The developmental stages in the acquisition of auditory language are shown schematically in Figure 16. As this figure illustrates the child first acquires meaningful experience. He does not first learn the words and then the meaning; meaningfulness and experience precede the acquisition of words to symbolize the experience. The relating of experience and symbol is the basis of *inner language*. As this process develops the child can think in words, he can use mental trial and error, he can group and classify his experiences, he can "talk to himself." A period of from six to nine months is required for the development of inner language before comprehension of the spoken word can occur.

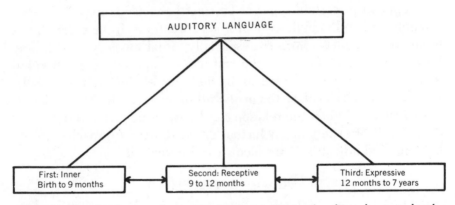

FIG. 16. The developmental sequence in the acquisition of auditory language by the normal child.

When inner language has been established to a minimal degree, the infant begins to comprehend. He now can internalize the word "Mommy" in a rudimentary way according to the *norm* for this symbol in his culture. At first he can do this only with words which symbolize basic experiences such as eating and motor functions. This process of relating the words he receives through audition to experience is the basis of *receptive language*. As shown in Figure 16 as inner language increases, receptive language is enhanced; a reciprocal "feed-back" process is established.

After minimal inner and receptive language have been established, the infant begins to use the spoken word expressively. This process begins genetically approximately three months after the initial comprehension. The child's first spoken words, like his first receptive language, are concrete, names of objects or specific acts. Using the spoken word to relate experience to others is the basis of *expressive language* of the auditory type. Again a reciprocality and "feed-back" are noted. As the child speaks, he enhances his receptive and inner language.

Developmentally we see that the pattern or sequence is for inner language to be acquired first, receptive language next, and expressive language last. Receptive language can develop only after inner language has been initiated, and expressive language can be accomplished only after comprehension has been established; *output follows input, so the child speaks only after he comprehends.* By two years of age he has considerable facility in auditory language. Not until at least five years later does he have comparable facility with read language. Therefore, as in phylogenetic development, ontogenetically the child requires more "evolution," growth, and maturity in order to learn to read and to write as compared to the acquisition of the spoken word. Moreover, evidence is accumulating which indicates that reading and writing are first learned by the superimposition of the read word onto the auditory word. Again, phylogenetic evidence and considerations are revealing. Western Man evolved an alphabet by relating visual "letters" to spoken sounds and words, the *phonetic system.* This resulted in a relationship between what the word looks like and what it sounds like. A similar evolvement did not occur in the case of Oriental Man. Therefore, such a relationship between the read and heard word does not exist in most oriental languages; their written language is non-phonetic. In Western languages, reading is acquired by relating what the word looks like to what it sounds like. Only the sophisticated reader can read without reference to how the words sound; even the sophisticated reader "regresses" and uses a "sounding out" process when he encounters a word which is difficult or with which he is unfamiliar.

A schema illustrating the developmental hierarchy of verbal language is presented in Figure 17. The fundamental basis of all language is experience and meaningful experience precedes the acquisition of the verbal symbol for the experience. Until the child has acquired at least a part of the *norm* of experience which is symbolized by the word "dog," he cannot use the word meaning-

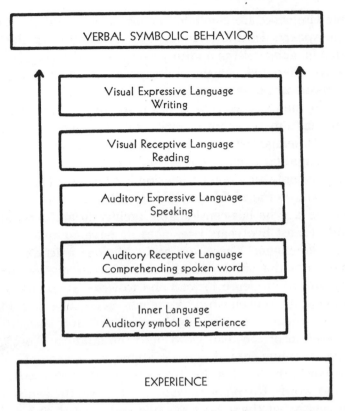

FIG. 17. The developmental hierarchy of Man's language systems.

fully. This is a fundamental concept in the psychology of language development. *Meaning* must be acquired before symbolization can occur. A word without meaning is not a word.

Evidence for the hierarchy of language systems suggested in Figure 17 is derived from various sources. Arieti[2] has shown that when experience is distorted, as in Schizophrenia, language disintegrates into "word salad." Individuals having experiential distortions from perceptual disorders due to neurological deficits also may have difficulties with the meanings of language. Likewise in sensory deprivation, one of the reasons the child having deafness from early life encounters a severe problem in acquiring language is that his *norm* of experience varies from the normal. It is more difficult for him to acquire the *meaning* to be associated with the word.

Likewise much has been learned about the hierarchy of Man's language systems from the study of aphasia, dyslexia, dysgraphia, and spelling disorders in children and adults. These findings will not be given here. However, as indicated by the schema in Figure 17, an individual might have a dysgraphia, thus be unable to write, without affecting his other language functions. This is possible because writing is the last language function acquired and, therefore, is superimposed on those which had been acquired earlier. In contrast, if auditory receptive language cannot be established because of deafness, then acquisition of all of the succeeding language functions will be impeded.

The point of view expressed here derives especially from the study of children deaf from early life. A century of experience on the part of educators of the deaf is consequential in this regard. One must inquire why impaired hearing from the prespeech age results in a generalized imposition on language development. It is evident that the child who does not hear the spoken word will not acquire auditory language. But why does he not learn to read normally at the expected age? Could we not assume that if there were no relationship between the spoken (auditory) word and the read (visual) word, the deaf child would learn to read as readily as the normally hearing child? In actuality, the child with deafness from infancy has a marked retardation in all aspects of language. Furthermore, no educational methodology known has been highly successful in overcoming this limitation. We must infer that when auditory language is lacking or seriously impeded, read and written language are restricted on a reciprocal basis. This concept of reciprocality, or feed-back, is useful in understanding the total hierarchy of language systems. At the auditory level we have stressed that reception must precede expression. This requisite holds also for reading and writing. As speech is the expressive phase of the reception of the spoken word, writing is the expressive phase of the visual word, that is, of reading. Stated differently, *one does not speak until he comprehends speech, and one does not write until he comprehends the written word, until he reads.* This is a major implication of the developmental hierarchy of Man's language functions. This concept is stressed here because of its significance in understanding the marked language problem found in deaf children. When hearing is lacking and the hierarchy of language functions is disturbed, it is necessary for the child to acquire verbal systems in some other manner; another type of hierarchy must be established. It is the task of every human infant to acquire the language of his culture. No child is born with language, but normally he is born with the capacity to acquire it without conscious effort. The deaf child, too, is expected to acquire language, but because of the importance of auditory language in Man's verbal symbol system, in doing so, he is confronted with one of the most difficult problems of learning known.

The intriguing problem of language acquisition in the presence of early life deafness requires further analysis. The inner and receptive language of the normal child is first auditory. In fact, for some time it may be considered as exclusively auditory because the read form is acquired much later. It is impossible for the deaf child first to have language which is auditory. His symbol system of necessity must be visual or tactual-kinesthetic, or presumably it might be a combination of these two. Verbal language has not been acquired through the sensory channels of olfaction and gustation; Cobb[9] suggests that these are nonsymbolic sensory avenues. That the visual channel can be used to learn language is obvious from the fact that Man learns to read. That the tactual avenue also can be used for this purpose is obvious from the fact that the blind learn to read Braille. A fundamental question in the psychology and education of the deaf is which sensory channel should be emphasized for language acquisition when the auditory avenue is of minor usefulness or cannot be used. From the history of the education of the deaf we see that a basic choice, or assumption, was made in this regard some time ago. It was assumed that both the visual and tactual avenues should be used simultaneously, leading to an emphasis on speech with speech development becoming a criterion for language development. In other words, the main emphasis has been on the development of the expressive spoken word, not on the development of inner and of receptive language. Furthermore, the stress has been on auditory language, not on the visual, except for the teaching of speechreading in a manner secondary to speech.

While the approach which emphasizes speech in the language development of the deaf child is logical, it has not been highly successful. Many studies testify to the fact that the individual with deafness from early life continues to have a marked limitation in language throughout his school life and thereafter. Why have not the methods for language training been more successful? It is likely that there are a number of reasons, some of which will be known only after many more years of scientific investigation and experimental study. A basic reason might be that undue emphasis has been placed on the expressive function (speech) without sufficient stress on the development of inner and receptive language. This possibility is viewed as being of importance and is considered in Chapter X and XI in relation to the data presented there. However, first we must analyze further what sensory channels would be used if inner and receptive language were to be given greater emphasis and if this training were to precede stress on expressive language. Consideration of this question is basic to our concept.

Vision is the residual distance sense and the deaf child's basic channel for monitoring. Moreover, it is one of the two sensory avenues through which Man characteristically acquires language. Therefore, although vision is a less suitable channel through which to acquire a basic language, we can assume that the deaf would acquire language receptively most readily if it were a visual symbol system. Because reading requires greater gowth and maturity, it does not serve the purpose of a symbol system which might be acquired in early infancy. The alternatives are speechreading and the manual language of signs. While the sign language has advantages for some deaf people, it cannot be considered comparable to a verbal symbol system; this is discussed further below. Therefore, although speechreading has limitations as compared to auditory language, we must assume that it is the most suitable receptive language system when deafness is present. *If speechreading were taught as the basic language the deaf child would learn to comprehend the spoken word through this means, and it would constitute his basic inner language symbol system.* He would "think" in words, but not in auditory words. Nor would he think in visual-tactual ideographic images such as characterize the language of signs. His inner language would consist of words as they appear on the lips when spoken. Instead of vowel and consonant sounds, instead of pitch, inflection, and intonation, his words consist of movement, form,

shape, color, and other visually observable characteristics and attributes. Although speechreading has not been taught as *the basic
language system,* there is evidence that it becomes such a symbol
system for many with deafness. Experience, substantiated by findings such as those given in Chapter X, indicates that the person
highly competent in speechreading is competent also in reading and
often even in speech. Furthermore, children who have speechreading aphasia do not acquire speech, despite the ardent efforts
of their teachers, until *they can internalize what the word looks like.*
This manifests that the deaf child, like the hearing child, does not
speak until he has internalized the word in some form; it must be
established as meaningful inner and receptive language before it can
be produced as meaningful expressive language. Our point of view
stresses that speech would be expected and emphasized only after
a minimum of inner and receptive language has been acquired. This
is shown schematically in Figure 18, and can be compared to the
schema for the normal child shown in Figure 16.

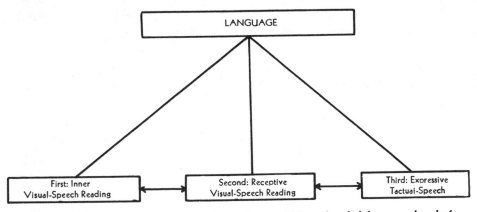

**FIG. 18. The developmental sequence in the acquisition of verbal language by deaf
children.**

As shown by these illustrations there is a fundamental difference
between the deaf and the hearing as to the processes involved in
acquiring the first basic language system. The hearing child acquires an *auditory* inner and receptive symbol system and uses the
same channel, audition, to monitor his first expressive language,
speech. In contrast, the deaf child, whose expressive language also
is speech, cannot monitor this function by using the same channel

through which he acquires his inner and receptive language. His visual symbol system, speechreading, must be converted into a tactual-kinesthetic system for speaking. In other words, *his spoken language must be monitored through a sensory channel other than the one used to monitor his receptive language.* This need to convert or to shift from one monitoring system to another in learning language seems to be unique to the person having profound deafness and may be one of the most difficult problems in learning encountered by Man. Not even those who are both deaf and blind encounter this problem; they receive language tactual-kinesthetically by placing their fingers on the lips of the speaker. Thus, both their receptive and expressive language are monitored by the tactual-kinesthetic channel. Perhaps this is the reason that some deaf-blind individuals acquire language facility which exceeds that of the deaf. Moreover, it may explain the preference of many deaf people for the manual sign language. This system is monitored visually both receptively and expressively; no conversion is necessary. The question before the scientist, the educators of the deaf, and before the deaf themselves is whether this advantage of the sign language outweighs its limitations as a language, as a symbol system.

For purposes of clarification an example is given of the shift in monitoring channels which must be made by the child having deafness. When he utters a vocalization to call his mother, he is not monitoring these vocalizations through hearing. He has learned that when he produces a kinesthetic sensation in his throat, he receives attention from his mother. Typically he has learned this by eight to ten months of age. However, kinesthetic monitoring of auditory utterances does not attain a high degree of accuracy, which explains the wide fluctuations of pitch and loudness characteristic of the speech of those having impaired hearing. Modulation and precise monitoring of one's speech is possible only when one has normal hearing. Even when the hearing loss is moderate and when hearing aids are highly beneficial, normal monitoring is difficult if not impossible.

We have indicated what appears to be the hierarchy of verbal symbol systems used by Man, referring also to the fact that this hierarchy is different when there is deafness, especially if the hearing loss is profound and exists from early infancy. Much study remains before the shift in monitoring channels and the hierarchy of symbol systems for the deaf can be fully explained. Also, the extent to which language training based on this frame of reference would be superior to other approaches remains to be ascertained. However, as a concept for language development it conforms to what has been learned about the perceptual organization, the monitoring processes, and the psychology of learning when the sensory deprivation of deafness is present. In order to illustrate further the monitoring problem and the hierarchy of symbol systems involved in the deaf child's acquisition of language, a schema is presented in Figure 19. This developmental hierarchy for the deaf can be compared to the one for the normal shown in Figure 17.

According to this frame of reference the deaf child, like the hearing child, *first* must acquire the *norm of experience* to be sym-

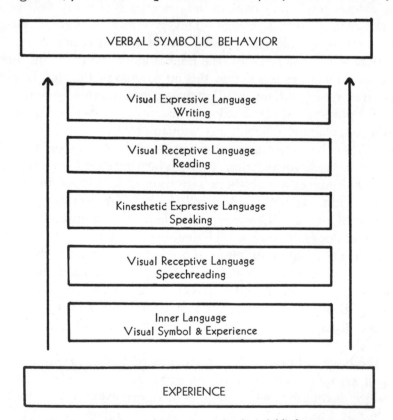

FIG. 19. The developmental hierarchy of the deaf child's language systems.

bolized by the word. To refer to the example used earlier, he must have gained the experience of "dog" before the word "dog" can have significance. Therefore, a fundamental consideration in language development for children deaf from early infancy is the difficulty which they have in gaining the expected norm of experience. All language systems disintegrate and become useless when the "expresser" and the "receiver" do not have a referent, a norm of experience for the words being used. In the case of the deaf child this problem is not so critical when the word refers to actual objects, when the words are nouns. An actual dog, a toy dog, or a picture of a dog can be used to indicate the experience intended for the word "dog." Even in this instance, however, we cannot assume a typical *norm* for the deaf child in comparison to the hearing child. A dog that runs, jumps, and wags his tail, but so far as the deaf child is concerned, does not bark, growl, and whine, must be viewed as being a *different* dog. The problem is increased when the deaf child encounters relational words such as, if, because, and unless. Since these are not nouns that he can see and feel, the norm of experience to be associated with them can be achieved only through long effort on the part of both the teacher and the child.

According to the point of view stressed here, more deliberate attempts must be made to assist the deaf child to gain the specific experiences to be associated with the word. Through speechreading he would then be given the visual symbol which is to be associated with the experience; an important factor in the total process is the proper timing of the events. *This is the basis of training for the development of inner language.* Expressive language would be stressed only after a minimum of inner and receptive language had been established. The visual symbol system of speechreading would be the basic inner and receptive language upon which reading and writing would be superimposed.

SPEECHREADING AND THE LANGUAGE OF SIGNS AS LANGUAGE SYSTEMS

Historically, the earliest efforts to educate the deaf were attempts to teach them to speak, followed by emphasis on the use of amplification. This early work recognized that the most direct effect of deafness is the restriction it imposes on communication, an awareness which has continued to the present time. In fact the problem of language has been stressed to such an extent that it has become a controversial issue. Several schools of thought have arisen concerning the most effective methods for developing language. These varying points of view will not be considered in detail. In general there are two major approaches: one the *Oral Method,* the other the *Combined Method.* The principal difference between the two is that the Oral Method does not use the manual sign language as an adjunct in language training, or as a supplement in teaching. The Combined Method uses both oral and manual means of communication in its approach to language training. From the point of view of language theory these differences are significant and warrant objective analysis.

Methods utilized for developing language in children with deafness are based on theory and experience rather than on scientific evidence. This is not surprising inasmuch as there is no way in which the methods used to teach any child can be completely verified. There continues to be controversy regarding *the* method for teaching reading to normal children. Therefore, the fact that the methodologies used with deaf children are based on opinion and experience is not a reflection on the greatness of the work done by educators in the past or in the present era. However, the need for scientific study must be clearly recognized. Many claims and counterclaims have been made regarding the effectiveness of a particular methodology. Only through objective study can such claims be evaluated.

The manual sign language, used by many deaf people, has a long history. It is an intriguing language although considerable controversy has centered around its role in the education of the deaf. The controversy which has been associated with it may have given rise to fallacious assumptions and argument. The advocates of the Oral Method have maintained that the use of the sign language deters and impedes the development of speech. This opinion is not supported by the statistical evidence given in Chapters X and XI. The problem of language behavior in children with deafness is more complex than is implied by the assumption of a simple, direct, inverse relationship between the use of speech and the sign language.

Claims made by the adherents of the Combined Method also

obscure basic questions. Usually these claims have concerned practical issues without consideration of the limitations of the sign language as a language system. Both speechreading and the sign language are visual symbol systems, and a visual system is most advantageous for the hearing impaired. However, while speech-reading is a verbal language, the sign language is not. The question of which is most effective must be determined in terms of which is *superior as a language*. All language systems have limitations. The phonetic system may be the most satisfactory yet evolved. How ever, this system is not directly applicable when deafness is present Therefore, the question becomes one of which language system is most adequate when hearing is impaired.

Study of Man's language development indicates that a sign-gesture method of communication preceded the acquisition of the spoken word. It is of interest that Man did not retain this means of communication but instead developed spoken, verbal language. Presumably, as Man evolved, the sign-gesture language became inadequate and did not meet his needs. Furthermore, the manual sign system restricted the use of his hands for other purposes imperative to his total well-being. It is apparent that over the centuries Man's language behavior has evolved and taken various forms. Clodd[8] has shown these evolutionary stages as follows:

  a. Mnemonic, the use of an object to convey a message
  b. Pictorial, a picture which conveys and communicates
  c. Ideographic, a picture which is representative and symbolic
  d. Phonetic, the letter, an arbitrary picture, which conveys the sound

The manual sign language used by the deaf is an Ideographic language. In Clodd's classification it falls under (c), a picture which is representative and symbolic. An Ideographic language characteristically uses a part of the object to represent the whole object. There are many examples of this in the sign language. Essentially it is more pictorial, less symbolic and as a system is one which falls mainly at the level of imagery. Ideographic language systems, in comparison with verbal symbol systems, lack precision, subtlety, and flexibility. It is likely that Man cannot achieve his ultimate potential through an Ideographic language, inasmuch as it is limited to the more concrete aspects of his experience. Comparatively, a verbal language is more abstract. Moreover, an adequate language system must include a written form. Although most Ideographic forms of language can be written, it is highly impractical to do so. In the case of the sign language it seems impossible to devise a written form. The manual sign system must be viewed as being inferior to the verbal as a language.

Speechreading as a language system is a modification of the phonetic system, point (d) in Clodd's classification. It is a verbal language. The Movements which are received visually supplant the sounds which the hearing person receives auditorially. As a language system it, too, has limitations. It requires close proximity to the speaker, somewhat closer than in the case of the sign language. Furthermore, all of the movements made in speaking are not visible on the lips. However, study of speech has shown that one need not hear all of the sounds in order to comprehend. It is evident from the number of individuals who can speechread with marked accuracy that likewise it is not necessary to see all of the speech movements. This does not mean that speechreading is equally as efficient as a system. It has been demonstrated that we can hear more speech sounds than is necessary for ordinary purposes of comprehension. It remains for scientific effort to clarify further this relationship in speechreading. Nevertheless, we cannot assume that because a number of speech movements are not observable, speechreading is more limited as compared to the sign language. On the contrary, although much scientific effort remains, it has advantages as a language system.

Speechreading and the sign language have common limitations in some respects because they both are dependent on reception visually. The marked difference between hearing and vision as sensory channels becomes most obvious through the study of language development. Because of the permissive nature of audition the hearing child hears language constantly. It is unnecessary for him to focus attention on what is being said; auditory reception is mandatory. In contrast, the young deaf child can receive what is being said, whether through speechreading or by the sign language, only when he can see the speaker.

The problem of input is more laborious and difficult to a remarkable degree. Thereby, the person dependent on vision for receptive language can communicate only with one person at a time. These limitations of vision as an avenue through which to receive language is common to both speechreading and the sign language. Only through the recognition of these problems is it possible to understand the difficulties encountered by those who have deafness.

When the advantages and disadvantages of speechreading and the sign language are considered, it seems that the verbal system, that is, speechreading, offers more possibilities and fulfills more of the requirements of an adequate language. This does not preclude the possibility that some persons with deafness may not be able to acquire this type of language with a high degree of facility. It must be emphasized that this is true of any group of persons, irrespective of the language system used. An important consideration is that only through a verbal language can we expect the human being to attain his highest potential.

REFERENCES

1. Allport, F.: Theories of Perception and a Concept of Structure. New York, John Wiley and Sons, 1955.
2. Arieti, S.: Interpretation of Schizophrenia. New York, Robert Brunner, 1955.
3. Bartley, S.: Principles of Perception. New York, Harper, 1958.
4. Brain, R.: The Nature of Experience. London, Oxford University Press, 1959.
5. Cantril, H.: The Nature of Social Perception. Trans. New York Acad. Science, 10, 142, 1948.
6. Cassirer, E.: The Philosophy of Symbolic Form, Vol. 1, 2, 3. New Haven, Yale University Press, 1953.
7. Ceram, C.: The Secret of the Hittites. New York, Knopf, 1956.
8. Clodd, E.: The Story of the Alphabet. New York, D. Appleton, 1900.
9. Cobb, S.: Borderlines of Psychiatry. Cambridge, Harvard University Press, 1948.
10. Friedrich, J.: Extinct Languages. New York, Philosophical Library, 1957.
11. Goldstein, K.: Language and Language Disturbances. New York, Grune and Stratton, 1948.
12. Hanfmann, M. and Kasanin, J.: Conceptual thinking in schizophrenia. Nervous, Mental Disease Mono., #67, 1942.
13. Hayakawa, S.: Language in Action. New York, Harcourt, Brace, 1941.
14. Heider, F.: The Psychology of Interpersonal Relations. New York, John Wiley and Sons, 1958.
15. _____ and Heider, G. Studies in the psychology of the deaf. Psychol. Mono., #242, 1941.
16. Korzybski, A.: Science and Sanity. Lancaster, Science Press, 1933.
17. Langer, S.: Philosophy in a New Key. Cambridge, Harvard University Press, 1957.
18. Leopold, W.: Speech Development of a Bilingual Child. Vol. 1, 2, 3, 4. Evanston, Northwestern University Press, 1954.

19. McCarthy, D.: Language development in children, in Carmichael, L. Manual of Child Psychology. New York, John Wiley and Sons, 1946.
20. Miller, G.: Language and Communication. New York, McGraw Hill, 1951.
21. Mowrer, O.: Learning Theory and Personality Dynamics. New York, Ronald Press, 1950.
22. Mowrer, O.: Learning Theory and the Symbolic Processes. New York, John Wiley and Sons, 1960.
23. Müller, M.: Science of Language. Vol. 1 and 2. New York, Charles Scribner's, 1887.
24. Nielsen, J.: Memory and Amnesia. Los Angeles, San Lucas Press, 1958.
25. Oléron, P.: Conceptual thinking of the deaf. Am. Ann. Deaf, 98, 304, 1953.
26. _____: Recherches sur le Développement Mental des Sourds-Muets. Paris Centre National de la Recherche Scientifique, 1957.
27. Penfield, W. and Roberts, L.: Speech and Brain Mechanisms. Princeton, Princeton University Press, 1959.
28. Piaget, J.: Language and Thought of the Child. New York, Harcourt, Brace, 1926.
29. Russell, D.: Children's Thinking. Chicago, Ginn, 1956.
30. Strauss, A. and Lehtinen, L.: Psychopathology and Education of the Brain-Injured Child. New York, Grune and Stratton, 1947.
31. Tagiuri, R. and Petrullo, L. (ed.): Person Perception and Interpersonal Behavior. Stanford, Stanford University Press, 1958.
32. Templin, M.: Certain Language Skills in Children. Minneapolis, University of Minnesota Press, 1957.
33. Vigotsky, L. S.: Thought and speech. Psychiatry, 2, 29, 1939.
34. Wells, H. G.: The Outline of History. Vol. 1 and 2. Garden City, Garden City Books, 1956.
35. Whitney, W.: The Life and Growth of Language. New York, D. Appleton, 1896.
36. Whorf, B. J.: Language, Thought and Reality. New York, John Wiley and Sons, 1956.
37. Yerkes, R.: Chimpanzees. New Haven, Yale University Press, 1943.

Suggestions for Further Study

Bloomfield, L.: Language. New York, Henry Holt, 1933.
Brown, R.: Words and Things. Glencoe, The Free Press, 1958.
Cassirer, E.: Language and Myth. New York, Harper, 1946.
Diehl, C. and England, N.: Mental imagery. J. Speech and Hearing Research, 1, 268, 1958.
Gelb, J.: A Study of Writing. Chicago, Univer. of Chicago Press, 1963.
Groht, M.: Natural Language for Deaf Children. Washington, The Volta Bureau, 1958.
Hogben, L.: The Wonderful World of Communication. Garden City, Garden City Books, 1959.
Kahne, H., Kahne, R. and Saporta, S.: Development of verbal categories in child language. International J. Am. Linguistics, 24, #4, 1958.
Ogden, C. and Richards, I.: The Meaning of Meaning. New York, Harcourt, Brace, 1923.
Mandelbaum, D. (ed.): Selected Writings of Edward Sapir. Berkeley, University of California Press, 1951.

Morris, C.: Signs, Language and Behavior. New York, George Braziller, 1955.

Revesz, G.: The Origins and Prehistory of Language. New York, Philosophical Library, 1956.

Spitz, R.: No and Yes: On the Genesis of Human Communication. New York, International Universities Press, 1957.

Travis, L. (ed.): Handbook of Speech Pathology. New York, Appleton-Century-Crofts, 1957.

Werner, H. and Kaplan, B.: Symbol Formation. New York, John Wiley and Sons, 1963.

Chapter X

SPEECHREADING AND SPEECH

SPEECHREADING IS THE PROCESS of comprehending the words of the speaker by associating meaning with the movements of his lips. It is a receptive language process used to some extent by everyone but of critical importance to those who have significant degrees of deafness. When the spoken word cannot be received through the usual channel, through audition, it is essential that some other avenue be used. As suggested in Chapter IV, the deaf are entirely dependent on substitute avenues while the hard of hearing might find it necessary to use such avenues only in a supplemental manner.

Speechreading is dependent upon the visual sensory channel. Emphasis on this form of communication in the education and rehabilitation of the deaf and hard of hearing has a history of many decades. Only rarely have other sensory avenues been tried as a fundamental means through which to develop competence in language. The work of Gault[5] is such an exception. He experimented with the possibility of using the tactual avenue as the lead or major sense through which to develop verbal language. This approach is again receiving attention from scientific workers, and possibly the tactual avenue could be used more effectively, especially as a supplementary sensory channel.

In the present discussion, as in Chapter IX, consideration is given to speechreading as a form of *receptive language*. It is not our purpose to give a critique of the various methods which have been developed. Rather, questions are raised regarding the nature of the speechreading process, and an attempt is made to analyze the psychological factors which might be involved in the development of this language system. The early work of Kitson[13] suggests that factors, such as the ability to synthesize, are important in achieving this skill. These abilities have been assumed by many teachers of the hearing impaired; however, most attempts to identify them have not yet met with success.

To achieve skill in speechreading is to develop skill in a

language system, in a type of verbal behavior. It assumes facility in identifying the symbol (word) from the speaker's lip movements and from other visual clues, and in internalizing the symbol with the appropriate unit of experience, attaching the correct meaning to the symbol. This process involves the ability to retain lip movements mentally while the speaker is speaking, the ability to sequentialize and properly group these movements, and then to associate them with experience. The psychologist concerned with language, especially with language as it pertains to deafness, is confronted with the task of objectively measuring these abilities. Only in this way can knowledge of the speechreading process be enhanced, making it possible to predict success and to indicate the methodologies which might be most effective in helping individuals to acquire this visual-verbal system of communication.

In addition to analyzing speechreading as a receptive language system, it is necessary to analyze the visual avenue as a channel through which to acquire and to use language. There is a critical difference between vision and audition as modalities for acquiring language. As emphasized in Chapter IV, hearing is mandatory and does not require direct attention. It is a sense which is projected in all directions simultaneously so that the hearing child hears speech within his auditory range whether or not he attends to it volitionally. Furthermore, he can hear in darkness, through walls, and around corners. By comparison, for acquisition of language, vision is a much less effective avenue. To speechread, the individual must see the face of the speaker and the speaker must face the speechreader. In some respects it can be compared to reading but speechreading presents a greater problem in this regard. In reading only one person, the individual himself, is involved but the speech-reader is dependent on the speaker's willingness to adjust to his needs and on the speaker's being in a situation where he can make such an adjustment. Because this form of communication is dependent upon vision, it is further restricted by the need of prox-imity, adequate lighting, and an unobstructed view between the persons concerned. Just as one cannot read while operating a power saw or while performing many other types of work, so the person dependent on speechreading cannot communicate with others while engaged in another activity. Essentially this is because of the nature of vision which does not readily fulfill the requisites for being a channel through which to acquire the basic language system. Perhaps this is an important reason for Man's finding it necessary to evolve a phonetic, auditory language system and for speech being Man's fundamental means of communication.

PSYCHOLOGICAL FACTORS AND SPEECHREADING ABILITY

Early investigators who studied speechreading include Story,[26] Nitchie,[19] Pintner,[21] Kitson,[13] Heider and Heider,[10] Morkovin,[17] and Mason.[16] While others have devised tests of speechreading, the most extensive and most widely used was developed by Utley.[28] Pintner found no relationship between speechreading and mental ability. Even on an empirical basis this seems illogical because it would be expected that learning such a verbal system would correlate with intelligence, as has been found in the study of other types of language behavior. In fact, it is now apparent from the work of Costello,[2] O'Neill,[20] and Simmons[25] that when measured appropriately, this language function is significantly correlated with various types of intellectual abilities.

The work of Costello is of considerable importance inasmuch as she studied speechreading as a receptive language. She devised a test consisting of isolated words and sentences, and established its validity through the use of teachers' ratings. She studied deaf and hard of hearing school children and related the scores to those from several psychological tests. The hard of hearing were superior to the deaf. There was no sex difference for the deaf, but the hard of hearing females were superior to the males. Sex differences in language abilities for normal children, favoring females, often have been reported.

The psychological tests selected by Costello to study factors which might be related to speechreading were: Knox Cube Test,[14] Digit Span,[1] Wechsler Picture Arrangement,[30] and Progressive Matrices Test.[24] To study the relationship between speechreading and reading, the Gates Reading Test[4] was used. Interestingly of the memory tests used, only the Visual Digit Span correlated significantly with the ability to speechread; this test consists of memory for symbols (numbers). As indicated in Chapter V, the Knox Cube Test entails memory for a sequence of movements, not symbols.

On the basis of these findings, memory for a sequence of symbols as a factor is related to speechreading ability. Conversely, should an individual have a limitation in this type of memory, he might be expected to find it difficult to learn this means of communication.

Scores on the Wechsler Picture Arrangement Test also correlated significantly with speechreading ability for both the deaf and the hard of hearing. This test measures the ability to perceive and to understand social situations; it might be considered a test of "social intelligence." It involves ability to empathize and to use insight, especially as it pertains to other people. Because scores on this test and on speechreading ability were significantly correlated, we must assume that the abilities measured by the Wechsler Picture Arrangement Test are involved in this visual-verbal process. Again, conversely, should an individual be low on the ability to perceive social situations, he might be expected to find it difficult to learn to speechread. The Wechsler Picture Arrangement Test does not involve verbal symbols and, thus, provides a measure of the nonverbal aspects of speechreading ability. That self-perception, person-perception, ability to maintain interpersonal relationships, and to empathize are a part of the matrix of speechreading ability is indicated also by the data on personality given below, and by the data on interest patterns presented in Chapter XIV.

Another provocative finding from the Costello investigation was a significant correlation between scores for speechreading and scores on the Progressive Matrices for the hard of hearing but not for the deaf. Furthermore, there was a relationship between scores in reading and speechreading, suggesting that the individual who achieves a high score on one type of verbal behavior achieves facility also in other language functions. The primary determining factor, therefore, may be the richness of inner language. In any event, the findings of Costello reveal that speechreading and certain factors of intelligence are related. Further studies are needed in this connection.

Speechreading and Intelligence

In our National Study of language development in deaf children, teachers rated each child on his ability to speechread. The rating scale consisted of excellent, good, average, fair, and poor.

Through statistical analyses these ratings were compared with the scores on the Draw-a-Man Test,[8] the Columbia Vocabulary Test,[3] and the Picture Story Language Test.[18] In all instances those subjects who were rated excellent-good-average were compared with those who were rated fair-poor.

The number of children rated excellent-good-average as compared to fair-poor in each school and by sex is shown in Table 54. The analysis disclosed that substantially more females than males were considered to have excellent-good-average speechreading ability. This was true irrespective of the type of school, that is, whether rated by teachers in Day or in Residential Schools. As in Costello's study, our findings strongly indicate a sex difference in ability to speechread. Perhaps this should be expected inasmuch as a number of investigators have shown sex differences for hearing children in verbal facility, females being superior to males. It is noteworthy that this same difference seems to exist for children having profound deafness.

TABLE 54.   The number of children rated high as compared to low in speechreading ability

| | Males | | Females | |
	Excellent-Good-Average	Fair-Poor	Excellent-Good-Average	Fair-Poor
Day	49%	51%	65%	35%
Residential	44%	56%	58%	42%

The Draw-a-Man Test scores for the speechreading groups as rated by teachers in each type of school are presented in Table 55. Interesting differences appeared from this comparison. In the Day School the males in the excellent-good-average category were superior in intelligence to the males rated as fair-poor and the differences were statistically significant. Moreover, in the Day School the total excellent-good-average group was superior to the total group rated fair-poor. While the data did not reveal a significant difference between the females in each category, it is clear that intelligence was an influential factor. Those children rated as excellent-good-average in speechreading by the teachers also were the more intelligent. Similar results were obtained for the Residential School group; however, no difference appeared on the basis of sex, a significant difference occurring only on the basis of total group comparison. Again the group rated excellent-good-average was superior to those rated fair-poor. These findings suggest that either the teachers rated the brightest children as being the best speechreaders or intelligence, as measured by the Draw-a-Man Test, is related to speechreading ability.

TABLE 55. A comparison of Draw-a-Man scores between those rated excellent-good-average and fair-poor in speechreading

	Males			Females			Total		
Day School	N	Mean	SD	N	Mean	SD	N	Mean	SD
Excellent-good-average	75	96.92	13.76	92	95.66	13.85	167	96.23	13.78
Fair-poor	76	89.16	14.36	50	91.46	11.35	126	90.07	13.25
Residential School									
Excellent-good-average	119	97.10	14.86	139	94.63	16.33	258	95.77	15.69
Fair-poor	151	94.71	15.60	101	87.93	16.02	252	91.99	16.09

SPEECHREADING, READ, AND WRITTEN LANGUAGE

In the discussion of Costello's findings it was suggested that the richness of inner language might be a critical factor in the development of receptive and expressive language; verbal facility may be a "g" (general) factor. On this basis we would expect that if an individual had superior ability in the comprehension of the spoken word, he would show superiority also in spoken, read, and written language.

Reading

To investigate the interrelationships of language functions further we compared the reading ability of those rated excellent-good-average with those rated fair-poor. The Columbia Vocabulary Test[8] was used as the measure of reading. The results of this comparison are shown in Table 56. The statistical analysis disclosed significant differences by sex and by total groups. The males who were rated good in speechreading scored higher in reading vocabulary than the males who were rated low. The same was true for the females and for the total groups irrespective of the type of school attended. These results definitely reveal a correlation between speechreading ability, as rated by teachers, and reading. Those children who were most successful in speechreading were found to be the best readers, which highlights the reciprocality between verbal systems, especially in relation to receptive language processes. These results are in agreement with the findings of Heider and Heider[10] and Goda.[7] The implication is that the principle of "feedback" should be stressed in the language development of deaf children. Emphasis on speechreading might enhance the level of reading with the opposite also being true; emphasis on reading might raise the level of function in speechreading.

TABLE 56. A comparison of Columbia Vocabulary Test scores for those rated excellent-good-average and fair-poor in speechreading

Day School	Males			Females			Total		
	N	Mean	SD	N	Mean	SD	N	Mean	SD
Excellent-good-average	78	8.04	9.26	99	10.23	9.23	177	9.27	9.28
Fair-poor	78	3.87	6.74	52	5.08	6.19	130	4.35	6.53
Residential School									
Excellent-good-average	91	7.69	8.09	120	8.24	8.60	211	8.00	8.37
Fair-poor	134	4.87	6.67	94	5.20	6.41	228	5.01	6.54

Written Language

Success in speechreading was related also to the ability to use written language. We devised the Picture Story Language Test as a measure of written language; this test is discussed in Chapter XI, Read and Written Language. The speechreading groups were compared on the basis of their scores on Sentence Length. The results are given in Table 57. Again, statistically significant results were obtained. The children rated as the most proficient in speechreading wrote the longest sentences. This was with the exception of the males in the Residential School where there was no relationship between the length of sentence written and speechreading ability. The verbal behavior of these males differed in various ways from that found for the other groups.

TABLE 57. The relationship between Sentence Length scores and ratings in speechreading

Day School	Males			Females			Total		
	N	Mean	SD	N	Mean	SD	N	Mean	SD
Excellent-good-average	76	5.96	3.40	99	6.22	3.17	175	6.11	3.26
Fair-poor	71	4.31	3.03	50	4.90	3.04	121	4.56	3.04
Residential School									
Excellent-good-average	100	5.56	3.44	124	6.44	2.92	224	6.05	3.18
Fair-poor	139	4.97	3.53	84	5.46	3.86	223	5.16	3.66

In addition to Sentence Length, the Picture Story Language Test is scored on Syntax, the extent to which the individual uses grammatically correct sentence structure in written language. The Syntax scores for those rated proficient and those rated fair-poor in speechreading were compared; the results are presented in Table 58. With the exception of the scores for the males in the Residential Schools, the differences between the groups were significant. For both the males and females in Day Schools and for the females in Residential Schools, there was a relationship between speechreading ability and competence in the use of grammatically correct written language.

TABLE 58. The relationship of Syntax scores to ratings in speechreading

	Males			Females			Total		
	N	Mean	SD	N	Mean	SD	N	Mean	SD
Day School									
Excellent-good-average	76	71	27	99	78	25	175	75	26
Fair-poor	71	56	26	50	60	28	121	58	27
Residential School									
Excellent-good-average	100	66	27	124	77	22	224	76	25
Fair-poor	139	62	29	84	63	28	223	62	29

A third score is derived from the Picture Story Language Test. An evaluation is made of the extent to which the individual uses Abstract-Concrete thought. The groups were compared to ascertain relationships between speechreading ability and conceptualization. The results are given in Table 59. While, again, this revealed no differences for the males in Residential Schools, for the other groups speechreading and abstraction were significantly related; those most proficient in speechreading used more abstract concepts. These results manifest that the greater the verbal facility of the

TABLE 59. The relationship of Abstract-Concrete scores to ratings in speechreading

	Males			Females			Total		
	N	Mean	SD	N	Mean	SD	N	Mean	SD
Day School									
Excellent-good-average	77	10.70	6.29	99	12.75	5.66	176	11.85	6.01
Fair-poor	70	7.58	5.49	49	9.35	6.03	119	8.31	5.76
Residential School									
Excellent-good-average	100	9.13	5.80	124	11.31	5.66	224	10.33	5.81
Fair-poor	139	8.06	6.11	83	9.47	6.20	222	8.59	6.17

deaf child, the more likely he is to use abstract ideas. It is interesting that such a relationship was not found for the Residential males.

Summary

Success in speechreading as revealed by teachers' ratings was found to be related to scores on the Draw-a-Man Test of intelligence; the more intelligent children were the most proficient speechreaders. In general, these results are in agreement with those of Costello[2] and Simmons[25]; they do not confirm the early findings of Pintner.[22] They disclose that intellectual abilities are a factor in the learning of the language system referred to as speechreading, just as mental capacity has been found to be related to other types of language systems. We can assume that general intelligence is a factor in the successful asquisition of speechreading, but it is evident that certain specific types of intellectual abilities are more directly related than others to such learning. More research on this problem using factor analysis might be expected to be highly rewarding.

The difference in intelligence between the "good" and "poor" speechreaders provides an explanation for the finding that those who are most successful in acquiring one language system also will be equally successful in acquiring other types of verbal facility. However, that these differences provide a complete explanation for some not being successful in speechreading seems unlikely. Given a certain degree of mental competence, and all of the groups in this study fell within normal limits of intelligence, other factors must be considered. This is illustrated strikingly by the findings for the Residential males. While the mean intelligence quotients for this group are equal to, or higher, than the mental test scores for the other groups, they showed no difference on the basis of speechreading ability. In this group the "good" and "poor" speechreaders were equally intelligent and were equally successful in acquiring other language facility, such as reading and writing. Hence, we see a variation on the basis of sex and the type of school attended. It is noteworthy that Costello, too, found sex differences, the males being inferior to the females, and the correlation with other factors varied on the basis of sex.

Although sex differences in learning to speechread seem to be present in deaf children, again we note that this is only a partial explanation of our results for the Residential males. The type of school experience also is a factor because the Day School males differed consistently when compared on the basis of "good" and "poor" speechreading proficiency. To explain this variability of the Residential males and to explore further the factors related to speechreading, we may draw from other evidence in the psychology of deafness. In Chapter V we noted that profound hearing loss affected functioning variously by sex, and in Chapter VI we indicated the differing effects on personality.

The findings on the Drawing of the Human Figure Test are especially relevant inasmuch as they are for the same population. Differences between the Residential males and the other groups also were obtained in this personality study. While all groups varied from the normal in body image, self-perception, and in some respects person-perception, it was the Residential males who deviated most. This group manifested the mental processes and altered psychological organization which most characterized the deaf organism. It is interesting that again, through this investigation of speechreading, we find an effect of deafness which varied by sex and according to the type of school attended. To be more successful in teaching speechreading, particularly to males in Residential Schools, it will be necessary to learn more about the effect of deafness and why Residential School experience seems to result in different learning and verbal behavior in males as compared to females. The implication is that the males use different mental processes, such as imagery, to a greater extent than the females, and that this natural difference by sex is increased and reinforced by Residential School experience.

Although much remains to be learned about speechreading as a receptive language system, in general, our findings for deaf children reveal a relationship between verbal systems; the greater the success in one type of verbal behavior, such as speechreading, the greater will be the success in other verbal systems. If facility in speechreading can be developed, facility in read and written language will be raised. An implication which might be of considerable importance is that the development of inner language is basic and fundamental to all other language behavior.

SPEECHREADING IN ADULTHOOD

A great deal can be learned about speechreading as a language system by investigating its use by deaf and hard of hearing adults. In our study of hearing impaired adults we asked each subject to rate himself as to his success as a speechreader. The rating scale consisted of *good, average,* and *poor,* and the number of subjects who rated themselves as having each of these levels of ability is shown in Table 60. As can be seen from these results, except for the hard of hearing males, there is a striking similarity between the groups. The same proportion of deaf males and females and hard of hearing females rated themselves as being good, average, or poor in speechreading ability. In agreement with the findings for emotional adjustment discussed in Chapter VI, the hard of hearing males rated themselves as being less proficient in speechreading as compared to the other groups.

TABLE 60.   The number of deaf and hard of hearing adults who rated themselves
as good, average, and poor speechreaders

	Deaf				Hard of Hearing			
	Males		Females		Males		Females	
	N	%	N	%	N	%	N	%
Good	31	30	24	26	11	25	20	25
Average	57	55	54	60	12	28	47	60
Poor	16	15	13	14	19	46	12	15

Sex differences did not appear for the deaf; both the males and females rated themselves as being of equal success or as being equally unsuccessful in speechreading ability. These self-ratings by deaf adults are not in agreement with the results of ratings of deaf children by teachers; the teachers rated the females as being the more proficient speechreaders. Moreover, Costello found the females to be more successful in this language function. Hence, it is interesting that the deaf male and female college students showed no difference in their self-ratings.

Definite differences by sex appeared for the hard of hearing. The females rated themselves as being substantially more proficient in speechreading. Almost one-half of the 42 hard of hearing males studied classified themselves as being poor speechreaders; this was three times the number in other groups who so appraised themselves. The sex difference for the hard of hearing adults is in the same direction as found by the teacher ratings of deaf children. Furthermore, it is in agreement with the findings of self-ratings of the extent to which deafness was found to be a handicap; the males rated themselves as being more incapacitated by a hearing loss.

Speechreading and Emotional Adjustment

To evaluate further the relationships between speechreading and psychological factors, the deaf adults who rated themselves "good" and those who rated themselves "poor" in speechreading were compared on the various categories of the Minnestoa Multiphasic Personality Inventory.[9] The results for seven of the Scales are shown in Table 61. The findings for the Depression and Hysteria Scales are treated separately because sex differences appeared on these categories. Sex differences were not found on the other Scales so the data in Table 61 include both males and females. The mean scores for those rating themselves "good" and for those rating themselves "poor" were markedly similar on Psychasthenia, Schizophrenia, Interest, Hypomania, Paranoia, Psychopathic Deviate, and Hypochondriasis; the differences were not statistically significant.

TABLE 61. Personality scores for deaf adults who rated themselves
"good" and "poor" in speechreading

Scale	Good N-53		Poor N-29	
	Mean	SD	Mean	SD
Psychasthenia	57.90	10.44	58.86	11.28
Schizophrenia	62.98	12.25	57.55	14.78
Interest	56.47	8.47	57.64	10.26
Hypomania	62.60	11.91	63.17	11.26
Paranoia	57.13	12.27	58.13	13.26
Psychopathic Deviate	52.52	10.33	55.58	10.50
Hypochondriasis	50.05	9.98	52.86	7.89

Personality factors, however, were found to be associated with self-ratings in speechreading proficiency. Significant differences were revealed on the Scales of Depression and Hysteria, but principally in regard to the males. The greater maladjustment was associated with the males, especially those who rated themselves "poor." A comparison between the males and females on the Depression Scale is shown in Table 62. The males were significantly

TABLE 62.   Comparison on Depression for deaf adults who rated
themselves "good" and "poor" in speechreading

	Good		Poor	
	Males	Females	Males	Females
N	31	22	16	13
Mean	54.68	48.86	61.12	49.92
SD	11.40	8.39	10.14	10.79

more depressed in comparison to the females, irrespective of whether they rated themselves "good" or "poor." However, the males who rated themselves "poor" scored as being the most depressed of all of the groups studied.

Despite the small samples involved, these data indicate that depression as a characteristic of adjustment might be an important factor in the successful use of speechreading in adulthood. Stated differently, it seems that a deaf adult who views himself as having poor speechreading proficiency might be unduly depressed. His feelings of worthlessness may cause him to rate himself as being incapable, or these feelings may impede his proficiency in speechreading. If the latter is the actual situation, attention to his problem of adjustment might increase his skill as a speechreader.

The personality characteristic of Hysteria also was found to be associated with self-ratings in speechreading, but again the relationship pertained only to the males. The males who rated themselves "poor" scored as being significantly more hysterical in comparison to those who rated themselves as being "good" speechreaders. Moreover, the males who rated themselves "poor" scored higher on Hysteria than the females who rated themselves as "poor." These results are shown in Tables 63 and 64. The samples are small

TABLE 63.   Hysteria scores for males who rated themselves "good"
and "poor" in speechreading

	N	Mean	SD
Good	31	51.26	8.85
Poor	16	58.06	7.18

TABLE 64.   Hysteria scores for males and females who rated themselves
"poor" in speechreading

	N	Mean	SD
Males	16	58.06	7.18
Females	13	50.08	6.38

and inferences must be drawn with caution. Nevertheless, these results again show the females to be more adequate and better adjusted than the males. Furthermore, for the males there was a significant relationship between Hysteria and self-ratings in personality; the "good" were distinctly more normal on this factor. These data suggest that the deaf male adult who rates himself as being a "good" speechreader can be expected to have more wholesome attitudes, to be more realistic and stable than the adult who rates himself as a "poor" speechreader.

The results of this analysis of the relationship between emotional adjustment and self-ratings in speechreading are intriguing and suggest the importance of further investigation. One implication is that emotional factors in relation to this language function are more influential in males than in females. Only further study can clarify this problem. There is the provocative possibility also that success in speechreading is a factor in the emotional adjustment of the adult deaf. At least to some extent these data indicate that inferior speechreading ability is related to greater emotional disturbance. As in other areas of learning, it can be assumed that acquiring proficiency in speechreading will be impeded by undue emotional conflict, whereas emotional stability will enhance such learning. Emotional factors in relation to speechreading seem to be of importance and warrant further investigation.

Speech and Expressive Language

Speech and writing are Man's basic verbal expressive language systems, but speech precedes writing developmentally by five or six years. Considerably more maturity organismically is required before writing can be accomplished. Speech is possible by one year of age, and as McCarthy[15] and Templin[27] have shown, increases rapidly until the age of five to six years in normal children. However, unless the child *receives* and comprehends the spoken word, speech, his spoken language will not ensue. The deaf child, because of his auditory deficiency, does not receive the spoken word; hence, he does not acquire speech. Except for the hard of hearing who can be aided by amplification, the hearing impaired child must receive verbal language non-auditorily through channels other than audition. To develop oral expressive language (speech), he must convert the symbol he receives through one sensory channel into another verbal system. The complexity of this problem has been emphasized in Chapter IX. Our purpose here is to consider speech in terms of spoken language and to relate it to other aspects of language development in children with profound deafness.

In the past more emphasis has been given to the mechanics of speech production, to factors influencing intelligibility, than to speech as expressive language. Speech production presents difficult and complex problems in children with severely impaired hearing but through workers such as Hudgins,[11] much knowledge has been gained. Less is known about speech as spoken language. Perhaps increased knowledge of speech as language will be beneficial also in connection with intelligibility.

In our National Study of language development in deaf children, the teachers were asked to rate the children's ability to use spoken language. The rating scale used was *excellent, good, average, fair,* and *poor*. For statistical analysis those rated excellent, good, and average were compared to those rated fair and poor. The per cent of the total number of children rated as having a high and a low level of ability in spoken language is shown in Table 65. These results, like those for speechreading, show that more females than males were rated as having good proficiency in spoken language, a difference which was true for both the Day and Residential groups. However, the variation by sex was less for those in Day Schools. More Residential males than any other group were rated as being "fair-poor" in speech. Nevertheless, there is agreement between Day and Residential School teachers that less than one-half of the males achieve average or above average proficiency in spoken language. The ratings are comparable also for the females although the Day School teachers rated more girls as being proficient. These findings are in agreement with those on speechreading in demonstrating a sex difference in deaf children in the

TABLE 65. The percent of children rated excellent-good-average and fair-poor in spoken language

	Males		Females	
	Day	Residential	Day	Residential
Excellent-good-average	44%	36%	56%	50%
Fair-poor	56%	64%	44%	50%

acquisition of language. Because of the consistency of these findings, it is apparent that this variation in successful learning must be further investigated and possibly different methods devised to meet the needs of each sex more effectively.

Spoken Language and Intelligence

It is of importance psychologically and educationally to ascertain the extent to which mental capacity is influential in the acquisition of spoken language by children having profound deafness from early life. That ability to communicate orally is related to intellectual development in normal children has been demonstrated by several workers.[6, 27]

The children rated excellent-good-average in speech proficiency were compared in intelligence with those who were rated fair-poor. The results are given in Table 66. As can be seen from the mean scores, the intelligence levels for the groups are very similar; statistical analysis revealed no significant differences. In contrast to the findings for speechreading, proficiency in spoken language as rated by teachers was found to be unrelated to intelligence as measured by the Draw-a-Man Test.

This result is provocative and challenging because it is difficult to find an explanation. It might be assumed that to some degree all language functions are related to mental capacity. The lack of such a relationship in our results may be due to the nature of the test used or to the type of ratings secured. The Draw-a-Man Test is essentially a *visual* mental test and speechreading is primarily a *visual* task, perhaps explaining the correlation found between intelligence and ability to speechread. By comparison, spoken language for the deaf includes kinesthetic factors. Therefore, by inference, correlation with mental ability as measured by the Draw-a-Man

TABLE 66. Relationship between ability to use spoken language and intelligence

	Males			Females			Total		
	N	Mean	SD	N	Mean	SD	N	Mean	SD
Day School									
Excellent-good-average	67	93.85	14.40	78	94.86	13.61	145	93.39	13.94
Fair-poor	84	92.34	14.71	64	93.36	12.60	148	92.78	13.80
Residential School									
Excellent-good-average	97	97.14	14.62	121	93.76	16.69	218	95.27	15.86
Fair-poor	172	94.99	15.65	120	90.08	16.31	293	92.98	16.08

Test would be lowered. If a test such as the Van der Lugt Motor Memory Test[29] were used, correlation with spoken language might appear. We cannot state that because a lack of such an association was shown by our results, intelligence is unimportant in the acquisition of oral language. Rather, further study using various types of mental tests might be expected to reveal quite the contrary.

Another consideration in connection with our findings is the extent to which speech per se was confounded with speech as spoken language. It is conceivable that the articulation of speech by deaf children is less related to intelligence than spoken language. Perhaps the ratings by the teachers, in a large measure, included intelligibility in which case it would be expected that correlation with intelligence would be lessened. In Chapter IX we stressed the complexity of the psychological, monitoring processes involved in the production of intelligible speech by deaf children. The nature of these processes, the learning and skills entailed, have not been studied extensively.

However, Brannon[1a] conducted an ingenious new type of investigation of the speech production of deaf children. With electronic techniques of the biomedical engineering type and using a control group of hearing children, he analyzed ways in which deafness alters speech. The procedure included a glossal transducer for conversion of tongue motions into a moving record which could be observed on an oscilloscopic screen. In essence this made it possible to provide a visual feedback of motor speech output. By observing the oscilloscopic record while talking, the deaf child could see the deviations of his pattern from that of the hearing inasmuch as both patterns could be observed simultaneously.

The findings reported by Brannon are revealing and indicate the extreme difficulty the deaf child has in monitoring his speech utterances by other than auditory means. In comparison with the hearing the tongue motions of the deaf were slower and more labored. Moreover, they made unnecessary glossal movements; as the length of the utterances increased, the number of excess motions became greater. There was no correlation between intelligence and success in producing intelligible speech, confirming the findings of our National Survey.

One of the more challenging aspects of this study is the manner in which it provided a ratio between input and output. A score was computed for input (speechreading and reading) and output (speech intelligibility). The hypothesis, based on the concept discussed in Chapter IX, was that in speaking the deaf child must convert a visual (input) into an auditory (output) verbal system. Brannon concluded that the conversion loss for speechreading to speech was 52%, and for reading to speech, 78%.

Such data make it possible to more specifically indicate the remedial training needs of the deaf child. Methods must be found to help him convert one type of information into another. Progress is being made in the development of both visual and tactile means for providing a feedback of the speech produced. When this can be accomplished more successfully and when the deaf child has learned to use this type of information, it seems reasonable to assume that he will find it possible to monitor his speech more effectively and thus speak more intelligibly.

Spoken Language, Reading, and Writing

In our investigations of language behavior in children having deafness as well as those having language disorders due to neurological deficits, we found an intercorrelation between language functions. Such relationships were shown to be present in the case of speechreading. To explore more fully the spoken word as a language process in deaf children, we compared their proficiency in oral language with their competence in reading and writing. The results, showing the relationship between spoken and read language, are presented in Table 67; the Columbia Vocabulary Test was used to measure reading achievement.

TABLE 67. Relationship between reading scores and ratings in spoken language

	Males			Females			Total		
	N	Mean	SD	N	Mean	SD	N	Mean	SD
Day School									
Excellent-good-average	69	8.32	10.21	85	11.00	9.50	154	9.80	9.88
Fair-poor	87	4.08	5.90	66	5.18	6.04	153	4.56	5.97
Residential School									
Excellent-good-average	76	8.62	9.00	105	8.34	8.92	181	8.46	8.93
Fair-poor	149	4.68	6.05	109	5.52	6.40	258	5.04	6.20

The differences between the mean scores were statistically significant in all instances. The children rated as having good proficiency in spoken language showed substantially higher reading ability in comparison to those who were rated low. Although both groups were retarded in reading as shown in Chapter XI, those with the greater competence in spoken language scored approximately twice as high in reading as those who were rated below average in speech proficiency. These results are further evidence that a deaf child who shows success in one type of verbal behavior is likely to show competence in other types. Furthermore, it highlights the reciprocality, the interdependence of symbol systems. As stressed in Chapter IX, although output follows input, expressive and receptive language are related, and proficiency in one enhances the level of function in the other. The richness of the inner language seems to be critically influential.

SENTENCE LENGTH: The ratings in spoken language were analyzed also according to the three scores obtained on the Picture Story Language Test, Sentence Length, Syntax, and Abstract-Concrete Thought. The results comparing the groups on Sentence Length scores are presented in Table 68. With the exception of the males in Residential Schools, the differences between the mean scores were statistically significant. Except for this male group, those rated as being most proficient in spoken language wrote sentences of greater length in comparison with those rated low in ability to communicate orally. For most of the population the expressive language functions of speaking and writing were associated. Success in one of these verbal functions was indicative of competence in the other.

TABLE 68. Relationship between ratings in spoken language and scores on Sentence Length

	Males			Females			Total		
	N	Mean	SD	N	Mean	SD	N	Mean	SD
Day School									
Excellent-good-average	69	6.17	3.74	86	6.39	3.02	155	6.29	3.15
Fair-poor	78	4.25	2.26	63	4.98	3.15	141	4.57	2.87
Residential School									
Excellent-good-average	80	5.90	3.86	109	6.40	3.18	189	6.19	3.48
Fair-poor	159	4.95	3.54	99	5.40	3.55	258	5.12	3.54

SYNTAX: Proficiency in spoken language was evaluated further in terms of its being associated with ability to use correct Syntax in written language. These results are given in Table 69. Again, the only group for which the differences were not statistically significant was the Residential School males. For all of the other groups the differences favored those who were rated most competent in spoken language, revealing that those most proficient in oral communication scored highest on Syntax, on use of correct grammatical construction when writing a story.

TABLE 69. Relationship between ratings in spoken language and scores on Syntax

	Males			Females			Total		
	N	Mean	SD	N	Mean	SD	N	Mean	SD
Day School									
Excellent-good-average	69	70	28	86	79	25	155	75	25
Fair-poor	78	56	25	63	61	26	141	58	25
Residential School									
Excellent-good-average	80	65	26	109	78	20	189	73	23
Fair-poor	159	61	29	99	63	27	258	62	28

The effect of deafness on the development of abstract mental ability was discussed in Chapter V. To investigate more specifically the relationship between abstract thought and verbal functioning, we devised a scale for quantifying the nature of the ideation expressed in writing a story; this scale is discussed further in Chapter XII. The speech proficiency groups were compared on the basis of their scores on this Abstract-Concrete Scale. As can be seen from the results in Table 70, significant differences were found for all but the Residential male group. Except for these males those having the greater competence in spoken language used a higher degree of abstraction than those who were rated low in ability to commu-

TABLE 70. Relationship between ratings in spoken language and scores on the Abstract-Concrete Scale

	Males			Females			Total		
	N	Mean	SD	N	Mean	SD	N	Mean	SD
Day School									
Excellent-good-average	69	10.44	6.11	86	13.26	5.45	155	12.01	5.46
Fair-poor	78	8.19	5.85	62	8.35	6.00	140	8.71	5.93
Residential School									
Excellent-good-average	80	9.45	6.04	109	11.61	5.63	189	10.70	5.89
Fair-poor	159	8.01	5.96	98	9.51	6.10	257	8.58	6.05

nicate orally. As in the case of speechreading, spoken language facility was associated with the use of abstract concepts. Apparently, although other factors seem to be involved, verbal facility cannot be separated from the development of this important psychological function.

SUMMARY: One of the revealing outcomes of the analysis of spoken language was the lack of relationship found between the verbal functions in the Residential male group. These results are in agreement with those for speechreading where this group also deviated from the characteristic pattern. While the reading scores were correlated with ratings in speechreading for these males, such a relationship was not found for the other verbal functions. Likewise, their ratings in spoken language proficiency correlated significantly with reading but not with Sentence Length, Syntax, or Abstract-Concrete behavior; the results for this group were consistent from one verbal function to another.

The Residential School environment apparently influences males in ways which do not pertain to the females. It is unlikely that factors such as intelligence, degree of deafness, or age of onset are important in the variation of verbal performance in this group. Rather, as indicated in the discussion of the speechreading results, one suspects that Residential School environment produces varying effects in the psychic structure and organization for males and females. In any event from this analysis of spoken language proficiency as rated by teachers, we find that the females are more successful than males in acquiring this type of verbal facility. While actual sex differences seem to be present, there is an indication also that the schools and the methods used in teaching the deaf are more suitable for the females; the Residential School environment favors the females in learning.

This analysis indicates further that it is of considerable consequence to view the deaf child's speech as spoken language. While factors which influence intelligibility must not be neglected, spoken language is an integral part of the child's total verbal facility. Because the symbol systems are interrelated psychologically, development of spoken language should be considered a part of the child's total language development.

AUDITORY TRAINING, DEGREE OF DEAFNESS, AND LANGUAGE DEVELOPMENT

Over a period of time workers such as Pintner[22] and Pugh[23] have investigated the relationship between language development and the factors of age of onset and degree of deafness. In our study data were gathered concerning the degree of the hearing loss, the number wearing hearing aids, as well as the number receiving auditory training. It is obvious that the more residual hearing, the less severe will be the problem of language acquisition. Costello[2] has shown that a relationship exists between speechreading and the degree of deafness, the hard of hearing being superior to the deaf. Nevertheless, unwarranted assumptions might be made. The significance of limited remnants of hearing as far as language development is concerned, and perhaps in other respects, seem to have been overestimated. Small remnants of hearing near the borderline for total loss audiometrically, on the basis of experience with auditory training, apparently are not of major advantage in the development of language. Exact limits or "cut-off" points audiometrically remain to be established. The work of Wedenberg[31] and Huizing[12] indicates progress in this connection.

To explore relationships between the degree of deafness and learning we classified the children into three groups and compared them on the basis of intelligence. The groups consisted of those having a hearing loss on the better ear of less than 65 db, between 66 and 85 db, and between 86 and 100 db. The results showing the mean IQ for each group on the Draw-a-Man Test are presented in Table 71. From these data it can be seen that the population studied fell into the category of profound deafness. Of the total, 54 per cent had a hearing loss of 86 db or greater, 30 per cent had a degree of deafness which fell between 66 and 85 db, and 16 per cent had a loss of less than 65 db; 84 per cent had a hearing loss of

TABLE 71. The relationship between degree of deafness and scores on the Draw-a-Man Test

| | 0–65 db | | | 66–85 db | | | 86–100 db | | |
	N	Mean	SD	N	Mean	SD	N	Mean	SD
Males	67	92.86	13.79	121	93.60	15.06	208	94.90	15.33
Females	52	91.73	14.70	108	91.80	15.31	207	94.73	15.58
Total	119	92.37	13.90	229	92.75	15.17	415	94.82	15.42

more than 65 db. When these groups were compared on intelligence no differences appeared; they were comparable intellectually as measured by the Draw-a-Man Test. Occasionally it has been assumed that if a child has a moderate deafness superimposed on mental retardation, he would be placed in a school for the deaf. This presumption is not supported by these findings.

The information secured regarding the use of amplification revealed that proportionately many more children in the Day Schools than in the Residential Schools were wearing hearing aids. Again the factor of intelligence was investigated; the results are given in Table 72. Statistical tests disclosed no significant differences in mean IQ scores for those wearing and those not wearing hearing aids. As far as these results are concerned, hearing aid use was unrelated to intelligence.

TABLE 72. Comparison of those wearing and not wearing hearing aids on Draw-a-Man Test scores

	Males			Females			Total		
	N	Mean	SD	N	Mean	SD	N	Mean	SD
Day									
Yes	65	92.66	16.56	77	96.27	14.29	142	94.62	15.42
No	82	92.83	13.44	68	93.47	11.35	150	93.12	12.50
Residential									
Yes	71	92.28	15.38	74	94.16	18.06	145	94.71	16.84
No	186	95.70	15.09	157	90.82	15.46	343	93.47	15.43

TABLE 73. Hearing aid use and success in reading as measured by the Columbia Vocabulary Test

	Males			Females			Total		
	N	Mean	SD	N	Mean	SD	N	Mean	SD
Day									
Yes	62	6.24	9.37	78	8.14	8.75	140	7.30	9.04
No	80	6.23	7.98	63	9.38	8.86	143	7.62	8.50
Residential									
Yes	60	6.58	8.66	67	5.36	5.99	127	5.94	7.37
No	159	5.97	6.95	143	7.75	8.55	302	6.82	7.78

The hearing aid users and non-users were compared also on the basis of their scores on the Columbia Vocabulary Test. These results are shown in Table 73. Statistically significant differences did not appear; those wearing and those not wearing hearing aids showed equal reading ability. While these findings are in general agreement with other workers such as Costello and Pugh, the implications are provocative and complex. The need to establish "cutoff" points for the limits of practical usefulness of hearing is highlighted. Further evidence is given in Chapter XII, because although many more Day School children wore hearing aids, they were not found to be superior in language. Therefore, the findings given in Table 73 and the results presented in Chapter XII are highly complimentary. Nevertheless, other considerations are necessary.

Perhaps the question of serviceableness of residual hearing is complicated by the *type* of language function under study. A certain remnant of hearing might be beneficial for the development of speech but be of minor value in the development of read or of written language. On the other hand this hypothesis must be used with caution and tested carefully because there are significant relationships between all types of language systems; success in one is related to success in the others.

From the point of view of objective evidence, these findings of no relationship between hearing aid use and reading, we cannot avoid the inference that there has been undue optimism in regard to the significance of limited remnants of hearing. Beyond a certain point, which has not been well established, apparently the degree of deafness is of substantially less consequence than the factors of intelligence, personality, and verbal aptitude. This might be anticipated on the basis of the frame of reference stated in Chapters IV and IX.

Psychologically the individual is "deaf," his behavior is altered, learning occurs through different channels even though his audiogram shows certain degrees of residual hearing. We have stressed that the person's alteration of behavior begins as soon as his hearing loss deprives him of background sound, usually when his impairment exceeds 40 to 50 db. Fortunately such a loss does not seriously interfere with language behavior. While it may be premature to speculate regarding the point beyond which hearing is of little value in the language development of a congenitally deaf child, present evidence suggests that it is not as close to the threshold for total loss as has been assumed. In other words such a child may have definite audiometric indications of hearing on the speech range but show no advantage in language acquisition. We anticipate that in the next decade much definitive information will be available concerning this important problem.

IMPLICATIONS FOR LEARNING AND LANGUAGE DEVELOPMENT

There are a number of implications of the material presented in this chapter. We have seen that an interrelationship exists between speech and speechreading and other language functions. In regard to the frame of reference given in Chapter IX, the data support the hypothesis that inner language is the basis of both receptive and expressive language. Furthermore, inasmuch as speechreading shows conjunction with the other verbal systems, it fulfills the requisites of an adequate receptive language. If inner and receptive language are established the other verbal systems of spoken, read, and written language can be expected to follow.

Intelligence was shown to be an influential factor in language learning. However, in the presence of marked degrees of deafness, the use of a hearing aid seems not to be related to success in language usage. The implication is that beyond a certain degree of deafness, the more consequential factors in addition to intelligence are personality and special aptitudes. From the results of the Residential School males there is a strong suggestion that sex and type of school experience also are of importance in the verbal behavior of the deaf child. All males were inferior to the females but the language behavior of the Residential males was different from that of the other groups. There is little question but that the symbolic processes used by this group were not comparable to those used by the other groups. It seems that the natural inferiority of the males, their greater limitation in verbal learning, is increased by the Residential School environment. There is an indication that current educational programs comparatively are more successful with females than with males. Further analysis of these sex differences is needed and additional consideration of this problem is given in Chapter XII.

REFERENCES

1. Blair, F.: A study of the visual memory of deaf and hearing children. Am. Ann. Deaf, 102, 254, 1957.
1a. Brannon, J.: Visual feedback of glossal motions and its influence upon the speech of deaf children. Unpublished doctoral dissertation, Northwestern University, 1964.

2. Costello, M. R.: A study of speechreading as a developing language process in deaf and in hard of hearing children. Evanston, Northwestern University, Unpublished Doctoral Dissertation, 1957.

3. Gansl, I. and Garrett, H.: Columbia Vocabulary Test. New York, Psychol. Corp., 1939.

4. Gates, A.: Manual of Directions for Gates Reading Survey. New York, Columbia University, Bureau of Publications, 1953.

5. Gault, R.: Touch as a substitute for hearing in the interpretation and control of speech. Arch. Otolaryng., 3, 121, 1926.

6. Gesell, A. et al.: The First Five Years of Life. New York, Harper, 1940.

7. Goda, S.: Language skills of profoundly deaf adolescent children. J. Speech and Hearing Research, 2, 369, 1959.

8. Goodenough, F.: Measurement of Intelligence by Drawings. New York, World Book, 1926.

9. Hathaway, S. and McKinley, J.: Minnesota Multiphasic Personality Inventory: Manual. (Revised) New York, Psychol. Corp., 1951.

10. Heider, F. and Heider, G.: Studies in the psychology of the deaf. Psychol. Monog., #242, 1941.

11. Hudgins, C. and Numbers, M.: An investigation of the intelligibility of the speech of the deaf. Genetic Psychol. Monog., 25, 384, 1942.

12. Huizing, H.: Assessment and evaluation of hearing anomalies in young children. Groningen, University of Groningen, Proceedings of International Course in Paedo-Audiology, 1953.

13. Kitson, H.: Psychological tests for lip-reading ability. Volta Review, 17, 471, 1915.

14. Knox, H.: A scale based on the work at Ellis Island for estimating mental defect. J. Am. Med. Assoc., 62, 741, 1914.

15. McCarthy, D.: Language development in children, in Carmichael, L. Manual of Child Psychology. New York, John Wiley and Sons, 1946.

16. Mason, M.: A laboratory method of measuring visual hearing ability. Volta Review, 34, 510, 1932.

17. Morkovin, B. and Moore, L.: Life-situation speech-reading through the co-operation of the senses. Los Angeles, University of California Press, 1948.

18. Myklebust, H.: The Picture Story Language Test. Evanston, Northwestern University. To be published.

19. Nitchie, E.: Synthesis and intuition in lip-reading. Volta Review, 15, 311, 1913.

20. O'Neill, J. and Davidson, J.: Relationship between lipreading ability and five psychological factors. J. Speech Hearing Disorders, 4, 478, 1956.

21. Pintner, R.: Speech and speech-reading for the deaf. J. Applied Psychol., 13, 220, 1929.

22. _____, Eisenson, J. and Stanton, M.: The Psychology of the Physically Handicapped. New York, F. S. Crofts, 1946.

23. Pugh, G.: Appraisal of the silent reading abilities of acoustically handicapped children. Am. Ann. Deaf, 91, 331, 1946.

24. Raven, J.: Guide to Using the Progressive Matrices. London, Lewis, 1938.

25. Simmons, A.: Factors related to lip reading. J. Speech and Hearing Research, 2, 340, 1959.

26. Story, A.: Speech Reading and Speech for the Deaf. Stoke-on-Trent, Hill and Ainsworth, 1915.

27. Templin, M.: Certain Language Skills in Children. Minneapolis, University of Minnesota Press, 1957.
28. Utley, J.: A test of lipreading ability. J. Speech Hearing Disorders, 11, 109, 1946.
29. Van der Lugt, M.: Psychomotor Test Series for Children. New York, New York University Press, 1948.
30. Wechsler, D.: The Measurement of Adult Intelligence. Baltimore, Williams and Wilkins, 1944.
31. Wedenberg, E.: Auditory training of deaf and hard of hearing children. Acta Oto-laryngol. Suppl. 94, 1951.

Suggestions for Further Study

Hardy, W., Pauls, M. and Haskins, H.: An analysis of language development in children with impaired hearing. Acta Oto-laryng. Suppl. #141, 1958.

Harris, G.: Language for the Preschool Deaf Child, Second Edition. New York, Grune and Stratton, 1963.

Hudgins, C.: Voice production and breath control in the speech of the deaf. Am. Ann. Deaf, 82, 338, 1937.

Myklebust, H.: Language training: A comparison between children with aphasia and those with deafness. Am. Ann. Deaf, 101, 240, 1956.

Numbers, M. and Hudgins, C.: Speech perception in present day education for deaf children. Volta Review, 50, 449, 1948.

O'Neill, J.: An exploratory investigation of lipreading ability among normal hearing students. Speech Monog., 18, 309, 1951.

Peterson, G.: Influence of voice quality. Volta Review, 48, 640, 1946.

Reid, G.: A preliminary investigation in the testing of lipreading achievement. J. Speech Hearing Disorders, 12, 77, 1947.

Stobschinski, R.: Lip-reading; its psychological aspects and its adaptation to the individual needs of the hard of hearing. Am. Ann. Deaf, 73, 234, 1928.

Templin, M.: Certain Language Skills in Children. Minneapolis, University of Minnesota Press, 1957.

Chapter XI

READ AND WRITTEN LANGUAGE

LANGUAGE HAS BEEN VARIOUSLY DEFINED. As emphasized in Chapter IX, we use the term *language* to designate the process of transforming experience into a system of verbal symbols; the system may be auditory (speech) or it may be visual (reading and writing). We have stated also that in the normal child reading initially is achieved by relating the visual word to the auditory and that writing is the expressive, reciprocal phase of read language.

When deafness is present and auditory language cannot be established, different psychological processes must be involved in learning to read. The evidence presented in Chapter X indicates a relationship between reading, speech, and speechreading. Knowledge regarding the nature of this association might have important implications for the psychology of reading in deaf children. We have suggested that for the deaf child speechreading is the basic inner and receptive language. In reading and in speechreading vision is the monitoring channel and the avenue of reception. If there is a direct relationship between the receptive language, speechreading, and the receptive language, reading, might it not be possible to develop a method for teaching reading based on the reciprocality of the two language systems? Can we assume that reading is related to speechreading as speech is related to comprehension of the spoken word? While this possibility exists, unfortunately the reciprocality between speechreading and reading seems more complex despite the fact that both are visual symbol systems.

Intelligence is a major factor in learning to read, a mental age of at least six years being required. That intellectual capacity is of importance in learning to speechread is revealed by the discussion in Chapter X. However, the minimum mental age necessary has not been established. Some hearing impaired children have been observed to begin speechreading by 12 to 18 months of age, considerably earlier than for reading. If we assume that a child has sustained speechreading facility by seven years of age, should he not then be able to relate the read word to the speechread word as the normally hearing child relates the read and the heard word? Such a possiblity warrants attention and possibly deliberate attempts at experimental verification.

To analyze further the process of learning to read when deafness is present from infancy, it is revealing to consider the neurological areas which might be involved. Comprehension of the spoken word is dependent primarily upon the temporal lobe while speaking is dependent chiefly upon the frontal lobe. Nature has provided a means whereby these areas can function in a coordinated manner in the auditory comprehending-speaking process. Likewise, neurologists have demonstrated that reading is vitally dependent upon the occipital lobe. The area of the brain chiefly responsible for the ability to speechread has not been determined definitely, but as indicated by the discussion in Chapter XIII there is evidence which suggests that the parietal lobe is of major importance. Therefore, if the read word is to be related to the speechread word initially and developmentally, integration of the occipital and parietal lobes seems to be essential. Since it is known that this occurs in Man's learning, it does not present a unique neurological prerequisite to the hearing impaired.

Psychologically there may be more complex and difficult problems. In Chapter IX it was suggested that normally letters are learned first as pictures of sounds and spoken words. The deaf child must relate the written word form to what the sounds *look* like when seen on the speaker's lips. That this is a more difficult learning process in comparison to relating the *heard* and written form is testified to by all who are experienced in the education of the deaf. Why it is more difficult remains to be ascertained specifically, but various factors may be involved. If the deaf child's inner and receptive language are not equivalent to the inner and receptive language of the hearing child, his acquisition of reading will be impeded. The problem here is the adequacy of the verbal-symbolic system acquired *first* because the read symbol system must be superimposed on the one acquired initially. The last acquired system is dependent on the fluidity, flexibility, and subtlety of the first.

Another consideration is the effectiveness of present methods and procedures for teaching language to children with profound deafness. Perhaps present experience is not a test of the hypothesis stated here. If speechreading were developed as the basic inner and receptive language and if reading were taught deliberately by procedures designed to foster association between the written and speechread forms of the word, perhaps the deaf child would be more successful in his total language development. Only further study can provide conclusive evidence, but with our present knowledge, it seems that major effort might be expended in this direction. In other words, to achieve his highest potential, it seems that the deaf child initially must learn to read by relating the written word to the speechread form of the word. As he becomes a competent reader he will learn to "by-pass" the speechread form as the hearing individual competent in reading learns to "by-pass" the auditory form. The individual with deafness would "regress" to the speechread form and "visualize it out" when he encounters a difficult, unfamiliar word as the hearing person regresses and "sounds out" the word under similar circumstances.

READING AND EDUCATIONAL ACHIEVEMENT

Many studies of reading and the general educational attainment of hearing impaired children have been made in the past few decades. The investigations of Reamer[25] and Pugh[24] are noteworthy examples. The most commonly used measure has been the standard achievement test. While the use of such tests has been of value, many educators have questioned their face validity when used with deaf children. As with other psychological tests, the assumptions of standard achievement tests are not always valid when used with an individual having sensory deprivation and a marked limitation of language. For example, many of the items are of the multiple choice type, involving a task in which the child is to choose the word that applies to a picture. Likewise, in word meaning the requirement might be to underline the proper word for the incomplete sentence, while in paragraph meaning the problem might consist of underlining the phrase that conveys the fundamental message of the paragraph.

The *assumption* is that if the child can choose the proper word or phrase, he *comprehends the meaning*. Such an assumption usually is valid for normal children, for children who have a wealth of language at their disposal; the judgments and the other psychological processes involved conform to assumptions made in standardizing the test. For the deaf child these assumptions usually do not hold and, hence, the validity of the test scores must be reappraised. Typically the child with profound deafness does not make his choice and respond on the basis of the total meaning of the sentence or of the paragraph; such a procedure is too difficult for him. Rather, he makes his choice by *matching* words from the possible responses with words in the sentence or in the paragraph. If he sees the words *father, mother,* or *town* in the paragraph, he chooses the response which most closely matches these words. He is not guided mainly by the meaning of the passage because usually he does not comprehend it. This process of matching might result in a correct response and in an erroneously high score. Many such artifacts seem to be occurring through the use of tests of this type.

Another source of error, of invalidity, is the opportunity for chance successes. If only two possible responses are provided for a test item, the child has a 50-50 chance of success irrespective of his language and educational attainment; if there are three possible choices, the chance factor is one out of three. Again, it must be stressed that limitations such as these are not critical when the tests are used with normal children. However, when used with deaf children these factors do become critical and often result in spurious test scores.

In general, there has been agreement amongst studies covering a period of years that children deaf from early life are retarded at least three years in educational attainment, corroborated recently by the investigations of Costello,[8] Blair,[5] and Fuller.[12] As part of our National Study of the psychology of deafness we included a test of reading. The intent was to appraise the relationship between reading and the other verbal symbol systems used by deaf children. Despite the limitations of standard achievement tests as discussed above, a test of this type was used. The one selected, the Columbia Vocabulary Test,[13] is simple to administer and provides a measure of reading vocabulary. To recapitulate, in our National Study in addition to obtaining ratings of both speechreading and speech, a measure was secured of the child's competence in read and written language. The reading test results are given in Table 74 and include the mean scores by age for the Day and the Residential School children as well as for the control group of normal children.

TABLE 74. Comparison between deaf and normal children on reading vocabulary

| | Deaf | | | Normal | | |
	N	Mean	SD	N	Mean	SD
Age nine						
Males	65	3.24	2.68	19	19.89	8.20
Females	73	3.18	2.10	24	22.67	7.01
Total	138	3.21	2.38	43	21.37	7.61
Age eleven						
Males	83	5.00	6.11	33	33.33	10.20
Females	81	7.15	6.84	27	33.52	11.01
Total	164	6.06	6.55	60	33.42	10.43
Age thirteen						
Males	67	9.32	10.42	24	42.12	8.35
Females	75	10.86	7.99	27	44.44	8.50
Total	142	10.13	9.22	51	43.35	8.34
Age fifteen						
Males	61	11.09	7.23	22	63.64	10.91
Females	59	11.57	8.05	25	63.00	12.91
Total	120	11.32	7.62	47	63.30	11.89

While norms are available for the Columbia Vocabulary Test, we administered it to our control group of normal children. The mean scores by age as shown in Table 74 are virtually identical to those secured by Gansl and Garrett[13] in their standardization. Therefore, these scores for normal children can be considered as being reliable and as providing a firm basis of comparison for the scores for the hearing impaired children. Statistical analysis disclosed no sex differences in the normal population. The males and the females showed marked growth in their reading vocabulary at each two year interval from nine through 15 years, the age range covered, with the greater increment falling between 13 and 15 years. There seems to have been more rapid progress in reading as the child became older, suggesting that reading maturity is dependent upon high levels of competence psychologically, a finding which supports the description of the hierarchies of symbol systems given in Chapter IX.

The comparison of scores for the deaf and the normal revealed that those with sensory deprivation were severely retarded, the differences being statistically significant at the 1 per cent level of confidence at all age levels and for both sexes. Furthermore, as

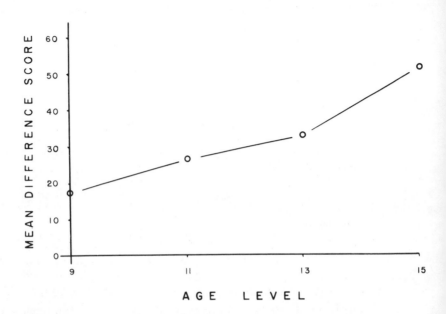

FIG. 20. Results showing retardation for deaf children in Read Language as age increases.

shown by Figure 20, the degree of retardation increased with age, a trend which was opposite to that found for the hearing. The data provided other indications of the severity of the read language deficit in deaf children. At nine years of age the mean score for the hearing impaired was 3.21 while for the normal at this age level, it was 21.37. At 15 years of age the mean score for the deaf was 11.32 while for the hearing it was 63.30. The total increment for the deaf was 8.11 points and for the hearing, 41.93. Comparatively, the child with profound deafness shows much less progression and growth in the acquisition of a reading vocabulary. As he reaches the age at which the hearing child completes high school, his ability to read is below that of the average nine year old child, or below the third grade level. These results indicate that when he completes his regular schooling, the deaf child is retarded seven to eight years in reading vocabulary. This does not mean that he is retarded in his general educational attainment to this extent, but because of its importance as a tool subject, this deficit in reading will greatly influence his academic progress. Although somewhat greater, the degree of retardation shown by our results is in general agreement with the findings of others.

Read Language in Day and Residential Schools

The comparison between the Day and Residential groups was considered important in the study of language behavior. Most of the children in the Residential Schools use the manual sign language for social purposes. While some Day School children also use this means of communication, as a whole they are more dependent on oral language. The manual sign language is the "native tongue," the inner language symbol system, in the case of many Residential School children; this can be presumed to be less true of children in Day Schools. Inasmuch as these groups did not differ in the degree of hearing loss, in the age of onset, or in intelligence, it might be postulated that any differences in verbal language behavior would be explicable on the basis of the effect of the sign language. We noted in Chapter X that there were no major differences in the Day and the Residential School children when rated by teachers on their success in speechreading or in speech; the trends were similar for both groups. Here the question of similarity is raised specifically in regard to read language. The mean scores on the Columbia Vocabulary Test by school, sex, and age are given in Table 75.

Statistical analysis revealed no clear superiority of either group; however, the significant differences favored the Day School children. The results show that there were no differences at the nine year level; at 11 years the Day School females and the total Day exceeded the total Residential group; there were no significant differences at the 13 year level; at 15 years the Day School females were superior to the females in Residential Schools, and the total Day exceeded the total Residential group. There were no statistically significant diffrences by sex, also true for the hearing, but the inferiority comparatively of the females in Residential Schools again was apparent. It must be recalled that this group showed inferiority in intelligence. In fact, at the 15 year level the differ-

TABLE 75.   Comparison between Day and Residential School children
on reading vocabulary

	Day			Residential		
	N	Mean	SD	N	Mean	SD
Age nine						
Males	37	3.78	3.37	28	2.53	1.02
Females	37	3.66	2.83	36	2.68	0.56
Total	74	3.72	3.09	64	2.61	0.79
Age eleven						
Males	23	7.54	9.23	60	4.03	4.08
Females	38	9.03	8.18	43	5.49	4.85
Total	61	8.47	8.55	103	4.64	4.48
Age thirteen						
Males	38	8.91	10.37	29	9.87	10.64
Females	38	12.53	8.84	37	9.14	6.71
Total	76	10.72	9.75	66	9.46	8.59
Age fifteen						
Males	21	12.86	8.72	40	10.16	6.24
Females	17	18.35	8.01	42	8.83	6.23
Total	38	15.32	8.75	82	9.48	6.28

ences between the Day and Residential groups seem attributable to this factor; the mean scores for the males were very similar.

If there were clear superiority of one group, one type of school over the other, it would be expected that significant differences would appear at each age level. Instead, no differences were found for the males; the deaf male was equally inferior in read language irrespective of whether he attended a Day or a Residential School. While differences appeared for the females, these seem to be due largely to the differences in intelligence between these groups. However, there is a possibility that the methods, procedures, and school environment of the Day School favors the female. So far as these results are concerned we cannot conclude that the Day School group is superior to the Residential in read language, suggesting that use of the sign language is not a major determining factor. To emphasize the use of signs as being a fundamental factor in the language retardation would obscure the much more important actuality of all deaf children being seriously limited in language acquisition, irrespective of the type of school or the methods and procedures used. The implication is that the sensory deprivation of deafness results in an alteration of learning processes which is fundamental and which serves as the basis of behavior. It is incumbent on workers in the psychology of deafness to further ascertain the nature of this behavior specifically as it relates to the acquisition of read language.

From the data on speechreading given in Chapter X and from the correlations presented in Table 87, it is apparent that reading is related to the other verbal symbol systems used by deaf children and as a language function, is of major importance to those with profound deafness. Hence, the psychologist and the educator are concerned with being able to predict success in reading. From the psychological appraisal of hearing impaired children, it is clear that all the good readers are not bright intellectually, and, conversely all poor readers are not mentally dull. It has been difficult to find nonverbal measures that are highly reliable indicators of verbal learning ability. Some performance tests show low correlation with academic success, as revealed by the work of Blair, Costello, and Fuller. They have demonstrated the usefulness of tests, such as the digit span, in the prediction of success in the learning of academic materials.

The findings of Farrant[10] are relevant in this connection. In a factor analytic study of the intellective abilities of deaf and hard of hearing children he found a predominant "verbal intelligence" factor. Relating this to read language, tests which significantly predicted success in reading were number ability, verbal reasoning, digit symbol, pictorial absurdities, and reasoning in figures. Through such studies a background of evidence and knowledge is being accumulated which the psychologist and educator can use to further understand the problem of read language as it relates to profound early life deafness.

WRITTEN LANGUAGE

WRITTEN LANGUAGE is the last symbol system acquired by the child and might be viewed as Man's highest level of verbal behavior. However, relatively little study has been made of the development of written language either in normal or exceptional children. In our study of language we included a measure of this verbal function so there were two indices of expressive language, spoken and written, and two indices of receptive language, reading and speechreading. It was of importance to have a measure of all of the levels of language indicated by the hierarchy of verbal symbol systems for the deaf in Figure 19. A measure of inner language could not be included. It was hypothesized that inasmuch as written language requires the highest degree of evolution and maturation and is the highest level of language used by Man, it might be an unusually revealing approach to the study of the language deficiencies resulting from deafness. Because a test with norms for hearing children was not available, The Picture Story Language Test was developed. This test consists of a picture about which the child writes a story. Among the criteria used in making the picture were: it should be of a school age child, it should show action, have a definite "figure" and "ground", and stimulate imagination. It should be appropriate and provide motivation for children from seven years through high school age and it should not be available for other purposes.

Norms for The Picture Story Language Test have been established developmentally for normal children as well as for the deaf. Data also are available for speech defective, reading disability, mentally retarded, and socially maladjusted children. Only results for the deaf in comparison with the hearing are presented here. Directions for using the test, as well as other data, can be found in the Manual for The Picture Story Language Test, by Myklebust[20]. In our studies of the deaf, group testing was done by providing a picture for each group of ten children. Three types of scores were derived. The first, *Productivity,* included the number of words written (Total Words), the number of sentences (Total Sentences), and the number of words per sentence (Words per Sentence. *Syntax,* the second score, was a measure of grammatical accuracy, the correctness of the language used, including punctuation. The third score was derived for the study of the relationships between language and thought, referred to as the *Abstract-Concrete Scale.* It is a measure of the extent to which the individual detaches himself from the stimulus. Only description of what appears in the picture, the observable, scores as marked concreteness, whereas use of imagination by giving the story a setting, a plot, or a moral, scores in the direction of abstractness. Grammatical constructions, Productivity, or other aspects of verbal facility are not included. Rather, the Abstract-Concrete Scale was devised for analyzing the relationship between facility in written language and thought processes. Because of the growing concern regarding the possibility that deafness from early life limits full development of potential for abstract behavior intellectually, this aspect of the investigation was considered important. We assumed that the results might be relevant to the question of whether deafness itself, because it limits experience, results in diminution of ability to use abstract thought or whether concreteness is primarily a function of the language deficiency.

Language Productivity

TOTAL WORDS: One of the ways in which verbal behavior can be studied is by the amount of language produced. The most common indices of Productivity are Total Words, Total Sentences, and Words per Sentence. These measures can be utilized in investigations of either spoken or written language. Templin[27] and McCarthy[18] have presented noteworthy results for spoken language, while the findings of Stormzand and O'Shea,[26] Heider and Heider,[15] Yedinack,[31] Thompson,[28] and Goda[14] are of importance in relation to written language. We compared deaf and hearing children on Productivity and the results for Total Words are shown in Table 76. Hearing children wrote longer stories at every age level except at

TABLE 76. Comparison between deaf and hearing children on Total Words

Age		Deaf			Hearing		
		N	Mean	SD	N	Mean	SD
7	Male	48	24.9	27.7	62	22.2	14.4
	Female	29	29.9	24.8	61	33.1	18.0
	Total	77	26.7	23.5	123	27.6	17.1
9	Male	83	32.5	36.5	61	83.1	43.1
	Female	78	40.7	43.0	62	97.6	58.1
	Total	161	36.5	39.9	123	90.4	51.5
11	Male	118	42.4	35.2	63	106.8	51.5
	Female	109	59.9	47.0	64	125.1	59.5
	Total	227	50.8	42.1	127	116.0	56.0
13	Male	80	68.5	59.9	63	143.5	64.3
	Female	85	86.9	63.1	62	156.0	75.5
	Total	165	78.0	62.0	125	149.7	70.1
15	Male	69	92.2	58.2	63	123.2	47.4
	Female	62	80.8	40.0	62	153.2	42.1
	Total	131	86.8	50.5	125	133.1	47.1
17	Male	25	88.0	33.1	61	158.5	61.3
	Female	26	112.2	39.9	63	164.2	62.8
	Total	51	100.3	38.3	124	161.4	61.9

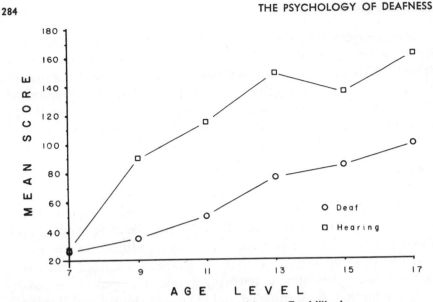

FIG. 21. Growth curves for deaf and hearing children on Total Words.

seven years. The equality at seven years can be attributed to the fact that all children at this age are just beginning to learn to use the written word. The hearing child makes rapid progress and greatly exceeds the deaf child in Total Words by nine years of age and he maintains this advantage throughout the age range studied. However, as shown in Figure 21, the growth curve for the hearing manifests a slight decrement at 15 years and then further maturation at 17 years. The same pattern appeared for the deaf females but not for the males; a decrement for the deaf males occurred at the 17 year age level. In both groups, hearing and deaf, the females showed the greater facility in written language, with the exception of the deaf males who at 15 years exceeded the deaf females.

To further analyze the differences between the deaf and the hearing, statistical tests of significance were applied; Student's t test. The differences between the groups at each of the age levels studied were highly significant with the exception of the seven year olds. The hearing exceeded the deaf at all other age levels. The F ratios tended to be high because of the large variances in each of the groups.

We also investigated whether each of the age groups was significantly superior to the one immediately below, permitting us to study in more detail the actual growth rate of the deaf in comparison with the hearing. The results were revealing in that for Total Words, the differences were statistically significant for the seven versus the nine year olds, the nine versus the 11's, and for the 11's versus the 13's. The differences between the 13's and the 15's and the 15's and the 17's were not significant. Therefore, although the mean scores increased at these upper age levels, the growth in Total Words after 13 years of age was slow and nonsignificant when considered in two year intervals. Growth occurs inasmuch as the mean scores for the 13 and 17 year olds were significantly different, but this represents an interval of four years. These results confirm the growth curve for the deaf shown in Figure 21, as the rise in the curve after 13 years is only slight and gradual. In addition, they are comparable to those found for the hearing in that the females showed no significant growth in Total Words after 13 years of age. The hearing males, on the other hand, showed significant progression from one age level to the next throughout the age range studied. In this statistical analysis of the differences between the deaf and the hearing, the outstanding result is that it reveals the slight growth of verbal fluency in the deaf after 13 years of age despite their serious inferiority. The implication is that educators give attention to the "slowing down" at this early age and attempt to have deaf children maintain growth even beyond the age where in the hearing verbal facility seems to have reached maturity.

From these findings it appears that deafness limits the amount of written language used in a given situation or circumstance. Even though progress is noted, the rate of maturation is significantly reduced and the evidence does not suggest that retardation is gradually overcome. The differences between the means for the total groups are: nine years, 53.9; 11 years, 65.2; 13 years, 71.7; 15 years, 51.3; 17 years, 61.1. While these mean differences vary by age level, they are consistent in showing a retardation of more than 50% in use of the written word. Another way in which to note the inferiority of the deaf is that at 17 years of age, their Productivity is comparable to a hearing child approximately 10 years of age.

In comparing the Day and Residential School children no consistent trend was found for one to be superior to the other; the Residential group showed a little greater facility at the 11 and 13 year age levels. Despite the inferiority of the females in Residential Schools, as shown by the Draw-a-Man Test, they wrote more words than the males at all age levels except at 15 years. The same trend appeared for the Day School females. This greater verbal facility on the part of females is in agreement with the findings for hearing children. It is of interest that this sex difference persists despite the impact of deafness.

TOTAL SENTENCES: Another way to evaluate productivity in verbal function is to ascertain the number of sentences used in the composition or story. In our developmental study of normal children we found a high correlation between Total Words and Total Sentences; the longer the story the more sentences used, a logical relationship. The findings for the deaf in comparison with the hearing, as shown in Table 77 and in Figure 22, are revealing and manifest a different pattern. While the deaf wrote fewer sentences at the early age levels, by 15 years of age their Productivity was equal to the hearing. Inasmuch as their stories were shorter, as evidenced by Total Words, rather than being long and complex, their sentences were short and simple. This is demonstrated also by the data on Words per Sentence discussed below.

TABLE 77. Comparison between deaf and hearing children on Total Sentences

Age		Deaf			Hearing		
		N	Mean	SD	N	Mean	SD
7	Male	48	3.9	6.3	62	3.6	2.5
	Female	29	5.6	5.8	61	5.0	2.8
	Total	77	4.5	6.1	123	4.3	2.7
9	Male	83	4.8	5.9	61	8.6	4.3
	Female	78	6.2	7.3	62	10.5	6.1
	Total	161	5.5	6.7	123	9.6	5.4
11	Male	118	5.9	5.4	63	10.1	5.2
	Female	109	8.4	6.9	64	11.5	6.7
	Total	227	7.1	6.2	127	10.8	6.0
13	Male	80	9.2	8.0	63	11.1	5.9
	Female	85	10.6	6.7	62	11.5	6.7
	Total	165	9.9	7.4	125	11.3	6.1
15	Male	69	10.9	7.0	63	8.4	3.8
	Female	62	9.8	4.6	62	10.9	4.5
	Total	131	10.4	6.0	125	9.7	4.4
17	Male	25	8.9	4.0	61	9.9	4.4
	Female	26	9.4	4.0	63	11.5	6.0
	Total	51	9.2	4.0	124	10.7	5.3

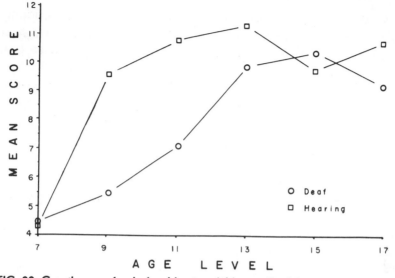

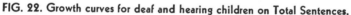

FIG. 22. Growth curves for deaf and hearing children on Total Sentences.

Statistical tests of significance were applied to the data on Total Sentences with the result that although the means showed progression through 15 years for the deaf, the differences from one age level to the next were significant only from nine to 11 and from 11 to 13 years. Again we note that the growth is slow and nonsignificant for the two year intervals of seven to nine, 13 to 15, and 15 to 17. These results are highly similar to those for Total Words, indicating only slight progress after 13 years of age; see Figure 22.

These findings, however, must be viewed in comparison with those for the hearing in whom the greatest increment found for a two year period was between seven and nine years of age; no difference at this age level appeared for the deaf. Moreover, in the hearing only the males showed significant growth at any two year interval after the age of nine; the females showed maturity in the number of sentences used at 11 years of age. The males showed an inexplicable decrement from 13 to 15 years. In general, both sexes plateaued markedly after nine years of age in the number of sentences written. In comparison, as measured by Total Sentences the deaf showed little growth until nine years of age, making significant progress between nine and 13 years of age, but no growth thereafter. In contrast, the hearing child showed rapid growth before nine years of age with little change in the years following. As shown by the

data on Words per Sentence, the length of his sentences continued
to show maturation beyond this age. As age increased he did not
write more, but rather, longer sentences. To some extent this also
was true of the deaf.

There was considerable variability within each age group for
both groups, especially for the deaf at the early age levels. By 17
years this variability had stabilized and was equivalent to the hearing. Only slight differences occurred by sex, with a tendency for
the females in both groups to write the most sentences. As far as
type of school was concerned, there was a nonsignificant trend for
the Residential group to use more sentences; variation occurred also
for Total Words. In general, this analysis of Total Sentences is in,
agreement with the other findings in showing a deficiency in deaf
children in the use of written language. Although they showed a
gradual increase in Total Sentences, but because an equivalent
increment in Total Words did not appear, this finding must be interpreted as indicating an undue use of short, simple sentences.

WORDS PER SENTENCE: Sentence length, an excellent measure of
verbal facility, has been used in studies of both the spoken and the
written word. Templin,[27] Davis,[9] and McCarthy[18] have presented
results for "length of remark" in their investigations of the development of spoken language. So far as written language is concerned,
Stormzand and O'Shea[26] conducted an early and interesting analysis
of the length of sentences used by average persons as well as by
professional workers. Sentence length also has been used as a
measure of complexity. Williams[30] reported a correlation of .80 and
Yedinack[31] a correlation of .88 and .93 between words per sentence
and complexity of the language used. In our study of the development of written language in hearing children, the mean for Words
per Sentence was highly similar to the mean scores obtained by
Stormzand and O'Shea and by Heider and Heider,[15] our mean
often falling between those reported by them. It can be assumed
that sentence length is one of the most reliable measures of Productivity and as shown by the results below, strikingly reveals the
language deficiency of deaf children.

The comparative results for deaf and hearing children are given
in Table 78 and in Figure 23. As they grow older both groups show

TABLE 78. Comparison between deaf and hearing children
on Words per Sentence

Age		Deaf			Hearing		
		N	Mean	SD	N	Mean	SD
7	Male	48	2.2	3.4	62	6.3	2.2
	Female	29	3.9	2.7	61	6.7	2.3
	Total	77	2.8	3.2	123	6.5	2.3
9	Male	83	3.7	3.2	61	9.9	2.5
	Female	78	3.9	3.0	62	9.5	2.5
	Total	161	3.8	3.1	123	9.7	2.3
11	Male	118	5.3	3.3	63	11.2	2.8
	Female	109	5.7	2.9	64	11.8	3.3
	Total	227	5.5	3.1	127	11.5	3.0
13	Male	80	6.4	3.6	63	13.8	3.6
	Female	85	7.7	2.7	62	14.2	3.2
	Total	165	7.1	3.2	125	14.0	3.4
15	Male	69	8.1	3.1	63	15.4	4.1
	Female	62	8.4	2.8	62	14.8	3.2
	Total	131	8.2	3.0	125	15.1	3.7
17	Male	25	11.5	6.2	61	16.8	4.1
	Female	26	12.0	5.3	63	15.4	3.8
	Total	51	11.7	5.7	124	16.1	4.0

a consistent, gradual increase in the number of words written per sentence and neither seems to have reached maturity by 17 years of age; a plateauing of the growth curves is not indicated. However, although parallel to the hearing, the rate of growth is much slower in the deaf. The differences between the means for the total groups are: seven years, 3.7; nine years, 5.9; 11 years, 6.0; 13 years, 6.9; 15 years, 6.9; 17 years, 4.4. The mean differences are almost identical from nine through 15 years but between 15 and 17 years, the deaf made a significant gain. Notwithstanding this increment their retardation was at least six years; at 17 years of age the mean length of the sentence written was equivalent to the average 11 year old hearing child. These results are remarkably consistent with those found for Total Words.

The differences between the deaf and the hearing were highly significant at all age levels. From seven through nine years the means for the hearing were approximately three times those for the deaf, while from 11 through 15 years they were about twice as large. Scores for the sexes for both groups were markedly similar, sentence length being one of the few measures of verbal facility on which the

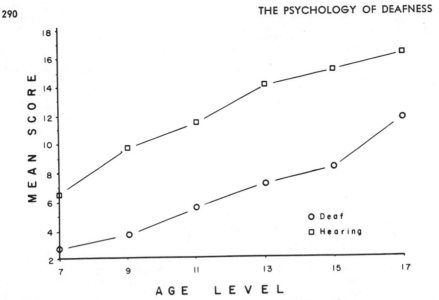

FIG. 23. Growth curves for deaf and hearing children in Words per Sentence.

females did not appear to be superior. So far as type of school is concerned these data corroborate the other findings from this study in that no differences appeared between the Residential and Day School groups.

The growth curves for both groups, hearing and deaf, are smooth and show a consistent increment from one age level to the next. However, the hearing showed very little maturation in number of Words per Sentence after 13 years of age. Although growth occurred after this age, the increments were small. On the other hand the greatest gain between any age level for the deaf was from 15 to 17 years and in contrast to the hearing, a plateau was not reached, indicating that language instruction even beyond the age of 17 years might be beneficial. Moreover, these results for Words per Sentence showed that the deaf made a significant gain at each of the age levels. As such this measure holds much promise as a reliable indicator of progress in written language. Educators should find it useful in evaluating and predicting success in the language development of deaf children.

Language Structure and Correctness

SYNTAX: Every language has its unique characteristics and its use assumes adherence to precedents which have evolved concerning a given symbol system. The rules which govern the use of language has been referred to as the parts of speech, sentence structure, and grammar. *Syntax,* referring to the patterns of formation and structure of sentences, is more inclusive. Through linguistics much has been learned regarding the structure of language, both ancient and modern. In the development of the Syntax score on The Picture Story Language Test we relied especially on the work of Perrin,[23] Thompson,[28] Fries,[11] Leopold,[17] and Carroll.[7] The classifications were suggested primarily by Perrin and Thompson and included *Carrier Phrases, Omissions, Substitutions, Additions, Word Order,* and *Punctuation.* Spelling was omitted. Errors of this type were scored as Syntax, the language correctness score obtained for each child. Also, an evaluation was made of the errors which characterized the deaf in comparison with the hearing.

The mean Syntax scores by age and sex for the deaf and hearing populations are presented in Table 79, and the growth curves shown in Figure 24. The findings for the hearing are interesting in that they reveal progression only through 11 years of age. Significant differences appeared between the seven and nine, and the nine and 11 year age groups but not at the older age levels. Apparently Syntax, as here measured, is comparable to that of the average adult by 11 years of

TABLE 79. Comparison between deaf and hearing children on Syntax

Age		Deaf			Hearing		
		N	Mean	SD	N	Mean	SD
7	Male	48	42.4	56.4	62	84.7	22.0
	Female	29	64.3	33.5	61	88.9	18.7
	Total	77	50.7	36.7	123	86.8	20.5
9	Male	83	53.8	34.3	61	94.3	7.9
	Female	78	57.5	32.7	62	96.4	4.7
	Total	161	55.6	33.5	123	95.4	6.5
11	Male	118	66.0	28.0	63	96.8	4.2
	Female	109	74.9	28.0	64	98.1	2.9
	Total	227	70.3	28.3	127	97.5	3.7
13	Male	80	73.7	26.9	63	97.4	2.7
	Female	85	83.9	19.4	62	98.0	3.1
	Total	165	78.9	23.8	125	97.7	2.9
15	Male	69	78.2	17.8	63	97.2	3.5
	Female	62	84.0	11.8	62	98.8	2.3
	Total	131	80.9	15.5	125	98.0	3.1
17	Male	25	89.4	9.2	61	97.9	3.3
	Female	26	83.1	17.2	63	99.9	12.8
	Total	51	86.2	14.1	124	98.9	9.5

age. In other words, in contrast to most other aspects of verbal behavior the ability to use the structure of language properly, to acquire the rules for using a given language is attained at an early age and long before ability to use sentences of adult length. These findings suggest that the structure of written language conforms closely to the spoken form. Inasmuch as spoken language developmentally precedes the written and, according to Templin[27] essentially is matured by seven years of age, apparently maturity in the syntax of written language is attained as soon as the child is able to read and has learned to write. From these results this is achieved by 11 years of age or when the child educationally is at the level of fourth to fifth grade.

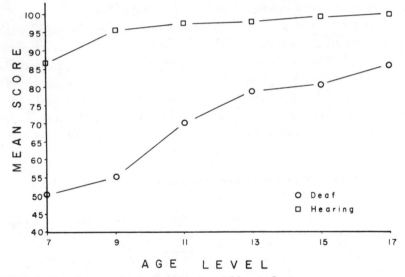

FIG. 24. Growth curves for deaf and hearing children in Syntax.

Lacking the basis of auditory language, the deaf child has great difficulty in acquiring the rules which govern the structure of his native tongue. They were inferior to the hearing at seven years of age and remained substantially so at each of the age levels studied; the differences were statistically different. We have seen that the deaf child is deficient in Productivity; he lacks fluency and an adequate vocabulary to express his ideas and feelings. However, it appears that the acquisition of Syntax is at least as great a problem and in some respects may be even more difficult when profound deafness is present from early life. Although progress is made show-ing maturation and although at 17 years the deaf males had attained equivalent facility, the females showed no growth after 13 years. On the other hand the deaf males continued to progress until 17 years of age though inferior to the females in early life. The growth curves by sex and total group therefore are not identical to those for the hearing. The females, plateauing at 13 years and showing early maturation of Syntax, are more comparable to the hearing. Because they have not attained normal function, an important consider-ation is why they plateau and do not show further growth in this aspect of language behavior. The deaf males made progress throughout the age range studied, showing noteworthy gain between 15 and 17 years. However, they required four additional years to attain the level of the females. We must assume that the effect of deafness on this aspect of language varies by sex. Both sexes are affected but not in an identical manner. The psychology of learning as it relates to Syntax seems to be different and needs further inves-tigation. Although by 17 years of age the level of attainment is equivalent by sex, it shows a marked retardation, the greatest we have encountered in studies of the effects of early life deafness on verbal behavior. At 17 years of age the deaf child's syntax facility is approximately equal to that of the average child of seven years; see the examples shown in Figure 44.

The means and standard deviations for the Day and Residential School groups were strikingly similar with no trends for either to be superior. Correctness of language usage, sentence structure, and grammar seem unrelated to type of school experience. As for most of the findings from this study, the implications are that although the child has daily associations with hearing children and with his parents as the Day School child has, there is little advantage as far as acquisition of Syntax is concerned. From the frame of reference used here and from an array of findings in the psychology of deaf-ness, this was not unexpected. Exposure to a world which uses auditory language is not of major benefit to the child who does not hear. Only through highly specialized procedures based on a psy-chology of learning which grows out of the effects of deafness can his severe language limitation be alleviated. *Emphasis must be given to his capacities, his potentials, his monitoring systems, and his total*

*psychological organization as a deaf child if he is to show greater
achievement in language as well as in other aspects of his behavior.*

TYPES OF ERRORS: To gain a thorough knowledge of the language problem resulting from early life deafness, it is necessary to know not only the magnitude of the deficiency but we must see the problem dynamically, the specific nature of this inadequacy. Only then can the most effective remedial procedures be developed. In other words, we need to know not only that the deaf are inferior in language but whether their errors show characteristic patterns. Experienced educators frequently comment to the effect that the language errors of deaf children are unique and refer to them as *deafisms.* If this is true, what is the nature of these errors which characterize their language? Heider and Heider[15] considered this question and analyzed samples of written language according to the types of sentences used, simple, complex, and compound. Thompson[28] used the method of studying the types of errors, a procedure which we followed in our investigation. Adhering to the plan of analysis used in studying the growth of written language in hearing children,[20] we computed the percentage of deaf children at nine, 11, 13, and 15 years of age who made each of the following errors: *Undue use of Carrier Phrases, Additions, Omissions, Substitutions,* and *Errors of Word Order.* While the use of a *Carrier Phrase* was not considered an error in a technical sense, it was necessary to study this phenomenon in order to determine its influence on the other scores; see examples in Figures 39 and 40.

The average number of errors per child by age, sex, and school are presented in Table 80. In comparison with the hearing the average number of errors made by the deaf was substantially higher. Moreover, as age increased the error scores for the hearing decreased whereas for the deaf they remained remarkably similar from one age level to the next. It appears that although the deaf child as he grows older achieves greater verbal facility, he does not show proportionate growth in accuracy of the language which he uses. Another observation deriving from this analysis pertains to the frequency with which each of the errors occurred. The most common error was *Omission;* essential words were left out. Next in order of occurrence was *Substitutions* followed by *Additions* and *Word Order.* While the implications for remedial training are summarized

TABLE 80. Percentage of total errors in each category by school, age and sex

Day School

Age	9		11		13		15	
	Male	Female	Male	Female	Male	Female	Male	Female
Omissions	72	70	67	73	60	56	48	48
Substitutions	19	13	16	17	23	23	24	28
Additions	5	11	12	6	12	14	25	21
Word Order	4	6	5	4	5	7	3	3

Residential School

Age	9		11		13		15	
	Male	Female	Male	Female	Male	Female	Male	Female
Omissions	56	62	60	59	54	58	59	51
Substitutions	28	22	18	26	33	26	23	28
Additions	12	7	17	10	13	13	14	19
Word Order	4	9	5	5	0	3	4	2

at the end of this chapter, we see that these data support the observations made by educators over a period of many years; that is, the written language of deaf children is characterized by certain types of errors, there are *deafisms*. Moreover, it appears that these can be analyzed quantitatively, in terms of magnitude and frequency as well as qualitatively, in terms of nature and type. Such analyses should constitute the basis of the methods used for language instruction.

The deaf and hearing were compared by ascertaining the number (percent) of children making each of these most commonly occurring errors. *Carrier Phrases* were used frequently by the deaf, particularly at the lower age levels. Undue use of Carrier Phrases consisted of a series of sentences which varied only in the noun, such as *I see a boy, I see a dog*, and *I see a baby*. The extent to which this stereotyped language structure was used is shown in Figure 25. The deaf children used Carrier Phrases much more frequently than the hearing. The hearing used virtually no language of this type after nine years of age whereas the deaf did not overcome dependency on this form until they reached the age of 15 years. Because to some extent Carrier Phrases are found only in the language of young hearing children, the deaf can be said to use immature language forms. The normal maturational pattern or sequence is disturbed by profound deafness from early life.

From the point of view of proper language structure, that is the correctness of usage, *Omissions* was by far the most frequently occurring error. This can be seen in Figure 26, which is an errorgram

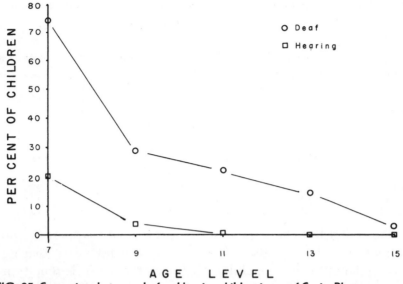

FIG. 25. Comparison between deaf and hearing children in use of Carrier Phrases.

showing the percentage of deaf and hearing children who omitted essential words. Examples of this type of error can be seen in the stories presented in Figures 39-44. The hearing children made this error only in early life when they were beginning to use the written language form, principally before nine years of age; a plateau appeared from 11 to 15 years. The pattern for the deaf was widely different. The seven year olds seemed most like the hearing but this is explained by the fact that almost all deaf children at this age used Carrier Phrases; see Figure 25. Approximately 75% of the deaf used this sentence form at this age level as compared to about 25% of the hearing. As soon as the hearing impaired began to use a less rigid sentence structure, approximately 90% of them omitted essential words and wrote sentences such as *A boy playing;* see examples in Figures 40, 41, 42, and 43.

The severe difficulty encountered by the deaf in overcoming this type of error is revealed by the comparison shown in Figure 26. More than 80% of the children continued to omit essential words even up to 15 years of age. As indicated above this analysis shows that Omissions is the most commonly occurring deafism. Furthermore, this error is highly characteristic of their written language and little progress is made in overcoming it during the period of their

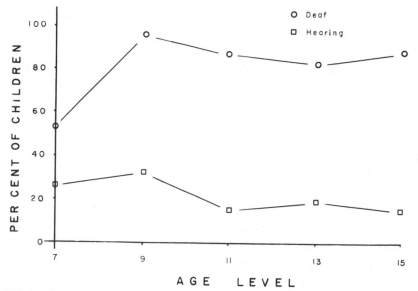

FIG. 26. Comparison between deaf and hearing children on errors of Omission.

schooling, signifying a great need to analyze this specific deficiency in detail. Why do children deaf from early life "forget" to include essential words in their expressive language? Does this problem derive from a generalized deficiency in vocabulary? This seems unlikely because the words omitted often are simple and well known to the child. Many questions of this type must be investigated and only when the true nature of this problem is known can properly focused remedial procedures be inaugurated. Investigation of these peculiarities of language structure so characteristic of the deaf offers a challenge to the educator, psychologist, and language pathologist.

The second most common error was *Substitution;* comparative results for the deaf and the hearing are shown in Figure 27. A substitution error consisted of using an incorrect word for the correct one. An example is, *A boy will playing,* in which *will* is substituted for *is.* Other examples can be seen in Figures 40, 41, 42, and 43. As with Omission errors the number of deaf children making this error remained essentially constant from nine through 15 years, whereas for the hearing as age increased there was an obvious decline in frequency. Between 50% to 60% of the deaf children made errors of Substitution at age nine and the same number continued to make these errors throughout the period of schooling, or at least until the age of 15 years. It appears that *deafisms* become firmly established, showing no trend to be relinquished on the basis of the remedial educational methods currently being used. Further study of this type of error, of the reasons for it being associated with deafness is indicated. Our data manifested that many of the errors derived from the wrong use of tense. While this constituted only one of the types of errors in this category, the suggestion is that if correct use of tense could be more firmly developed, Substitution errors would be largely eliminated. It seems appropriate therefore to raise the question of why deaf children find the proper use of tense so difficult. Inasmuch as tense is related to time, to the past, present, and future, conceivably this particular language error is to some extent a function of their sense of time; see Chapter V. Ausubel[2] and Mowrer[19] have indicated that there is a psychology of verbal learning. It is this psychology specifically as it relates to the deaf child that is in need of further investigation. *It is the child who is deaf, not his language.* If his problem of verbal learning is approached psychodynamically by relating it to the organismic impact of deafness, further language growth may be fostered.

The third most common error was Additions, such as *A boy is be playing.* This error consists of using, of adding an unnecessary

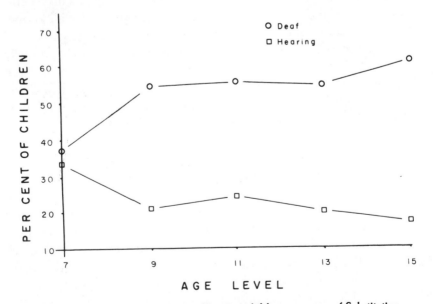

FIG. 27. Comparison between deaf and hearing children on errors of Substitution.

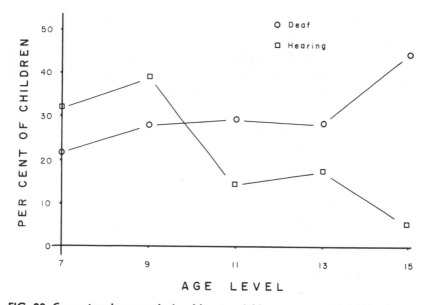

FIG. 28. Comparison between deaf and hearing children on errors of Addition.

word. The percentage of deaf in comparison to the hearing children who made this error is shown by the errorgram in Figure 28. Addition errors was the only instance in which at certain age levels the hearing made more errors than the deaf. This occurred at the ages of seven and nine years. In fact, errors of this type were made by more hearing children than any of the other incorrect usages studied, especially at the two lower age levels. However, there was a definite decline with very few children adding unnecessary words after 11 years of age. Inasmuch as the hearing served as a control group, we must assume that the deaf made less than the average number of errors of this type at the ages of seven and nine years.

As in the case of Omissions, comparatively they used many more Carrier Phrases than the hearing and this precluded the use of added words. It is not clear what other factors might be involved. In any event in contrast to the hearing, the deaf did not show a trend of overcoming this language error as they became older; an inexplicable increase in the number of children adding words appeared at 15 years of age. While less characteristic, it is noteworthy that deaf children both omit and add words which are incorrect. Analysis of the types of words omitted in comparison with those which are added might be enlightening. Presumably errors of Omission and errors of Addition could be related and constitute a single factor in the psychology of language development and usage in deaf children. Nevertheless, until further evidence is available, it should be stressed educationally that while the far greater problem is Omission, both the leaving out and the adding of words must be dealt with if more adequate language facility is to be achieved.

The fourth type of error in order of frequency was *Word Order;* comparison between the groups can be seen in Figure 29. An error of Word Order consisted of placing the words of a sentence in the wrong order, such as *A boy playing is,* not of omitting, substituting, or adding words incorrectly. Other examples can be found in Figures 41, 42, 43, and 44. Except at seven years of age, the earliest period of learning to use written language, hearing children did not make this type of error while they were common to 10% and 20% of the deaf children at each of the age levels. However, except at 15 years, they tended to make less errors of this type as they became older. This was the only deafism which seemed to diminish as a result of greater maturity and additional educational training.

Summarizing the data on types of errors, we find that at seven years of age 75% of the deaf children used Carrier Phrases but by 15 years this stereotype had been essentially overcome. Approx-

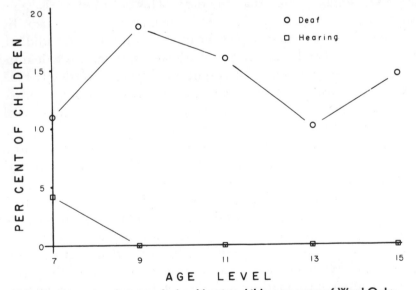

FIG. 29. Comparison between deaf and hearing children on errors of Word Order.

imately 85% omitted necessary words and only slight progress was noted in this respect as they became older. At least 55% substituted incorrect for correct words and this problem too persisted without improvement throughout the entire age range. About 25% added words which were inappropriate and this ratio also continued despite language training and advancement in age. From 10% to 20% used incorrect Word Order with most of these errors occurring before the age of 13 years. Moreover, this was the only deafism that tended to be overcome as age increased.

In addition to these errors the ability to use correct punctuation and capitalization was scored and analyzed statistically. Three types of punctuation scores were obtained: *Errors of Addition, Omission, and Substitution.*[20] The results showed the deaf to be superior to the hearing on all three scores. In errors of adding unnecessary punctuation and of substituting improper for proper punctuation, there were only slight differences between the deaf and the hearing. Both groups made more errors of Omission, not using the necessary punctuation. However, the hearing made many more such errors than the deaf and never attained an equal degree of accuracy; the difference was statistically significant.

It is difficult to explain this better facility with punctuation on the part of the deaf. Perhaps it is because they learn language visually and punctuation is predominantly a visual phenomenon. Except through accent, inflection, and other variations auditorially, punctuation per se does not appear in spoken language. From this we might infer that the deaf child being essentially visual, attains this skill more readily. On the other hand, the hearing child who is basically auditory in his language behavior experiences difficulty in acquiring this aspect of written language. From these results errors of punctuation cannot be considered a type of deafism.

TYPES OF ERRORS BY SCHOOL: The Day and Residential School children were compared according to their characteristic errors in written language. The percentage of the total errors falling into each category was computed and the results are shown in Table 80. No differences appeared by school, age, or sex which corroborates the findings given above for the total deaf group in comparison with the hearing. The order of magnitude was the same for both school groups: Omission, Substitution, Addition, and Word Order. Further-more, except for Word Order, the category in which the least number of errors fell, the scores did not diminish by age. The characteristic errors, the deafisms, appeared with equal frequency for males and females and by school group. So far as written language is concerned the Day and Residential School children were equal. It seems that it is the factor of deafness which is of importance, not the type of school nor the variation in methods of teaching.

Conceptualization and Abstract Thought

As indicated by the discussion in Chapter V, one of the primary concerns of students studying the effects of sensory deprivation has been the possible relationship between these handicaps and develop-ment of ability to use abstraction. Moreover, philosophers and psy-chologists for generations have been curious about the ways in which abstract thought might be dependent on language. Abstraction has been said to be a result of ability to use words. Because of the im-portance of this question psychologically and educationally, in The Picture Story Language Test we devised a means whereby facility with written language and the use of abstract ideation might be compared.[20] The measures of *Productivity* (Total Words, Total Sen-tences, and Words per Sentence) and of *Syntax* were viewed as indices of the extent to which language had been acquired. The *Abstract-Concrete Scale* provided a measure of the extent to which imagination and conceptualization was used in writing a story. In obtaining this score, verbal facility and accuracy of language usage were ignored. Hence we could evaluate the degree of abstraction irrespective of the adequacy of the language used.

The criteria evolved for determining the level of abstraction were similar to those suggested by Oléron.[22] The more the child described only what could be seen in the picture, the more "stimulus-bound" he was, the more he scored in the direction of concreteness. For example, if the story described only objects which were observ-able, it was scored as being concrete while if there was a plot, if a moral were drawn, or if imagination were shown in other ways it scored as being abstract. The Scale provided for a continuum of five levels, from extreme concreteness to marked abstraction of ideas and thought: (1) *Inappropriate*, (2) *Concrete-Descriptive*, (3) *Con-*

crete-Imaginative, (4) Abstract-Descriptive, (5) Abstract-Imagina-
tive. The reliability of this Scale was found to be comparable to
other standard tests of achievement and capacity.[20]

The results for the deaf, Day and Residential groups combined,
compared with the hearing are presented in Table 81. These data disclose a progression by age for both groups in the use of abstraction.
However, the deaf were inferior to the hearing at all age levels as
is shown by Figure 30. The significance of these differences was
determined by applying Student's t test which affirmed that the
Abstract-Concrete scores for the deaf were significantly inferior at
the 1% level of confidence at all age levels. It seems noteworthy
that the deaf gained and attained more normal scores as they became
older. Not considering the seven year age groups where use of
abstraction was minimal, the mean differences were as follows: nine
years, 7.0; 11 years, 6.8; 13 years, 5.2; 15 years, 5.7; 17 years, 3.6.
At least to some extent the tendency was for the deaf to overcome
their limitation, the inferiority in ideation which was portrayed in
their stories.

The differences in the growth curves for the deaf and the hearing can be seen in other ways. The hearing females showed no
increment after 15 years of age but the hearing males made signif-

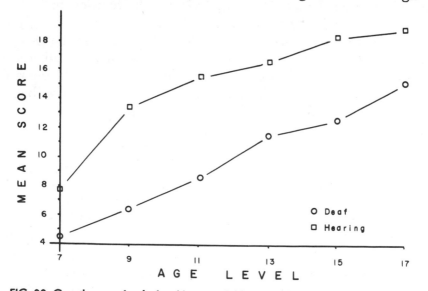

FIG. 30. Growth curves for deaf and hearing children on Abstract-Concrete

TABLE 81. Comparison between deaf and hearing children on Abstract-Concrete

Age		Deaf			Hearing		
		N	Mean	SD	N	Mean	SD
7	Male	48	3.9	3.6	62	7.3	3.5
	Female	29	5.6	3.5	61	8.4	2.9
	Total	77	4.5	3.6	123	7.8	3.2
9	Male	83	6.1	4.6	61	13.0	5.1
	Female	78	6.8	4.5	62	13.8	4.8
	Total	161	6.4	4.5	123	13.4	4.9
11	Male	118	7.7	4.8	63	14.8	5.2
	Female	109	9.8	5.2	64	16.2	4.4
	Total	227	8.7	5.1	127	15.5	4.8
13	Male	80	10.0	5.4	63	16.5	4.3
	Female	85	12.8	5.7	62	16.9	4.5
	Total	165	11.5	5.7	125	16.7	4.4
15	Male	69	11.8	4.4	63	17.4	4.6
	Female	62	13.8	5.3	62	19.5	3.6
	Total	131	12.7	4.9	125	18.4	4.3
17	Male	25	14.4	4.8	61	19.5	3.7
	Female	26	15.8	4.5	63	18.2	4.3
	Total	51	15.2	4.6	124	18.8	4.0

icant progress between the years of 15 and 17; earlier maturation occurred in the females. In the deaf both sexes continued to show growth through the age level of 17 years. The females, both deaf and hearing, tended to be superior to the males. Statistical analysis showed that only at the age level of 13 to 15 years was the growth made in a two year interval nonsignificant. At each of the other age levels the progress made was highly significant, including the interval from 15 to 17 years. These findings show that growth was being made beyond the age where verbal functions in general had ceased to show progress.

Use of abstraction as a mental process acquired developmentally and as measured here cannot be considered synonymous with intelligence. The growth pattern and the differences by sex are not typical of those for mental development. The hearing males did not achieve full maturation inasmuch as a plateau was not reached by 17 years of age and neither sex in the deaf group had reached maturity by this age. Ability to engage in abstract thought was developing more slowly in the deaf but they and the hearing males apparently would show increased ability beyond the age level included in our study.

The extent to which the deaf might show greater gain in comparison with the hearing is not divulged by these data. Therefore the retardation denoted cannot be interpreted as a final manifestation of the effects of deafness on the levels of abstraction which might be attained. Nevertheless, the level of function attained by the deaf at 17 years of age was essentially equivalent to the level achieved by the hearing child of 11 years. This degree of retardation is comparable to that found for written language but seems more optimistic in that the tendency was for the deaf to gain, to overcome their concreteness as they became older.

While equivocal, and it is unlikely that the inferiority is fully overcome, these data do not support the opinion that ability to engage in abstract thought is synonymous with verbal facility. Nonetheless, as suggested in Chapter V, a relationship between deafness and use of abstract ideas, abstract thought, and conceptualization was found. A marked auditory deprivation from early life apparently restricts development of this important aspect of Man's psychic capacities. A greater dependency on the observable prevails. Whether this limitation is principally a result of verbal inferiority or whether both verbal and nonverbal facets are involved remains undetermined. These data suggest that the deaf child's abstract abilities can be developed further and perhaps more effectively by utilizing approaches which stress both verbal and nonverbal aspects of mental processes.

ABSTRACTION IN RELATION TO SCHOOL AND SEX: Only one sex difference appeared in the standardization study; the females exceeded the males in the use of abstraction at the 15 year age level. In contrast, the deaf females were significantly superior to the males in this ability at all age levels except at nine years. Again we encounter the curious circumstance of the effects of deafness operating selectively by sex. Ostensibly this sensory impairment restricts the development of abstract thought and the use of conceptualization in males to a greater extent than in females. If abstract ability is closely associated to verbal facility, this advantage of the females might be explained by their better command of language.

The development and the use of abstraction seemed unrelated to the type of school experience; only one significant difference occurred in that the Day School children exceeded the Residential School children at the age level of 11 years. In general, the Day and Residential School groups were equally inferior and equally successful in the extent to which they engaged in abstract, imaginative thought processes. These results are in agreement with the pattern which appeared throughout this investigation, showing the equivalency of the groups by school.

ABSTRACTION AND THE PARTS OF SPEECH: In the study of language development a relationship has been found between mental growth and the types of words and sentence structure used. As McCarthy[18] and Templin[27] have shown, in spoken language the child does not first acquire the more difficult parts of speech, such as an interjection. He first acquires the names of objects, nouns, and only gradually begins to use the more complex verbal forms. From this developmental point of view and from experience with individuals who have language disorders, the parts of speech might be classified on a continuum from the more concrete to the more abstract. Although the psychology of language acquisition is more complex, on such a continuum the normal child first acquires concrete language and attains ability to use the more abstract forms only as he matures.

Because nouns are acquired first, can we assume that they represent a concrete level of language usage? Because interjections and conjunctions are acquired later, does their usage signify a higher level of abstract behavior? Inasmuch as they occur later developmentally, apparently we are justified in assuming that mastery of such forms requires a higher level of mental capacity. Empirically it is evident that words vary in difficulty of meaning. Some, especially nouns, refer to concrete, often observable objects or experiences. Verbs refer to actions, but as Fries[11] has emphasized, some verbs and even some adjectives are "names" as much as are some nouns. Nonetheless verbs can be said to refer to meanings which are to some extent less observable than nouns. Even greater differences between words can be seen when we compare nouns with prepositions, articles, interjections, conjunctions, and especially adverbs.

From the data presented in Figure 37, adverbs more than any other word type reveal the psychology of language development as it relates to the parts of speech. Manifestly each of the parts of speech assumes more complexity of language usage as well as of meanings, ideation, and thought processes. From this point of view the most abstract form of language usage is the metaphor. Interesting discussions of the relationship between use of metaphor and abstraction have been presented by Langer,[16] Asch,[1] and Brown.[6] When we use the expression "a chip on your shoulder" none of the words used can be taken literally because the idea being conveyed is a feeling of anger, hostility, or resentment; experienced teachers of the deaf know how difficult it is to teach metaphors to deaf children. Perhaps there is a range of abstract behavior, varying from the concrete noun to the adverb and to the metaphor. Though this possibility requires further study we pursued the analysis of some of our data accordingly.

A special analysis was made of a sample of the stories written on The Picture Story Language Test. Using a random selection procedure, 200 stories written by deaf children were compared with 200 written by hearing children. The subjects who wrote the stories were matched on chronological age and intelligence. Forty children, 20 of each sex, deaf and hearing, were selected at each of the age levels, seven, nine, 11, 13, 15 years. Of the deaf, one-half were selected from Day Schools and one-half from Residential Schools. Every word in each of the 400 stories was counted and classified according to the parts of speech. Common classifications were used, largely on the basis of the discussion by Perrin.[23] Scores were derived on the basis of the percentage of the total number of words written, comparable to the procedure used by Templin[27] for spoken language. Because of the extreme range of scores for the deaf and the numerous zero scores, medians were used instead of means. Hence the scores derived were median percents for each of the parts of speech analyzed.

Nouns. The most frequently used part of speech by both the deaf and the hearing was *nouns*. However, as shown in Figure 31, the hearing impaired used more nouns than the normal at all age levels, using approximately twice as many at seven years. While from seven through 15 years of age the hearing used essentially the same number of nouns in their written language, the deaf found it

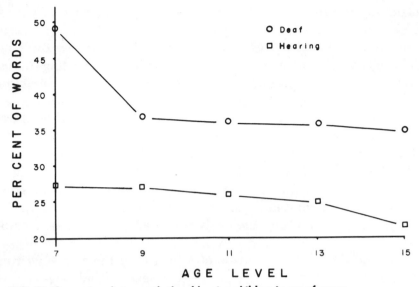

FIG. 31. Comparison between deaf and hearing children in use of nouns.

necessary to use proportionately many more words of this type. As they progressed in language acquisition the use of nouns by the hearing impaired diminished but they did not overcome their dependence on this simple type of language usage; we have referred to this as the *naming level* of verbal behavior. The range of scores is interesting; at seven years of age some children, both deaf and hearing, wrote only names of objects, giving them a score of 100 percent for nouns. No hearing child wrote only nouns after seven years of age. In contrast 100 percent noun scores occurred with some frequency through 11 years for the deaf, and even at the 13 and 15 year age levels some had noun scores of over 90 percent. This naming level type of written language persisted into the later school age and if noun usage is taken as the criterion, the language of the deaf is substantially more concrete than that used by the hearing.

Verbs. The second most commonly used part of speech by both the deaf and the hearing was *verbs;* the median percentage scores by age are given in Figure 32. These results are complementary to those for nouns in that because the deaf used so much *naming level* language, they used fewer verbs in comparison with the hearing. At seven years the hearing used approximately twice as many "action" words. From nine through 15 years the median scores for the two

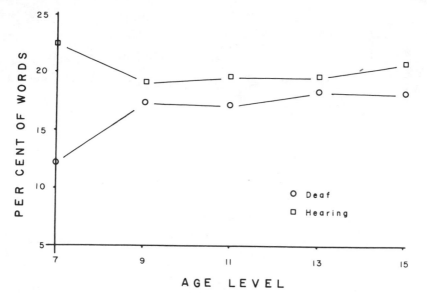

FIG. 32. Comparison between deaf and hearing children in use of verbs.

groups were comparable but more deaf children at all age levels had zero scores; they used no verbs. Such scores appeared at all age levels for the deaf but only up to nine years of age for the hearing.

Articles. Following nouns and verbs, *articles* were used most frequently by both groups; these results are presented in Figure 33. In comparison with the hearing, the deaf at seven years used very few articles but from nine through 15 years they exceeded the normal in the use of this part of speech. Evidently as soon as the child with deafness learns to write, he engages in frequent use of articles, in the use of *a, an,* and *the.* Does this mean a greater use of abstract words? In view of the total findings this appears unlikely. The deaf child is drilled in writing expressions such as *a boy* and *the baby;* it was from sentences of this type that the high incidence of articles occurred. Furthermore, learning words is not easy for children having deafness from early life and *they might use most frequently those that are least difficult.* The articles are one, two, and three letter words, readily combined with a noun or a verb to form a short sentence. Because the hearing impaired child used more nouns, more naming level language than the normal, he also used more articles.

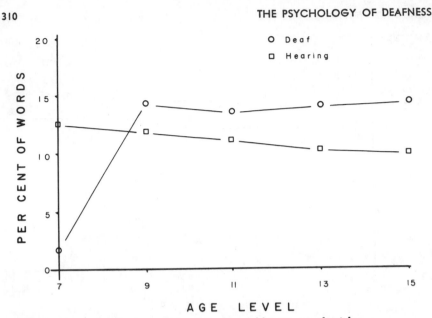

FIG. 33. Comparison between deaf and hearing children in use of articles.

Pronouns. In frequency of usage *pronouns* were fourth in order for both groups; these data are shown in Figure 34. The hearing used pronouns with a certain frequency (about 12% of all the words they wrote) at seven years and maintained this ratio in comparison with other words at all of the age levels. The deaf found it virtually impossible to use this part of speech until after nine years of age. From nine to 13 years they showed rapid progress in acquiring pronouns but from 13 to 15 years further growth was not attained although the level of function was below that of the hearing. As in the case of nouns, verbs, and articles the deaf acquired the use of pronouns but at a much later age and with less facility in comparison with hearing children. Moreover, some deaf children at all age levels up through the age of 15 years wrote stories in which no pronouns appeared. No such stories were written by the hearing after the age of nine years.

Because of the intercorrelations found among spoken, read, and written language we can assume that the deaf child is restricted in his use of pronouns irrespective of the form of language he uses. Psychologically this may be of consequence because he lacks words for personal reference. Words such as *I, me, he, she, they, you, him,* and *her* must be of unusual importance in assisting the child in identifying himself, in distinguishing between hmself and others. Perhaps all verbal development in early life is concomitant with psychological development, mentally and emotionally. Use of pronouns may be closely allied with ego development. Another possibility is that inadequate use of pronouns such as *he, she, him,* and *her* are associated with limited and delayed differentiation between the sexes. If so, we should expect a rather direct association between these specific deficits of language and the personality characteristics which have been found to be allied with deafness.

Prepositions. Fifth in frequency of usage were *prepositions.* As shown in Figure 35, none of the deaf children at seven years of age used this part of speech. However, in contrast to the other parts of speech studied, facility in the use of prepositions was acquired on a developmental basis; as they became older usage increased until by 15 years it was equal to the hearing. Also, this was the only instance in which the deaf children showed growth of verbal function to the extent that they overcame the marked limitation which was apparent at the age of seven years.

Because this is an unusual phenomenon in the study of language

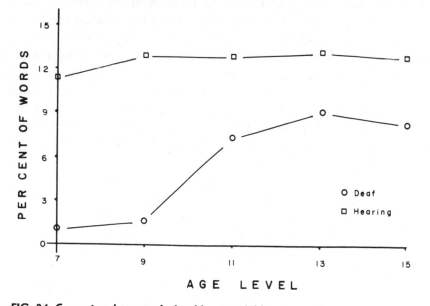

FIG. 34. Comparison between deaf and hearing children in use of pronouns.

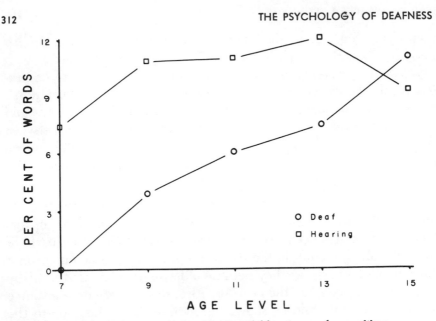

FIG. 35. Comparison between deaf and hearing children in use of prepositions.

acquisition by the deaf it warrants further study. One cannot but be curious as to the reasons for a deaf child being able to acquire normal facility with prepositions and not with the other parts of speech. Why are the language teaching techniques being used more effective with prepositions? In our studies of language behavior we have been impressed with the possibility that the psychological factors involved are different for the various parts of speech. It is this possibility which prompted this discussion of abstraction in relation to this aspect of verbal behavior. Stated another way, it seems that the psychology of learning a noun or a verb is not equivalent to that of learning a pronoun, preposition, adjective, or adverb and that each of these again is different from each of the others. Another possibility is that they not only vary psychologically but also neurologically. When one deals with persons who have involvements of the brain resulting in dysnomia, an inability to remember nouns, or formulation aphasia, an inability to form normal sentences syntactically, one must be impressed with the way in which the parts of speech are related to specifics of brain function. It is in these terms that more must be learned about the psychology of deafness and its relationship to verbal learning. On the basis of our results, deafness affects the learning of the parts of speech selectively, not uniformly. It affects acquisition of certain types of verbal proficiency more than others.

Adjectives. Sixth in order of frequency was use of *adjectives;* the results for the deaf and the hearing are shown in Figure 36. Psychologically and educationally it is important to note that developmental growth in the hearing occurred chiefly with prepositions, adjectives, and adverbs. For the other parts of speech, nouns, verbs, articles, and pronouns and to some extent conjunctions, adult proficiency existed at seven years and did not show significant change as age increased. In contrast the deaf typically were highly deficient at seven years, made progress but with the exception of prepositions, did not overcome their limitation. Taking the growth patterns found for the hearing as our guide, we see that prepositions, adjectives, and adverbs require greater maturation developmentally before full proficiency can be achieved; this is especially true of adverbs as discussed below. Perhaps this indicates that these parts of speech require greater mental ability and hence a greater degree of abstraction. If this is true, then we must conclude that deafness has more deleterious effects on the abstraction involved in learning adjectives and adverbs than it does in learning prepositions.

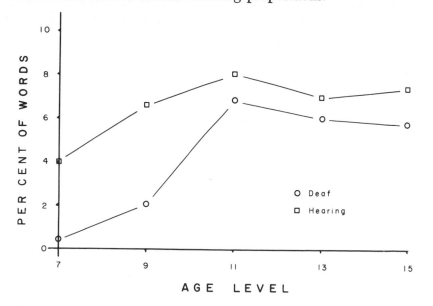

FIG. 36. Comparison between deaf and hearing children in use of adjectives.

From Figure 36 we see that the deaf children used very few adjectives until after nine years of age, which was comparable to their use of pronouns and conjunctions. Adverbs were more delayed and nouns, verbs, articles, and prepositions were less so. Again we see the variable effect of deafness on the parts of speech. By 11 years the median scores for the deaf and the hearing were nearly alike but this apparent adequacy on the part of the hearing impaired may be misleading. A number of the deaf throughout the age levels studied used no adjectives in their stories. In fact, more 15 year old deaf children than nine year old hearing children did not use this part of speech.

Adverbs. Of the parts of speech studied, *adverbs* presented the greatest difficulty for deaf children and showed the most unusual growth or frequency curve for the hearing. In the hearing the acquisition of facility in use of adverbs was closely related to developmental maturation; as the child became older he acquired fluency in use of adverbs, growth continuing to 15 years of age, the highest age level studied. No other part of speech showed this degree of relationship with chronological age. The deaf showed greater retardation, greater delay in attaining even rudimentary use of adverbs than in any of the other parts of speech. From Figure 37 we note

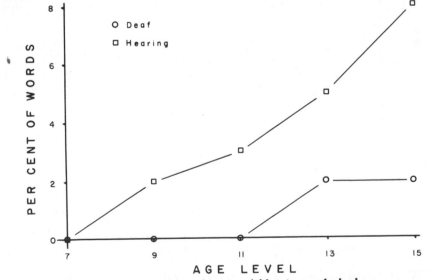

FIG. 37. Comparison between deaf and hearing children in use of adverbs.

that the deaf used no adverbs until after 11 years of age and then usage was extremely limited.

From these findings it appears that learning to use adverbs, at least as far as written language is concerned, presents somewhat of a special circumstance to both the deaf and the hearing. To some extent adverbs manifest most clearly that the psychology of verbal learning may not be identical for the various parts of speech. The question we face is, Why is adverb learning closely related to maturation for the hearing and apparently the most difficult of the common parts of speech for the deaf? Is abstract ability especially involved in proper adverb usage? This possibility cannot be overlooked when we consider that adverbial terms refer to qualifications and relationships. These words are used principally to qualify or limit a verb and to express "some relation of place, time, manner, attendant circumstance, degree, cause, inference, result, condition, exception, concession, purpose, or means.[3]" Such usage seems to entail abstract aspects of intelligence and may be related to Templin's[27] findings regarding the differences between deaf and hearing children in reasoning ability. Further study of the variables in acquiring facility in the use of adverbs by the deaf as well as by the hearing, promises to be revealing in relation to the psychology of language acquisition in general. Investigations of this type should provide greater insight into the specific nature of the problems encountered by deaf children in acquiring verbal facility.

Conjunctions. Next in order of frequency of the parts of speech was *conjunctions;* the results from this analysis are given in Figure 38. This part of speech was acquired by the hearing at nine years of age but did not appear in the language of the deaf until 11 years. It was then used but not with so great a frequency as by the hearing. After 11 years all of the hearing included conjunctions whereas a number of the deaf even at 15 years of age did not use this part of speech.

Interjections. Only a few children, deaf or hearing, used *interjections* in writing their stories. This type of expression was not used frequently even by hearing children but they began using interjections by nine years of age. Ostensibly, the stimulus picture did not provide ample opportunity for use of this part of speech but it was

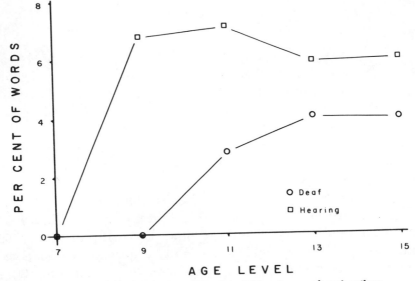

FIG. 38. Comparison between deaf and hearing children in use of conjunctions.

apparent that its usage was very difficult for deaf children. Because of the large number of zero scores occurring in both the deaf and the hearing groups, these data are not presented.

SUMMARY OF PARTS OF SPEECH AND ABSTRACTION: Interesting differences between the deaf and the hearing appeared in the developmental patterns for written language. The hearing child's production consisted primarily of nouns, verbs, articles, and pronouns while the deaf child's to a greater extent was made up of nouns, verbs, and articles. Use of pronouns, prepositions, adjectives, and conjunctions was markedly delayed in the deaf and only rudimentary use of adverbs was attained by 15 years of age.

While inferences must be tentative, it appears that developmentally there is some relationship between maturation of intelligence, abstraction, and use of the parts of speech. However, in written language except for prepositions, adjectives, and adverbs usage of the parts of speech is well established in the hearing child by seven years of age, that is as soon as he is capable of writing. The pattern for the deaf child is widely different with usage being delayed until the age of nine or later. Moreover, those parts of speech which are more closely related to intellectual development appear to be the most difficult for the deaf to master.

Our purpose in making this analysis was to gain further information concerning the language learning problem encountered by deaf children and to note whether the retardation in language was associated with limitations in ability to use abstraction, to engage in abstract thought. It would be of considerable benefit psychologically and educationally if we could demonstrate whether the deaf child becomes concrete and thus is reduced in the use of language, or whether he is deficient in language and thus becomes concrete. In other words, is the concreteness *cause* or *effect*. Extensive study will be necessary before conclusions can be reached regarding this question which pertains not only to the psychology of thought processes in the deaf but also to the psychology of language and concept formation in general.

As far as our results are concerned, it must be stressed that the outlook appears hopeful. The deaf child in comparison with the hearing finds it necessary to use more naming level, more concrete language but the evidence does not denote that he lacks concepts, that he is without ability to engage in abstract thought. Rather, the indications are that he uses abstract ideas to the extent that he has words for their expression. Conceivably the deaf child's language is more concrete than his mental processes. He may, however, show concreteness in comparison with the hearing because, as mentioned in Chapter V, even certain nonverbal behavior could be more verbal than we have assumed.

Perhaps this does not greatly simplify the learning and adjustment problem confronting those with profound deafness from early life. Nor does it notably simplify the problem for those concerned with the education of the deaf. Possibly it projects the impact of deafness in a somewhat clearer perspective so that remedial procedures of various types can be planned more directly, more specifically in terms of the nature of the deficit. For example, in contrast to many individuals with brain involvements, those who have psychoneurological learning disorders of the type discussed in Chapter XIII, the deaf seem to have more concepts than they can use effectively. They lack the language required for more successful expression of the abstractions of which they are capable. From the point of view of remedial education the implication is that they would develop greater fluidity of thought, more imaginative ideation and conceptualization, if limitation in verbal behavior could be further alleviated. It is conceivable that stress on a vocabulary, especially for abstract concepts, based on developmental levels as shown by studies of the normal would aid the deaf in actualizing their abstract abilities more effectively. This would not obviate the need to emphasize concepts and abstractions in and of themselves both verbally and nonverbally.

Correlation Between Language Functions

The theoretical frame of reference or model which we have used for many of our studies of language behavior has been discussed in Chapter IX. This construct hypothesizes that relationships exist between the verbal systems used by Man. It postulates that in the hearing auditory language is acquired first, preceding acquisition of reading. Moreover, reading must be established before the beginning of written language. Another aspect of this point of view is that inner language is basic to the development and normal function of all of the verbal systems. We assumed that these language functions are interrelated. To some extent this was found to be true of speechreading; these data were presented in Chapter X.

Now we consider this question further through reviewing the results for written language. An analysis was made of the correlation between the five scores on The Picture Story Language Test as well as of the correlation between these scores and reading and intelligence. In all instances these findings were compared with those for the hearing.

Total Words: The correlation between Total Words and the other measures of written language are presented in Table 82. As for the hearing the relationship to Total Sentences was high for the deaf; the more words written, the greater the number of sentences. The results for Words per Sentence, however, differed from those obtained for the hearing where there was virtually no correlation between the number of words written and Words per Sentence. Sentence length showed consistent growth from seven through 17 years irrespective of the length of the stories written; see Figure 23.

For the deaf there was a definite association between Words per Sentence and story length at all age levels for both sexes with the exception of the 17 year old males. In other words, when deafness was present there was a substantial correlation between Total Words

TABLE 82. Correlation between Total Words and other measures
of written language by age and sex

Age	Males							Females					
	7	9	11	13	15	17		7	9	11	13	15	17
TS	.82	.92	.89	.93	.79	.55		.96	.93	.93	.90	.81	.27
WPS	.29	.54	.51	.44	.38	.27		.37	.50	.47	.50	.43	.71
A/C	.36	.72	.68	.68	.58	.27		.44	.64	.60	.63	.63	.55
Syn	.60	.49	.52	.53	.21	.09		.49	.53	.43	.36	.15	.40
N	47	77	114	77	69	23		29	74	103	82	61	25

	Total					
Age	7	9	11	13	15	17
TS	.87	.93	.92	.91	.80	.42
WPS	.33	.52	.48	.48	.38	.47
A/C	.40	.68	.65	.66	.54	.51
Syn	.56	.51	.49	.47	.17	.20
N	76	151	217	159	130	48

TS—Total Sentences A/C—Abstract-Concrete
WPS—Words per Sentence Syn—Syntax

and both of the other measures of Productivity. It seems that Productivity, verbal facility and fluency in written language is more of a general factor in the deaf. Unless fluency, such as manifested by the number of words written, is developed or exists at a given level, it impedes normal growth of the number of words used per sentence. Hence the more words the deaf could write in a sentence, the more words they wrote in the story. These findings are in agreement with those on Productivity as shown in Tables 76, 77, and 78. The lack of generalized verbal facility is again conveyed as a basic problem when profound deafness is present from early life.

Another major difference in the correlations for the deaf in comparison with the hearing is that which occurred for Syntax. While the trends for these findings were the same for both groups, important variations could be seen. We have noted that Syntax showed early maturation for the hearing with the females manifesting the more rapid growth. Therefore the only association between this factor and Total Words appeared at the early age levels, mainly before nine years of age. The deaf also showed the greatest relationship between these factors of written language in early life, with a gradual diminution as age increased. However, significant correlations appeared up to 15 years, revealing the slower growth of Syntax in the deaf. Presumably, difficulty with the structure of language was a factor in impeding development of normal facility with words.

A finding not anticipated was the consistently high interdependence between Total Words and Abstract-Concrete behavior. A definite relationship between these factors was found for both the deaf and the hearing for both sexes and at all age levels. It is curious and perhaps of unusual importance that of the measures of Productivity, only Total Words showed this degree of relationship with use of abstraction. As discussed below this was not true for Total Sentences nor for Words per Sentence. It appears that the more words written as measured by The Picture Story Language Test the more imagination is used, the more that which is written tends to include ideas which are not stimulus bound. To some extent general fluency and use of abstract ideas are mutually associated, one enhancing the other. This relationship exists whether or not deafness is present.

Total Sentences: As stated above there was a close and consistent relationship between Total Words and Total Sentences; the longer the stories, the greater the number of sentences used in writing the stories. For the hearing a negative association was found between Total Sentences and Words per Sentence with the correlations being statistically significant at 11, 13, 15, and 17 years. At these ages the more words included per sentence, the fewer the number of sentences written per story. While this trend appeared also for the deaf, the pattern varied substantially from that seen for the hearing; see Table 83. From seven through 13 years for both sexes the correlations were positive and statistically significant; the longer the sentence the more sentences written. Only after 15 years of age did this association change and show the pattern found for hearing children; the more words per sentence the fewer the number of sentences written. Until verbal fluency of a degree is acquired, the deaf child is confronted with a general problem of limited language and manifests a handicap both in the number of sentences he uses and in the number of words he writes per sentence. Only after 15 years of age does he have sufficient command of language so that he can write sentences of a length which permits him to express ideas independently of the number of words he uses in writing a story. While these findings again show the limitation in verbal facility associated with early life deafness, they are hopeful in that the growth pattern eventually conforms to that found for the hearing.

TABLE 83. Correlation between Total Sentences and other measures
of written language by age and sex

Age	Males						Females					
	7	9	11	13	15	17	7	9	11	13	15	17
TW	.82	.92	.89	.93	.79	.55	.96	.93	.93	.90	.81	.27
WPS	.37	.58	.44	.28	.07	−.59	.39	.57	.46	.22	−.14	−.46
A/C	.36	.77	.68	.68	.60	−.05	.42	.64	.63	.60	.53	.16
Syn	.76	.61	.65	.52	.31	−.18	.59	.64	.55	.35	−.05	−.13
N	47	77	114	77	69	23	29	74	103	82	61	25

Total						
Age	7	9	11	13	15	17
TW	.87	.93	.92	.91	.80	.42
WPS	.39	.57	.45	.27	−.00	−.52
A/C	.40	.70	.66	.64	.51	.06
Syn	.70	.62	.61	.46	.19	−.17
N	76	151	217	159	130	48

TW—Total Words   A/C—Abstract-Concrete
WPS—Words per Sentence   Syn—Syntax

A similar circumstance appeared in connection with Syntax. For the hearing Total Sentences and Syntax were correlated but only in early life, at seven years for the females and at seven, nine, and 13 years for the males. These findings were interpreted as showing different maturational rates by sex. In the deaf these factors were significantly related up through 15 years for the males and through 13 years of age for the females. The pattern of correlation, therefore, was the same for the deaf as for the hearing, the difference being that the pattern evolved later in life for the deaf. In terms of the development of written language, the general significance is that while the impact of deafness is evident, it does not alter the nature of the relationships between the factors of Total Sentences and Syntax.

Total Sentences was associated with Abstract-Concrete behavior but the relationship was different from that found for Total Words in both the deaf and the hearing. Total Words correlated with use of abstraction at all ages for both groups while Total Sentences was associated with Abstract-Concrete behavior only through 13 years for the hearing and through 15 years for the deaf. Comparing these results with those shown in Figure 22, we may infer that there is a correlation between Total Sentences and use of abstraction up to the point where the number of sentences ceases to mature developmentally, at approximately 15 years. These findings then are in agreement with those for Abstract-Concrete development in suggesting that use of abstract ideation seems to mature beyond the level of the verbal functions studied. While the verbal functions attain maturity, Abstract-Concrete behavior does not. Hence, the lack of correlation at the upper age levels. This pattern emerges whether or not deafness is present. Even though the deaf show a retardation, the implication is that they may develop proficiency in the use of abstraction beyond the level of their verbal facility.

Words per Sentence: We have indicated that the number of words written per sentence is a rather independent and reliable measure of the development of written language; see Table 78 and Figure 23. Except for being correlated with Abstract-Concrete and Syntax in the males and with Syntax at seven years in the females, the only consistent relationship found in the hearing group was with Total Sentences; the longer the sentence the fewer sentences written. In contrast, in the deaf Words per Sentence was highly related to all of the other measures of written language, the pattern of relationship being widely different from that found for the hearing; see Table 84. The correlations between this factor and the four other measures were highly significant for both sexes at all age levels from seven through 13 years, and only a few exceptions appeared at the ages of 15 and 17 years. Perhaps the most unusual findings in comparison with the hearing occurred in the relationships with Syntax. In the

TABLE 84.   Correlation between Words per Sentence and other measures
of written language by age and sex

Age	Males						Females					
	7	9	11	13	15	17	7	9	11	13	15	17
TW	.29	.54	.51	.44	.38	.27	.37	.50	.47	.50	.43	.71
TS	.37	.58	.44	.28	.07	−.59	.39	.57	.46	.22	−.14	−.46
A/C	.81	.83	.65	.61	.37	.42	.69	.78	.64	.38	.24	.44
Syn	.70	.87	.76	.78	.55	.20	.83	.91	.81	.61	.37	.41
N	47	77	114	77	69	23	29	74	103	82	61	25

Age	Total					
	7	9	11	13	15	17
TW	.33	.52	.48	.48	.38	.47
TS	.39	.57	.45	.27	−.00	−.52
A/C	.78	.81	.64	.53	.31	.43
Syn	.76	.88	.78	.74	.48	.28
N	76	151	217	159	130	48

TW—Total Words   A/C—Abstract-Concrete
TS—Total Sentences   Syn—Syntax

hearing Words per Sentence and Syntax were correlated only at the age of seven years. In contradistinction, for the deaf these functions were highly associated at all age levels except for the males at 17 years of age.

As the deaf child became older the length of his sentences were less and less related to his ability to use correct language structure. This trend is comparable to results found for the hearing inasmuch as the only significant relationship between these variables occurred at the early age levels. Presumably as the deaf achieve greater facility syntactically, the correlation with Sentence Length diminishes. This trend existed irrespective of sex and the type of school attended. Similarly, the number of words written per sentence was related to Abstract-Concrete behavior; the longer the sentences written, the more abstract was the ideation. For hearing children this correlation was slight. If we view Words per Sentence as a basic indicator of verbal facility, we must conclude as measured by this criterion that for the deaf sentence length is closely associated with all of the other verbal functions as well as with use of abstraction. Previously we have seen the marked limitation in the use of sentences of normal length by the deaf; see Table 78 and Figure 23. This particular limitation seems to be critically related to development of other factors of verbal facility as well as to the use of imagination and abstract ideation.

Words per Sentence must be considered as an important means for disclosing the effects of early life deafness on the development of language and on thought processes. The significance and consequences of this finding are considered further below.

Syntax: Another instance in which the pattern of correlations for the deaf and for the hearing was highly deviate was in Syntax. The only consistent findings for the hearing appeared at seven years, with a few occurring also at nine and 11 years for the males. The pattern was one of reflecting early maturation, with the growth rate being most rapid in the females; see Figure 24. The results shown in Table 85 are in distinct variation with this trend. For the deaf Syntax was closely associated with all of the other scores for both sexes at all age levels from seven through 13 years; for the males this was true also at 15 years with the exception of Total Words. In other words, when deafness is present Syntax is a far more critical factor

TABLE 85. Correlation between Syntax and other measures
of written language by age and sex

			Males						Females			
Age	7	9	11	13	15	17	7	9	11	13	15	17
TW	.60	.49	.52	.53	.21	.09	.49	.53	.43	.36	.15	.40
TS	.76	.61	.65	.52	.31	−.18	.59	.64	.55	.35	−.05	−.13
WPS	.70	.87	.76	.78	.55	.20	.83	.91	.81	.61	.37	.41
A/C	.70	.82	.62	.70	.31	.37	.60	.80	.67	.42	.14	.03
N	47	77	114	77	69	23	29	74	103	82	61	25

			Total		
Age	7	9	11	13	15	17
TW	.56	.51	.49	.47	.17	.20
TS	.70	.62	.61	.46	.19	−.17
WPS	.76	.88	.78	.74	.48	.28
A/C	.68	.81	.66	.60	.26	.16
N	76	151	217	159	130	48

TW—Total Words   WPS—Words per Sentence
TS—Total Sentences   A/C—Abstract-Concrete

in relation to the development of verbal facility and thought processes than when hearing is normal and language is acquired naturally. Again we see the high relationship between the more technical aspects of language and the more general measures of verbal facility. As with Words per Sentence, Syntax is unusually critical as a determinant of language proficiency in other respects. These results loom as being of even greater consequence when we recall that syntactical facility is essentially fully matured by nine years of age in the hearing. In the deaf it is limited and impedes other verbal functions, as well as use of abstraction, until at least 15 years of age. It should be noted, however, that in all instances this relationship diminishes by age. As the child becomes older Syntax is less critical in its association with other indicators of language acquisition and growth. If the deaf child could achieve adequate use of Syntax earlier, at a more normal age, conceivably his language development in other ways would be more adequate.

These findings highlight the frame of reference we have outlined in Chapter IX inasmuch as it indicates that auditory language serves as the basis for the read and written forms. When auditory language is not acquired it is extremely difficult to learn even the syntax of one's mother tongue, an aspect of verbal behavior which the hearing child learns naturally and easily early in life. There is a need to further explore the means whereby syntactical usage can be better developed in deaf children.

TABLE 86. Correlation between Abstract-Concrete behavior and measures of written language by age and sex

Age	Males						Females					
	7	9	11	13	15	17	7	9	11	13	15	17
TW	.36	.72	.68	.68	.58	.43	.44	.64	.60	.63	.63	.55
TS	.36	.77	.68	.68	.60	−.05	.42	.64	.63	.60	.53	.16
WPS	.81	.83	.65	.61	.37	.42	.69	.78	.64	.38	.24	.44
Syn	.70	.82	.62	.70	.31	.37	.60	.80	.67	.42	.14	.03
N	47	77	114	77	69	23	29	74	103	82	61	25

Age	Total					
	7	9	11	13	15	17
TW	.40	.68	.65	.66	.54	.51
TS	.40	.70	.66	.64	.51	.06
WPS	.78	.81	.64	.53	.31	43
Syn	.68	.81	.66	.60	.26	.16
N	76	151	217	159	130	48

TW—Total Words   WPS—Words per Sentence
TS—Total Sentences   Syn—Syntax

Abstract-Concrete: To study the thought processes of the deaf in comparison with the hearing, the Abstract-Concrete scores were correlated with the measures of written language. The pattern of results differed substantially from those obtained for the groups of hearing children on whom The Picture Story Language Test was standardized. For the hearing group the principal correlations with use of abstraction occurred between Total Words and Total Sentences. Words per Sentence and Syntax were largely unrelated to abstract behavior except at the lower age levels.

By comparison, use of abstraction by the deaf was highly correlated with all of the measures of verbal facility through 13 years for the females and through 15 years for the males. The association with Total Words and Words per Sentence reached significance for both sexes at all age levels; see Table 86. We must conclude that in the deaf imagination, use of ideation which is not bound to the observable, is more dependent on all aspects of language than in the hearing. When Syntax and sentence length are attained normally, then use of abstraction is more closely related to verbal fluency only, that is, to Total Words written. However, when language is limited, when vocabulary is meagre and Syntax is poor, then these too are interrelated with the development of abstract thought.

It appears from these results that the psychology of thinking, the nature of the thought processes in the deaf is not necessarily identical to that found for the hearing. While the problem is complex, there is reason to assume that if the verbal level of the deaf could be raised their use of abstraction would be increased. Supposedly this would be true whether their verbal facility were fostered through developing greater fluency, greater sentence length, or through increased syntactical ability. In general, we cannot avoid the conclusion that in children deaf from early life there is a greater inherent relationship between verbal facility and use of abstract thought than there is in the hearing.

We have indicated that for the hearing abstract ideation was correlated principally with the Productivity measures of Total Words and Total Sentences; little association was found with Words per Sentence and Syntax. While for the deaf all four of the scores for written language correlated significantly with Abstract-Concrete behavior, the most outstanding relationships were with Total Words and Words per Sentence. The most consistent results were those obtained for Total Words; for both groups the interdependence of number of words written and facility with abstract ideas was pronounced. Whether or not deafness was present the longer the story, the more the child engaged in thought processes which were not bound to the stimulus, the more he detached himself from the observable and employed ideas which entailed fantasy, conceptual integration, and creative imagination. Ostensibly, the more fluency with the written word, the more the child found it possible to use abstraction.

With the hearing group the least association with Abstract-Concrete behavior was with Words per Sentence, followed by Syntax. In view of the excellence of Words per Sentence as a measure of language growth and acquisition, this finding is of interest. In the hearing child it is not the adequacy of his verbal behavior as determined by the length of his sentences which is influential as far as the use of abstract thought is concerned. Instead it is more the manner in which he uses this facility to produce a composition of adequate length. Taking the opposite point of view, a child might have developed verbal facility at least at the average level but if he has a poverty of ideas, if he does not have fluidity of thought and ideation, he writes a short story despite the adequacy of his language ability in terms of Words per Sentence or Syntax.

When language proficiency is limited as a result of deafness, circumstances are altered. Ideas still are critical because association with story length persists in being of great importance. Nonetheless, because of the poverty of language, use of abstraction now is correlated with all aspects of verbal facility, with productivity as well as with structure syntactically. When deafness is present, not only the length of the story is critical but also the length of the sentence and the ability to use proper structure, parts of speech and tense, in fact all aspects of grammar. We should mention that except for Total Words these associations between verbal facility and Abstract-Concrete behavior diminish with age. Moreover, these results were consistent irrespective of the type of school attended.

The Relationships Between Reading and Writing

To analyze the interrelationships between verbal functions in detail the scores for visual receptive language, reading, were correlated with the scores for expressive language, writing; the scores on the Columbia Vocabulary Test were correlated with each of the measures on The Picture Story Language Test. The results are presented in Table 87. These findings indicate a number of significant relationships between input and output functions, between receptive and expressive language. Total Sentences showed the least correlation with read vocabulary whereas the associations were high with

TABLE 87. Correlation between scores on read and written language by age and sex

Age	Males 9	11	13	15	17	Females 9	11	13	15	17
TW	.17	.54	.32	.35	.11	.30	.27	.31	.19	.44
TS	.17	.37	.14	.09	−.16	.25	.18	.09	−.11	−.37
WPS	.37	.49	.68	.60	.36	.28	.37	.71	.48	.65
A/C	.40	.38	.38	.19	.38	.30	.31	.16	.22	.19
Syn	.31	.31	.35	.41	.47	.29	.34	.43	.48	.58
N	77	144	77	69	23	74	103	.82	61	25

Total Age	9	11	13	15	17
TW	.24	.40	.33	.27	.34
TS	.21	.28	.14	.01	−.25
WPS	.33	.43	.70	.55	.49
A/C	.35	.36	.30	.21	.29
Syn	.31	.34	.40	.44	.51
N	151	217	159	130	48

TW—Total Words   WPS—Words per Sentence   Syn—Syntax
TS—Total Sentences   A/C—Abstract-Concrete

Total Words, Words per Sentence, Syntax, and Abstract-Concrete behavior. In comparison with the hearing more correlations were found for the deaf and in general were of greater magnitude.

These results support the point of view that receptive and expressive verbal functions are interdependent. Although the statistical results do not reveal which is more critical initially, which must be acquired first, as we have stated in Chapter IX empirically it is logical to assume that input must precede output. If this is true then these results manifest the reciprocal manner in which the limitation in reading restricts facility in written language. Inasmuch as reading ability is far below the norm for the hearing, written language also is seriously deficient. Perhaps one of the most beneficial and effective ways to improve the level of written language is to raise the level of read language. Evidence on the processes whereby language is acquired suggests that the feedback principle is of importance. After a degree of receptive function has been established then output, expressive function, enhances the input; writing the words one has learned to read fosters efficiency in reading which in turn fosters efficiency in writing. Therefore, written language also must be emphasized in the total program of language development. Recognition of these relationships and the processes which must be assumed might form the basis of a new emphasis, a new approach to the problem of language acquisition in the deaf.

The correlation between reading and writing was analyzed by school and there was a slight trend towards earlier use of written language in relation to reading in the Day School, shown by the association found between the Columbia Vocabulary scores and Words per Sentence. Besides, minor differences appeared in the correlations between reading and Syntax; in the Day School group there was a gradual decrease and in the Residential group a gradual increment by age. In general the patterns were consistent in showing a close relationship between ability to read and facility with the written word from nine through 13 years of age for both sexes. At the ages of 15 and 17 years the most significant affiliations were with Total Words, Words per Sentence, and Syntax.

To summarize, respectively it is first the speechread symbol, then the read word that are the basic verbal systems in deaf children. The correlation data reveal an interdependence of the various language systems, receptive and expressive, which highlights the importance of inner language. Moreover, all types of verbal proficiency are related to the use of abstraction by the deaf; verbal and abstract behavior cannot be separated. If the deaf child's verbal competence could be fostered more successfully, an improvement in abstract capacity would be expected. The opposite may be equally true; if greater facility in the use of abstraction could be developed, increased language adequacy might be the result.

LANGUAGE AND INTELLIGENCE

Many investigators have reported a correlation between intelligence and language capacities. Binet[4] showed this relationship in the development of his classic mental test and it has been demonstrated also by the work of Wechsler.[29] More recently Templin[27] found a relationship between intelligence, developmental age, and measures of spoken language. The data presented in Chapter X disclosed a correlation between mental ability and proficiency in speechreading. To explore the verbal processes in deaf children, correlations were computed for the Draw-a-Man scores and the scores on The Picture Story Language Test. These results are shown in Table 88.

No association appeared between facility in written language and intelligence at the age level of seven years with the exception of Words per Sentence for the females, perhaps because ability to write was so meagre at this age. Substantial relationships between these factors was found at the ages of nine and 11 years with all five measures of written language being significantly correlated with intelligence. In most instances, however, the coefficients showed a decrement with age; hence, the relationships above 13 years were scattered and varied by sex. The most consistent trends occurred with Total Words, Words per Sentence, and Syntax; use of abstraction was related to intelligence in the males only at the age levels of nine, 11, and 13 and in the females only at nine and 11 years.

Templin[27] also reported a decrement by age in the correlation between intelligence and language. While in our findings as in hers this might be a function of the tests used, it appears that as verbal ability matures, the relationship to intelligence diminishes. A similar result was found for the hearing in our developmental study of writ-

TABLE 88. Correlation between measures of written language and intelligence

	Males						Females					
Age	7	9	11	13	15	17	7	9	11	13	15	17
TW	−.07	.32	.26	.26	.24	.08	.33	.25	.33	.23	−.12	.40
TS	−.19	.31	.27	.28	.16	−.11	.29	.30	.32	.24	.19	−.35
WPS	.04	.47	.27	.19	.28	.26	.37	.29	.44	.17	.09	.60
A/C	.05	.42	.25	.30	.12	.31	.26	.37	.37	.13	.08	.24
Syn	−.02	.43	.29	.29	.27	.48	.23	.33	.41	.29	.09	.05
N	47	77	114	77	69	23	29	74	103	82	61	25

	Total					
Age	7	9	11	13	15	17
TW	.10	.27	.26	.24	.09	.21
TS	.00	.29	.27	.26	.02	−.23
WPS	.19	.38	.33	.17	.18	.40
A/C	.17	.38	.27	.21	.07	.25
Syn	.12	.37	.32	.27	.17	.24
N	76	151	217	159	130	48

TW—Total Words   WPS—Words per Sentence   Syn—Syntax
TS—Total Sentences   A/C—Abstract-Concrete

ten language. It is our presumption that most types of verbal facility mature at a more rapid rate than mental ability and reach a plateau at an earlier age. This seems to be true of spoken language as studied by Templin, and of written language as shown by our studies. Such a trend in deaf children may be seen, especially when a nonverbal measure such as the Draw-a-Man Test is used to measure intelligence. Nevertheless, there is little question but that at the early age levels, mainly through 11 years of age, a correlation exists between facility with written language and mental capacity; the intellectually competent acquire language more successfully.

The findings relative to the use of abstraction are interesting. It might be assumed that Abstract-Concrete behavior was more closely associated with mental ability. Although the measure of abstraction was not viewed as being a type of intelligence test, it has been generally predicated that abstract ability was eminently affiliated with intellectual capacity. In view of the findings for the deaf, we must assume that the results are influenced by verbal facility; development of abstract behavior is impeded by the limitation verbally and therefore the correlation with intelligence is altered.

In order to not over-simplify or over-generalize however, we should stress that the relationships between intelligence and language acquisition are far from perfect. Beyond a certain limit of intellectual brightness, other factors may be of greater importance. Teachers of the deaf are aware that the most intelligent children are not always the most proficient in speech, speechreading, reading, or in use of the written word. Individual differences such as degree of residual hearing, age of onset of deafness, and special aptitudes play an important role. Another notable factor is the teacher herself. Teachers vary in aptitudes, with some being more successful than others in helping deaf children master the difficult problem of acquiring language.

In contrast to most of the other findings, the type of school attended also played a role. The association between intelligence and use of abstraction was found to be closer in the Residential group than in the Day. A sex difference appeared in the Day School children in that the correlation for the males was significant at all ages except at 15 years whereas for the females, significance was reached only at nine years of age. Sex differences were not found for the Residential group or for the hearing. These deviations on the basis of school, found only rarely in our study, may be due to psychodynamic factors such as those disclosed by the projective analysis of the Draw-a-Man Test and presented in Chapter VI.

Reading and Intelligence: The relationships between reading and mental ability also were investigated and these findings are given in Table 89. We have noted that intelligence correlated with speechreading (see Chapter X) and with written language. For reading the association with mental ability varied by age, the greatest degree of correlation occurring at 11 and 17 years of age; none of the coefficients were high. While some of the relationships were significant, the Draw-a-Man Test seems less useful as a predictor of success in reading than of certain other verbal functions.

From the results of this test presented in Chapters V and VI, we might expect that the findings would vary by school and by sex. In the Residential School group significant relationships were found for both sexes at 15 and 17 year age levels but not at the age levels of 11 or 13. In contrast, for the Day School group significant correlations appeared at nine, 11 and 13 years but not at 15 years. Also, for those in Day Schools the relationship diminished by age while for the Residential School children it remained constant or diminished.

TABLE 89.   Correlation between scores on the Columbia
Vocabulary and Draw-a-Man Tests

Age	N	Males	N	Females	N	Total
9	77	.16	74	.24	151	.19
11	114	.20	103	.27	217	.22
13	77	.13	82	.17	159	.14
15	69	.06	61	.06	130	.14
17	23	.49	25	.56	48	.51

In agreement with other findings of the investigation, especially for
the Draw-a-Man Test, the psychological processes entailed are not
identical for the two groups and in addition, the verbal behavior of
the Residential School males deviated from the general trends for
the deaf group as a whole.

IMPLICATIONS FOR TRAINING, LEARNING AND ADJUSTMENT

In this chapter we have considered the problems of acquiring
read and written language when deafness is present from early life.
There is an extensive relationship between these verbal functions
and sensory deprivation; deaf children are markedly retarded in
reading and in use of the written word. Analysis of their written
language disclosed characteristic errors. In order of frequency of
occurrence these were:

1. Productivity   5. Word Order
2. Omissions   6. Undue use of nouns and articles
3. Substitutions   7. Deficiency in use of adjectives,
4. Additions   conjunctions, adverbs, and interjections

For the psychologist and the educator there is an urgent need
for further knowledge regarding the psychology of language development in deaf children. We must ascertain the nature of the specific deviations encountered and then evolve educational methods
for alleviating them. Basic questions are why the deaf child omits
words and perhaps certain types of words more than others, why he
substitutes inappropriate for appropriate words, why he adds unnecessary words, and why he places the words of a sentence in the
wrong order.

Students who pursue these questions may wish to explore
whether the omission and addition of words constitutes a single
factor, a unitary deficiency in the language behavior of deaf children.
If so, what techniques might be most effective in assisting them to
overcome this error which is so characteristic of their language.

A related finding is that deaf children learn to use prepositions more successfully than any other part of speech and comparatively, one of the more difficult for them is the adverb. We have suggested that this may be because adverbs are used primarily to qualify and limit verbs, whereas prepositions principally are words placed before nouns to show their relation to other words in the sentence. These differences, these hierarchies of difficulty in verbal learning as found in the deaf provide a basis for developing new approaches to language teaching and training.

Verbal deficiences became apparent in other ways. In comparison with the hearing, deaf children are grossly deficient in Productivity, especially in writing fewer Total Words as well as less Words per Sentence. The need to develop a more extensive vocabulary and a more fluent use of language is obvious. Language structure, Syntax, also is decidedly inferior and together with Productivity was found to be closely related to Abstract-Concrete behavior. For more successful language development in deaf children, careful consideration should be given to both Productivity and Syntax.

Despite his limitations verbally the deaf child reaches a plateau in language development. In some aspects of language he shows virtually no progress beyond 11 years of age. Of major importance is the development of ways to keep him progressing in language growth even beyond the age at which verbal maturity is attained by the hearing. That specialized techniques and methods, now applied mainly at the early age levels, should be devised and stressed in later school years is clearly evident.

While the deaf child's deficiency in language is not mainly one of immaturity, the concepts of mental age and emotional growth must be used in conjunction with new approaches to language development. These approaches now can be more *child oriented* than in the past because more knowledge has been gained relevant to the total maturation of all children, deaf and hearing. The traditional educational techniques devised for deaf children have been more *method* than child oriented. Because more objective evidence is becoming available, new procedures can be originated which are firmly based on the concept of developmental age, on the characteristic problems of learning associated with deafness and on the specific deficiencies found in the language of deaf children.

It would be premature to outline such a system in detail because this can be done only through experimental work covering a period of several years. However, new methodologies for language training are indicated even now by the evidence before us. As suggested in Chapter IX these should take cognizance of the hierarchy seen in Man's verbal behavior. Inner language would be stressed first, followed by emphasis on Receptive and Expressive Language. Though based firmly on the psychology of deafness, on the input, output, and monitoring systems available to the deaf, the procedures in early life would be informal with formal techniques predominating as the child becomes older. The system which might be most beneficial is one which provides for self-correction by *alerting* and *reminding* the child of his errors. The feedback system would be devised to provide self-corrective information especially in regard to the errors characterizing his language. While it can be assumed that pre-programmed, automated approaches using electronic instrumentation will be available and beneficial in such training, the teacher can now inaugurate programs of this type. For example, giving the child the benefit of feedback as quickly as possible after an error has been made, she might use a system as follows:

O = Omission Error	Ad = Use adjectives
S = Substitution Error	Con = Use conjunctions
A = Addition Error	Adv = Use adverbs
WO = Word Order Error	Int = Use interjections
N = Undue use of Nouns	Pro = Use more words, phrases, sentences,
Art = Undue use of Articles	longer compositions, etc.
	CP = Do not use Carrier Phrases

Much effort remains before systems like these can be fully developed. But already the ingenious teacher might want to try this method, especially at the middle and upper school ages, by adapting it to flash cards or even by making a set of slides which could be shown on a screen one at a time by pushing a button. Because deaf children like such techniques, soon they would want to push the button themselves while trying to find their errors. The teacher who adds an error counter to the equipment, simply and automatically would have the basis for securing learning curves on the children in her classes. Through such procedures progress will be made and the characteristic problems of learning and adjustment associated with deafness will be minimized.

ILLUSTRATIVE STORIES: Deaf and Hearing

Although statistical analysis adds greatly to knowledge and clarifies questions which have been raised scientifically, it is also important to make observations clinically and empirically. Many educators and other professional workers must make qualitative judgments daily regarding the types of errors and successes which characterize the efforts of the children with whom they are working. For this reason Illustrative Stories are presented which reveal growth in the development of written language in both deaf and hearing children.

A typical story, one falling close to the mean for each group was selected; none was far below or far above the average for the age level which it represents. A sample story for both sexes is given for each of the age levels; see Figures 39 through 44. In studying the differences among these stories, whether by age or by group, it will be helpful to refer to Tables 76, 77, 78, 79 and to Figures 21, 22, 23, and 24.

Inspection of these sample stories clearly indicates differences between the deaf and the hearing, shown also by the statistical analysis. At the seven and nine year levels those written by the deaf are characterized by Carrier Phrases and hence consist of a series of generally unrelated sentences. Those for the hearing, even at this early age, express what is assumed to be happening in the picture which they are viewing; there is consistent fluency and sequence such as is expected when telling a story.

It is apparent that the stories written by the deaf are considerably shorter than those written by the hearing. For example, the Total Word score for the deaf females at nine years is 41 and for the hearing female it is 98; these scores are almost exactly at the respective means for the groups as shown in Table 76. This difference in Productivity can be seen throughout the examples shown.

Likewise, the differences in sentence length are striking but perhaps the most obvious deviation between the groups is in Syntax. Even at 17 years of age the problem of syntactical structure is vividly apparent. For example, the deaf male at this age level made errors in tense, in use of articles, in Omission, in Substitution, and in Word Order. The fifth sentence of his story typifies the language errors of deaf children. The idea being expressed is of high level and manifests use of abstraction; it is not observable. Written correctly, what

a Boy had some toys.
And he was playing house.
He had a little chair to put a
little girl on it.

Hearing, Male

I saw car,
saw shoe,
saw dog,
saw baby,
saw Father,
saw Mother,
saw boy,
saw girl,
saw books,
saw box,
saw Father,
saw ball,
saw eya,

Deaf, Male

I see 4 books.

I see a big chair

I see boy.

I see a car.

I see a doll.

I see a shoes.

I see two little chairs.

I see two table.

Deaf, Female

The Boy is playing
with toys. in his roob.
one is new. He has a lot of toys.
He is play with some dolls.
He likes to play with all of the toys.

Hearing, Female

FIG. 39. ILLUSTRATIVE STORIES: Seven years of age

This is a cripple child playing
with dolls. He is about 6 years
old. He is play house with the
dolls. the dolls are made of wood.
They are eating breakfast. the
baby is crying so the mother is
going to pick her up. the boy is
going to school. the father is
just getting done so he is going
to push his chair in. the
girl is just getting finished and
getting out of her chair.

Hearing, Male

A boy is playing on bed

He is sitting on chair.

He is playing on car.

He is sitting on table.

He is sitting on ball

He is sitting on books.

He is sitting on shoes!

He is playinggirl.

He is playing mani

He is

Deaf, Male

1. The boy play with doll house.
2. He put on the table.
3. The boy have many toys.
4. He have tables.
5. He have cars.
6. He have chairs.
7. We have mother and father.
8. We have books.
9. He have shoes.
10. He have a new shirt

Deaf, Female

One day I was in my room. First I play with my little doll family and their little furniture. Next I read one of my story books. I like to read books. It is fun to look at the pictures some of the pictures are funny. There is a little table and two chairs for me. I have a car in my room. I have a ball. I play with my ball outside mother wouldn't let me play ball in side. There is a place to keep my games.

Hearing, Female

FIG. 40. ILLUSTRATIVE STORIES: Nine years of age

Hearing, Male

The little Elis

Once upon a time there was a little boy named Stanley we called him Stan for short. The things he loves the most was his books and his little toys. One night he couldn't sleep he got so upset down near his paint book called ... his blocks and toys were near him but all of a suddenly they all came to life and they started to play. Stanley came and sing happy songs they were very happy but Stan's mother came in and broke the spell and then he just put their playing with him the toys that really came to life

Deaf, Male

A boy played a table and chair on the toy. A boy looked a books on the wood. A boy picked a chair many on the box. A boy looked a car and shoe on the wood.

I saw a picture of a boy. A boy playing some toys. He is playing house of people on the table. He sat on the chair near the cupboard. He has a neat the clothes. He has brown hair, and blue eyes. He has on yellow sweater, brown suits, and white shirt. Many books are on the cupboard and gray rugs on the floor.

Deaf, Female

This story is about a little boy who seems to be in a playroom playing with some toys and doll and furniture. It looks as if the family, he is playing with, is just sitting down to eat. The girl doll whose name could be Jane is being settled into her chair and Jother is just about to sit down also. Mother is lifting baby from his walker and is putting him in his highchair. But what is the boy doll Jack doing? Just as usual, he is saying to the dog; Come on old sport! I want some of my food? Of course the dog replied quickly, You see Jack isn't a very good eater but his pal Sparki, Jacks family though is very proud of him because he is very alert and good in school.

Hearing, Female

FIG. 41. ILLUSTRATIVE STORIES: Eleven years of age

Hearing, Male

When I Was Six

If I was during playtime in 1st grade. I was play house with the furniture and toy people. I finished to set up the furniture the way that I thought best. The chairs were not the right size for some of the stuff but it didn't really matter. I was very disappointed in the limit because it opened and closed.

I had set the table for the family to eat dinner. I had the silver ware and the plates, meat and potatoes. The little baby was on her scooter by the table hungry. I set the girl at the table, her parents were coming to the table with her brother.

After dinner they all retired to the living room. Baby in her scooter, father in his chair, brother playing with his new dog, then dog, mother was cleaning off the table. It was time to quit playtime so I cleaned off the table and put the toys away.

Deaf, Male

The boy is playing house on the table. There lot of toy on the table put the girl on the chair and little toy to play with little dog and Mother is play with little baby and father come home to see children, mother, baby, and it time supper. We put family on table and eat. We put rest of the toy on the chair. It almost time for supper him.

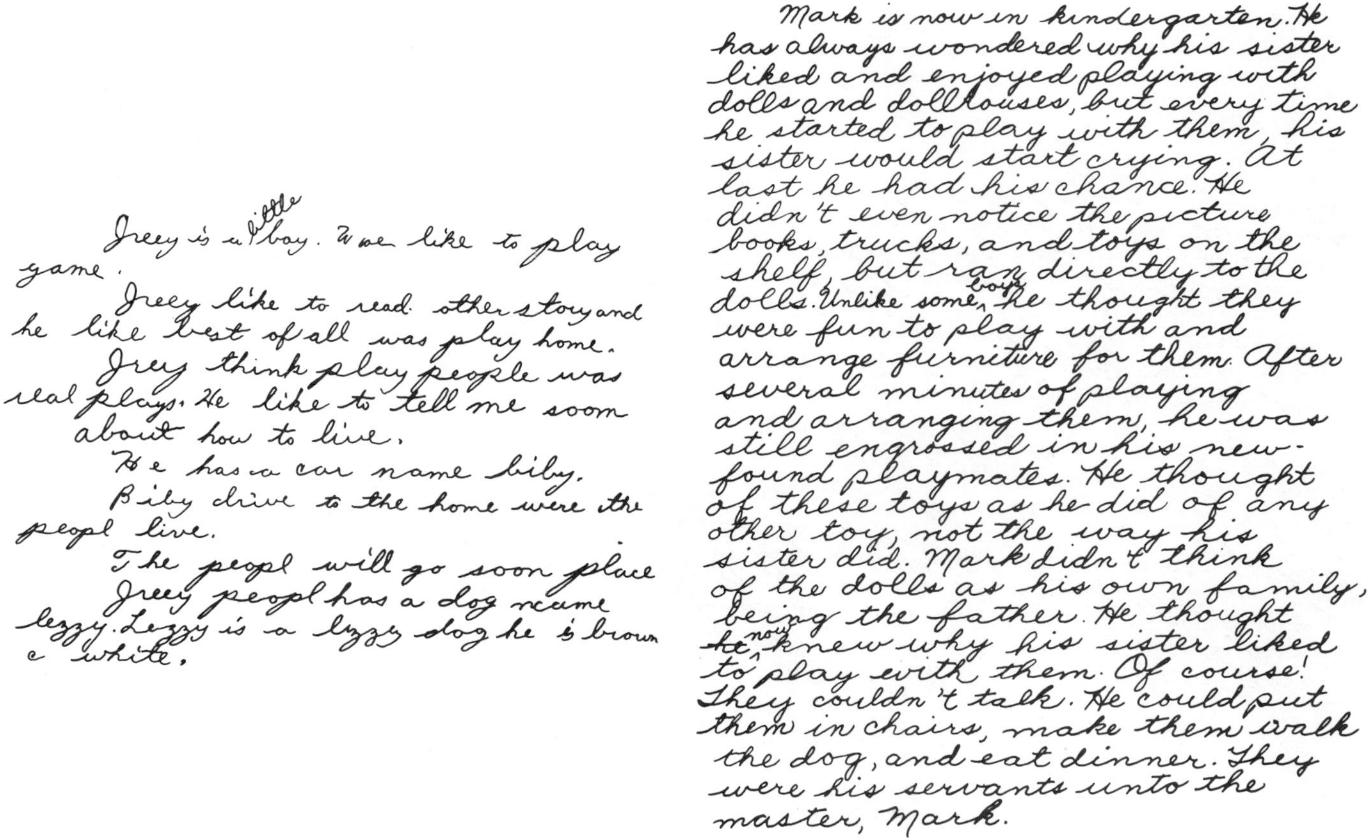

Hearing, Female

Mark is now in kindergarten. He has always wondered why his sister liked and enjoyed playing with dolls and dollhouses, but every time he started to play with them his sister would start crying. At last he had his chance. He didn't even notice the picture books, trucks, and toys on the shelf, but ran directly to the dolls. Unlike some, he thought they were fun to play with and arrange furniture for them. After several minutes of playing and arranging them, he was still engrossed in his new-found playmates. He thought of these toys as he did of any other toy, not the way his sister did. Mark didn't think of the dolls as his own family, being the father. He thought to know why his sister liked to play with them. Of course they couldn't talk. He could put them in chairs, make them walk the dog, and eat dinner. They were his servants unto the master, Mark.

Deaf, Female

Grey is a boy. I we like to play game. Grey like to read. other story and he like best of all was play home. Grey think play people was real play. He like to tell me soon about how to live.

B e has a can name lily.

Baby drive to the home were its pepol live.

The pepol will go soon place Grey pepol has a dog name Leggy. Leggy is a loggs dog he is brown a white.

FIG. 42. ILLUSTRATIVE STORIES: Thirteen years of age

Hearing, Male

This is the boy's first day at Kinder-garten. He is sitting in a little chair by the teacher, apart the other students since he does not know most of them, that is why he is sitting quietly in the backroom playing by himself.

His stepfather has put his best clothes on him, he has a new pair of his shoes are newly things because his mother wants him to look his best.

Surrounding him are many books and toys and on the shelves are many pieces of paper and many more toys and books.

Right now he is probably wishing he could be home playing with the gang or watching TV. But he realizes to will have to be content for a longer more hours.

Deaf, Male

I saw a little boy play with his toy in the picture. He play with his toy on the table. He had a hole a chair on his right hand. He had a little girl on his left hand. He had 5 family father stand behind the table and a little boy follow his boy. other little boy watch the boy. He had book, why boy ball and chair with a house. he inside. with a toy on the other chair. A little boy like to play with his toy.

A small boy is sitting down in the chair, and still playing with his toy furniture. He is changing them. I think he is about five years old. He is playing with his toys perhaps in his mother's kitchen. He has lots of toys to play with. Those toys are about toy dolls, toy chairs, tables, cupboards, etc. and books, and a car, ball, toy-shoe. I think he joined his toys very much. He wears a suit. His hair is brown. I think his eyes are brown, too.

Deaf, Female

from a rather regular day of school. It was raining and he was unable to think of a way to amuse himself. His older sister Sally was at a friend's house and his mother was very tired and upset over his bad day.

While pondering over an idea Johnny's eye suddenly caught sight of a small box tucked in the corner of his den. He approached it curiously. Upon seeing that it only contained old plastic furniture and people which Sally had cast aside, he turned away. However, in a moment's time curiosity got the best of him, and he carried the box over to a table.

As fast as Johnny kept watching to see if anyone was around to see him, soon he was so engaged in this new experience that he forgot all else. The dolls walked, sat, and moved various ways with the slight use of his hands. Here he had found amusement in a simple and different form. Would you have tried it?

Hearing, Female

FIG. 43. ILLUSTRATIVE STORIES: Fifteen years of age

Deaf, Male

A boy put some furniture, and he put the loaf on top the table and put the chair on his table. He put it some many furnitures on the table and he wide make some things for the dining room. The furniture boy sit on the chair. A boy wants to learn the furnitures. How to put some dining room on the table. The looks have many wands to learn in school. The toy car, wooden ring toss, wooden stars from books, and ball on the cabinet. The furnitures have the chair, armchair, dresser, table, dog, floor lamp, baby carriage, baby high chair, and cupboard cabinet.

Hearing, Male

A little boy can do many things in one day. On a rainy day all the need we do is very out a few toys and he may soon be on an airplane pilot setting a new record for an own country flight. We can do so in general carrying his things in the little time. First he whirls his things to a point, then he stacks. So the bookcauges on and over the wooly haunting counts stack on his important flock. Thirdly he turns ruplements and implements to the area. Often a touzzle of a few minutes de soon a dozen book, when they is seal at the ground also record an important ready to the case if picture. That go the little ground, there are not over, there will be many and bottle, just as option or just as agentorgoto him. There will be many and adventures for one toy and his toys.

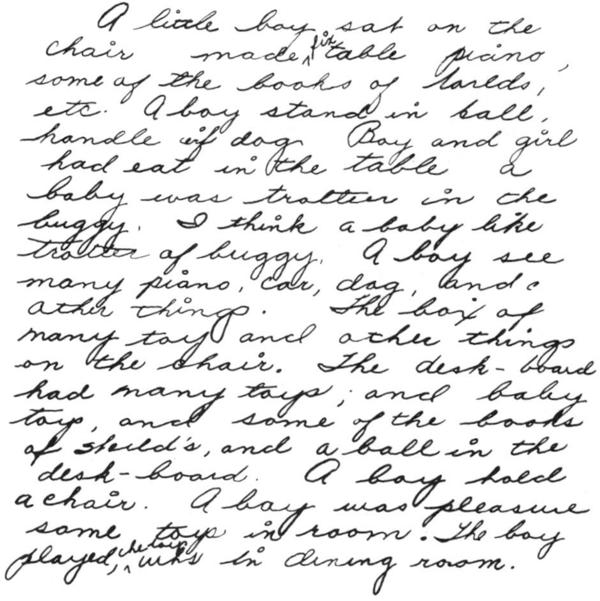

A little boy sat on the chair made of table piano, some of the books of Canada, etc. A boy stands in ball. Handle of dog. Boy and girl had eat in the table. A baby was trotten in the buggy. I think a baby like bottle of buggy, cat, dog, and a many piano, cat, dog, and a many toys and the things on the chair. The desk had had many toys, and baby top, and some of the books of stick's, and a ball in the dust-board. A boy had a chair. A boy was pleasure some toys in room. The boy played with in dining room.

Deaf, Female

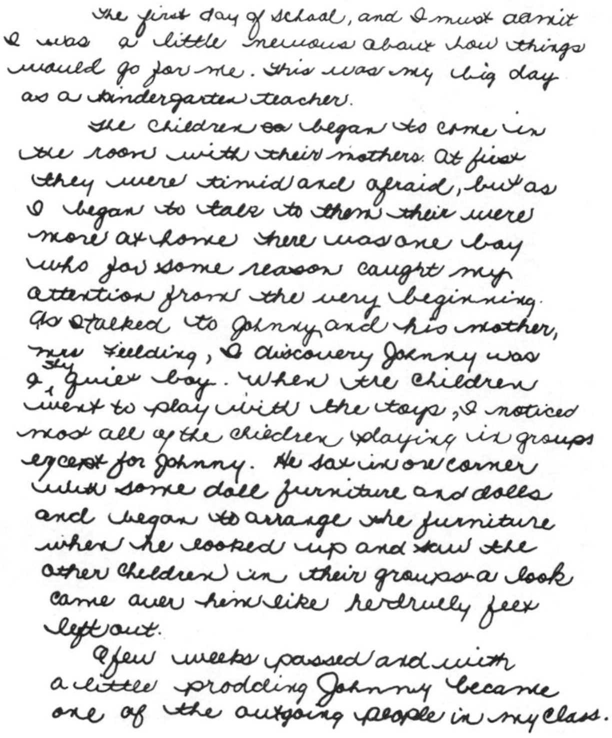

The first day of school, and I must admit I was a little nervous about how things would go for me. This was my big day as a kindergarten teacher.

The children began to come in. We soon knew their mothers. At first they were timid and afraid, but as I began to talk to them, their were many at home there was one day who for some reason caught my attention from the very beginning. As I talked to Jenny and his mother, my feeling, I discovery Jenny was a quiet boy. When the children went to play with the toys, I notice most all of the children playing in groups except for Johnny. He saw in corner with some doll furniture and dolls and began to arrange some furniture. When he looked up and would see other children in their group a look came over him like restlessly few left out.

A few weeks passed and with a little prodding Johnny became one of the outgoing people in my class.

Hearing, Female

FIG. 44. ILLUSTRATIVE STORIES: Seventeen years of age

he intended to say was, *The books have many words in them which should (must) be learned in school.* Examples of this type of error can be found in the other stories.

The subtlety of abstract thought which underlies the typical story written by the hearing is especially obvious. In some instances the entire story is based on a hypothetical, imaginative plan or plot. The deaf tend to write more about the actual circumstances portrayed in the picture, more about what can actually be observed. This is the reason the difference between the deaf and the hearing in the use of abstraction appears as it does in Figure 30.

REFERENCES

1. Asch, S.: The metaphor: a psychological inquiry, in Tagiuri, R. and Petrullo, L. (ed.) Person Perception and Interpersonal Behavior. Stanford, Stanford University Press, 1958.
2. Ausubel, D.: The Psychology of Meaningful Verbal Learning. New York, Grune and Stratton, 1963.
3. Barnhart, C.: The American College Dictionary. New York, Random House, 1952.
4. Binet, A. and Simon, Th.: The Intelligence of the Feeble-Minded. Baltimore, Williams and Wilkins, 1916.
5. Blair, F.: A study of the visual memory of deaf and hearing children. Am. Ann. Deaf, 102, 254, 1957.
6. Brown, R.: Words and Things. Glencoe, Illinois, The Free Press, 1959.
7. Carroll, J.: The Study of Language. Cambridge, Harvard University Press, 1953.
8. Costello, M. R.: A study of speechreading as a developing language process in deaf and hard of hearing children. Evanston, Northwestern University, Unpublished Doctoral Dissertation, 1957.
9. Davis, E. Mean sentence length compared with long and short sentences as a reliable measure of language development. Child Developm., 8, 69, 1937.
10. Farrant, R.: A factor analytical study of the intellective abilities of deaf and hard of hearing children compared with normal hearing children. Unpublished doctoral dissertation, Northwestern Univer., 1960.
11. Fries, C.: The Structure of English. New York, Harcourt, Brace, 1952.
12. Fuller, C.: A study of the growth and organization of certain mental abilities in young deaf children. Evanston, Northwestern University, Unpublished Doctoral Dissertation, 1959.
13. Gansl, I. and Garrett, H.: Columbia Vocabulary Test. New York, Psychol. Corp., 1939.
14. Goda, S.: Language skills of profoundly deaf adolescent children. J. Speech and Hearing Research, 2, 369, 1959.
15. Heider, F. and Heider, G.: Studies in the psychology of the deaf. Psychol. Monog., #242, 1941.
16. Langer, S.: Philosophy in a New Key. Cambridge, Harvard University Press, 1957.

17. Leopold, W.: Speech Development of a Bilingual Child. Vol. 1, 2, 3, 4. Evanston, Northwestern University Press, 1954.
18. McCarthy, D.: Language development in children, in Carmichael, L. Manual of Child Psychology. New York, John Wiley and Sons, 1946.
19. Mowrer, O. Learning Theory and the Symbolic Process. New York, Grune and Stratton, 1964.
20. Myklebust, H.: Manual for the Picture Story Language Test. New York, Grune and Stratton, 1964.
21. Neyhus, A.: The personality of socially well-adjusted adult deaf as revealed by projective tests. Unpublished doctoral dissertation, Northwestern Univer., 1962.
22. Oléron, P.: Conceptual thinking of the deaf. Am. Ann. Deaf, 98, 304, 1953.
23. Perrin, P.: Writer's Guide and Index to English. New York, Scott, Foresman and Company, 1942.
24. Pugh, G.: Appraisal of the silent reading abilities of acoustically handicapped children. Am. Ann. Deaf, 91, 331, 1946.
25. Reamer, J.: Mental and educational measurements of the deaf. Psychol. Monog., 29, #3, 1921.
26. Stormzand, M. and O'Shea, M.: How Much English Grammar? Baltimore, Warwick and York, 1924.
27. Templin, M.: Certain Language Skills in Children. Minneapolis, University of Minnesota Press, 1957.
28. Thompson, W.: An analysis of errors in written composition by deaf children. Am. Ann. Deaf, 81, 95, 1936.
29. Wechsler, D.: Wechsler Intelligence Scale for Children. New York, Psychol. Corp., 1949.
30. Williams, H.: An analytical study of language achievement in preschool children. Iowa City, University of Iowa Studies, Child Welfare, 13, 9, 1937.
31. Yedinack, J.: A study of the linguistic functioning of children with articulation and reading disabilities. J. Genetic Psychol., 74, 23, 1949.

Suggestions for Further Study

Anderson, I. and Dearborn, W.: The Psychology of Teaching Reading. New York, Ronald Press, 1952.
Brill, R.: Prognosis of reading achievement of the deaf. Am. Ann. Deaf, 86, 227, 1941.
Hofsmarksrichter, R.: Do the deaf see more than those with all their senses? Am. Ann. Deaf, 78, 113, 1933.
Kendall, B.: A note on the relation of retardation in reading to performance on a memory for designs test. J. Ed. Psychol., 39, 370, 1948.
McCarthy, D.: Language development in children, in Carmichael, L. (ed.) Manual of Child Psychology. New York, John Wiley and Sons, 1946.
Russell, D.: Children's Thinking. Chicago, Ginn, 1956.
Strayer, L.: Language and growth. Genetic Psychol. Monog., 8, #3, 1930.
Thompson, H.: An experimental study of the beginning reading of deaf-mutes. New York, Columbia University, T. C. Contrib. to Ed., #254, 1927.
Young, C. and McConnell, F.: Retardation of vocabulary development in the hard of hearing child. J. Except. Child., 23, 368, 1957.

Part Four

Other Handicaps, Special Abilities, and Aptitudes

Chapter XII

SEEING AND HEARING

VISION IS THE RESIDUAL DISTANCE SENSE for those with deafness. Despite the critical importance of seeing when hearing is impaired, only meager study has been made of the visual capacities of the auditorially impaired. In this chapter we raise the question of whether there is a relationship between auditory and visual deficiencies. As in the case of motor abilities or intelligence, a relationship between these sensory capacities may exist on two primary bases. The disease which caused deafness might also cause defective vision. For example, a child who has a hearing loss due to maternal rubella might also have impaired vision, both hearing and seeing having been affected by the disease. If this were true generally, we would expect that those having exogenous deafness would have more visual impairments than the endogenous. Present evidence, however, does not support this hypothesis.

Visual and auditory dysfunctions conceivably may be interrelated on another but more complex basis; that is, the effect of deafness on visual processes. Does deafness affect such visual functions as simultaneous vision, fusion, or stereopsis? In this case we are concerned about disturbances in vision resulting from the lack of normal stimulation auditorially. A number of workers have noted that auditory sensation affects the judgment of what is seen, or the process of seeing. Bartley[1] in his discussion of intersensory facilitation emphasizes that stimulating a second sense while the first is being stimulated, alters the response of the first modality, reducing or raising the threshold. This has been referred to as

heteromodal reciprocity.[14] Harris[6] has stressed the neurophysio-
logical mechanisms which may explain these sensory relationships.
That auditory stimulation alters visual responses in certain specific
respects has been demonstrated by the work of Kravkok,[11] Brogden,[3]
Jenkins,[10] Hartmann,[7] and Serrat and Kerwoski.[18] Werner,[22] Gesell,[5]
and Hebb[8] have emphasized the importance of synesthesia in the
total development of the organism. From the findings of these
various workers, we can assume that lack of auditory stimulation
would be related to visual behavior. Visual function may be altered
because of lack of intersensory stimulation, implying that certain
neural mechanisms mainly responsible for vision are, at least, partially dependent on auditory stimulation for maximum development
and efficiency. Another possibility is that visual perceptual processes are influenced by the lack of heteromodal reciprocity occurring
in the presence of deafness. Although research evidence is slight
and inferences must be made with caution, there are findings which
support each of these possibilities. Therefore, the visual behavior
of individuals having deafness seemingly may be altered both because the disease which resulted in a hearing loss has also caused
lack of normal intersensory facilitation neurophysiologically, and
visual perceptual deficiencies deriving from an imposition of heteromodal reciprocity.

In a study of the visual perception of deaf children Myklebust
and Brutten[14] found them to be deficient in specific functions; this
was not a generalized inferiority. These findings were supported
by the data on intelligence discussed in Chapter V, and to some
extent by the results of the Drawing of the Human Figure Test
given in Chapter VI. Deprivation of hearing deters and impedes
visual perceptual functioning in some respects, but it may cause
such functioning to be enhanced in other respects. In either case
an effect, an alteration, has occurred. It is apparent that possible
associations between deafness and visual deficiencies must be explored both in terms of sensory defects and altered visual perceptual behavior.

Visual Defects in Deaf Children

One of the first systematic studies of the vision of deaf children was made by Braly.[2] He studied 422 children between five

and 21 years of age, the total population of a Residential School, using the Snellen Chart Test of Visual Acuity. His hypothesis was that diseases which caused deafness might simultaneously impair vision. Braly found that 38 per cent of the population had visual defects, and concluded that in comparison to the normal the incidence of such deficiencies was considerably greater in deaf children.

The most intensive study of the vision of children with deafness has been made by Stockwell.[21] Her sample included 960 children who, when examined, were attending a Residential School. She, too, used the Snellen Chart Test but in addition each child was examined ophthalmologically. Her findings were that 45.5 per cent of the population had deficient vision to the extent of requiring refraction. She contrasted her results with those from a similar study for normal children in which it was found that 15 per cent were in need of refraction. Stockwell concluded that there was a considerably higher incidence of defective vision in deaf children.

To explore further the possibilities of a relationship between auditory and visual impairments, we studied children in attendance at a Residential School for the Deaf; the population was comparable to those used by Braly and Stockwell. In an attempt to investigate various aspects of seeing, we used the Keystone Visual Survey Tests, including the following types of visual functioning: Near and Far Point Vision, Monocular and Binocular Vision, Simultaneous Vision, Vertical Imbalance, Stereopsis, Lateral Imbalance, Fusion, and Visual Efficiency. These tests are administered through a Telebinocular; a procedure for nonverbal administration had been devised previously.

Many of the same problems are found in the study of vision that are encountered in the evaluation of other aspects of human behavior, such as intelligence or auditory capacities. An individual may show disability or inferiority for a number of reasons. He may be developmentally immature in terms of the measure being used, he may have perceptual disorders and fail for this reason, he may show incapacity for reasons of emotional disturbance and mental incompetence, or he may have sensory defects. We ascertained through a pilot investigation, using the Keystone Visual Survey Tests, that they could be given to deaf children at six years of age.

Our sample did not include children who were significantly emotionally disturbed or mentally deficient. However, the results cannot be interpreted as indicative only of sensory defects. The Keystone Visual Survey Tests, as do many tests, assume integrity of perceptual functioning. They measure chiefly oculomotor capacity, fusion, and visual efficiency in terms of acuity. The fusion and acuity tests especially assume normal perceptual abilities; failure may indicate either sensory or perceptual disabilities. This does not necessarily detract from these tests because a visual deficiency is of significance irrespective of its nature. If incapacities are indicated, further study should be made. Through a combined psychological, neurological, and ophthalmological appraisal usually a distinction can be made between sensory and other types of defects. Such distinctions are important in all cases but become critical in the presence of deafness.

The evidence of visual deficiencies in deaf children as revealed by our study is shown in Table 90. These findings disclose a higher incidence of visual defects in comparison to normal children; the incidence for normal public school children is reportedly between 10 per cent and 20 per cent, with a mean of approximately 15 per cent. When the criterion of one or more deficiencies is applied to the total group the findings are more similar to those of Stockwell than to Braly's. This is true when viewed either by total groups or by sex. Both Stockwell's and our study showed the females to have more visual disorders than the males. Stockwell found 42 per cent of the males, 49 per cent of the females, and 45 per cent of her total group to have visual defects needing correction. Comparatively in our study, 44 per cent of the males, 59 per cent of the females, and 51 per cent of the total sample had one or more visual deficiencies. These results are strikingly similar. Braly did not report findings by sex; he reported an incidence of 38 per cent of visual disorders for his total group.

TABLE 90. The incidence of visual deficiencies in deaf school children

	N	One or More Deficiency		Two or More Deficiencies	
		N	%	N	%
Males	109	48	44	32	29
Females	82	49	59	37	44
Total	191	97	51	69	30

When the criterion of two or more visual deficiencies is used, our results are in closer agreement with those reported by Braly. Inasmuch as Stockwell made diagnostic examinations in contrast to the screening techniques used by Braly and by us, apparently the criterion of one or more deficiencies is the more accurate indication. Therefore, the incidence of visual disorders in deaf children seems to be between 40 per cent and 50 per cent, considerably higher than that reported for hearing children.

Visual Defects by Age and Etiology

The incidence of visual deficiencies was computed by age, permitting appraisal of whether effectiveness of visual functioning varied on this basis and whether maturational factors were involved. These data are presented in Table 91. No statistically significant

TABLE 91. The incidence of visual deficiencies by age in deaf children

	6	7	8	9	10	11	12	13	14	15	16	17	18	19	20	21	Total
Age / N	10	18	20	12	21	18	11	16	9	10	14	11	12	5	2	2	191
Far Point																	
Simultaneous Vision		2	5	1	2	1	0	1	2	3	0	2	2	2			23
Vertical Imbalance						1	0	0	0	0	2	0	0				3
Lateral Imbalance	1	3	1	2	3	1	3	2	2	1	3	2	4	1			29
Fusion		3	3	2	7	2	2	1	2	2	3	3	3	1			34
Right Eye Efficiency		2	1			6	0	3	0	0	1	2	2	2			19
Left Eye Efficiency		5				5	0	0	0	0	0	2	2		1		15
Stereopsis				5	5	0	2	2	1	3	2	3	1			1	25
Near Point																	
Lateral Imbalance	1	2	1		2	2	2	1	0	2	3	2	3	2	1	1	25
Fusion		2	3			1	1	0	0	0	2	3	2	3	1	1	19
Right Eye Efficiency	1		6	1	6	6	3	3	2	0	2	1	1	1			33
Left Eye Efficiency	1	1	5		8	6	3	4	1	1	3	3	1	1			38
Total	4	13	31	7	34	36	13	17	11	12	23	21	24	12	1	4	

differences occurred by age level; there was an equal number of deficiencies for each of the functions measured for the children below and above 12 years of age. This held true for the individual tests and on the basis of the total number of deficiencies. These findings are in agreement with those of Braly. He found no difference in the incidence of defects for children between the ages of five and ten, 11 and 15, and 16 and 21 years.

The data in Table 91 reveal that the only visual function measured on which the deaf were "highly normal" was Vertical Imbalance, which is consistent with clinical experience. Of the oculomotor disorders measured by this test, Lateral Imbalance is the more common; this condition is referred to as *exotropia.*

The visual functions on which the highest number of deficiencies were found are Lateral Imbalance, Visual Efficiency, Stereopsis, and Fusion, all commonly associated clinically. The most prevalent single condition was hyperopia which agrees with the findings of Stockwell. As in the case of hearing, the infant is not born with his seeing capacities fully developed. Gesell[5] has shown that some visual processes do not attain maturity until at least seven years of age; distance vision is an example. The normal infant is farsighted with a gradual reduction of hyperopia occurring until approximately seven years of age. The findings for deaf children indicate that this maturational process does not occur normally in the presence of profound hearing loss from early life. Moreover, from the data it appears that in many instances the hyperopia remains. While there were more children below 12 years than above 12 years who were hyperopic, the difference was not statistically significant. We must assume that there is a higher incidence of hyperopia in deaf persons even into adulthood.

Stockwell attributed her findings of more hyperopia to a marked delay in developmental processes, including growth changes. This is a provocative suggestion and, if true, has far-reaching implications. Does marked deprivation of one sense, such as hearing, affect the maturation and development of another sense, such as vision? Unfortunately experimental evidence is meagre, consisting mainly of the studies of perceptual behavior in children who are deaf or blind.[14, 23] While it is difficult to separate sensory and perceptual capacities, we cannot assume that these are identical functions. Furthermore, Myklebust and Brutten used the Keystone Visual Survey Tests to eliminate those children who had visual defects so the differences they found in visual perception cannot be explained by the higher incidence of visual deficiencies in deaf children. Hence, a necessary presumption is that if profound deafness is sustained in early life, both visual perceptual disorders and visual defects are more common in comparison with the normal.

Another function, in addition to distance vision, which is known to show maturation is stereopsis or depth perception. As far as can be determined stereoscopic vision is not present in early infancy but shows gradual maturation and development and, according to the studies of Gesell, reaches maturity in the average normal child between seven and eight years. A test of stereopsis is included in the Keystone Visual Survey Tests, and we administered it to all of the deaf children, beginning at six years of age. None of the six or seven year olds was successful on the test, whereas, nine of the 20 subjects eight years old showed normal stereopsis, as did all of the 12 nine year olds.

These results show an obvious developmental pattern with maturation being attained between eight and nine years of age. If we accept seven to eight years as the norm for hearing children, it seems that deafness might also cause some delay in the development of stereopsis; definite conclusions in this connection must await further investigation. Results for the total sample studied manifest a higher incidence of disorders in depth perception in comparison to the normal. In a study of deaf children having special problems in learning, Myklebust[13] found that nine out of 21 had little or no stereoscopic vision.

The factor of etiology becomes an important consideration in the relationships between visual and auditory defects. Braly found a higher incidence of visual deficiencies in the congenitally deaf than in the adventitiously deaf, and the difference was statistically significant. He concluded that the greater problem of visual defects was unrelated to a specific etiology or to age of onset. Stockwell also considered possible relationships with etiology. She found that 47 per cent of the congenital, 45 per cent of the acquired, and 37 per cent of the unknown had visual deficiencies.

In our study the number of visual deficiencies was ascertained on the basis of whether the deafness was endogenous, exogenous, or unknown. The results are given in Table 92. Statistical tests revealed a significant difference between the endogenous and exogenous on Visual Efficiency for both eyes at Near Point. This is an interesting finding in that it discloses the greater incidence of hyperopia in the endogenous, revealed also by the further analysis given under the Visually Impaired in Chapter XIII. No other significant differences were found by test or by comparing the exogenous and endogenous on the total number of deficiencies. These results

TABLE 92. Incidence of visual deficiencies in deaf children by etiology

Far Point	Number of Deficiencies		
	Exogenous	Endogenous	Unknown
Simultaneous Vision	8	9	6
Vertical Imbalance	2	0	1
Lateral Imbalance	9	14	6
Fusion	9	16	9
Right Eye Efficiency	6	11	2
Left Eye Efficiency	4	9	2
Stereopsis	9	15	1
Near Point			
Lateral Imbalance	9	13	3
Fusion	9	5	5
Right Eye Efficiency	8	20	5
Left Eye Efficiency	8	24	6

are in agreement with those of Braly, showing more visual defects in children with deafness that dates from birth.

The evidence on the visual capacities of deaf children does not support the presumption that their greater problem in seeing is due to the disease factors which caused the deafness. On the contrary the studies are in agreement that, although those having acquired deafness also have more visual defects than the average, comparatively the problem is greatest in those having deafness from birth. In our study the congenitally deaf had endogenous deafness. In view of these results we must conclude that lack of hearing from birth causes the greatest delay or imposition on maturation of certain visual functions. Another possibility, which seems less adequate as an explanation, is that deafness and certain visual defects are genetically linked. Shoemaker[19] showed that retinitis pigmentosa is more prevalent in deaf children and that a genetic factor was involved. A relationship of this type has not been demonstrated for visual functions, such as hyperopia, stereopsis, or fusion. A more tenable explanation seems to be that when hearing is deprived from early life, there is a reciprocal maturational effect on certain aspects of seeing, suggesting a lack of normal intersensory facilitation and synesthesia. Hetermodal reciprocity is reduced because of the deafness, and the effect is that visual functioning remains less fully developed.

The extent to which the visual deficiencies of deaf children finally can be attributed to a reciprocal involvement of lack of hearing will be learned only through intensive investigation. Sensory deprivation experiments, such as those conducted by Riesen[17] and his associates, may provide valuable evidence on this question. They have shown that basic shifts take place, both behaviorally and structurally, when a chimpanzee is raised in darkness for varying periods of time. In some instances irreversible changes occur in the retina and in the ganglion cells. One of their conclusions was that the health of a cell is dependent on appropriate stimulation; understimulation or overstimulation might cause deterioration of cell function. Work of this type provides a basis for the assumption that if a sensory channel cannot be stimulated, changes in the nervous system involved must be expected. This might explain the greater incidence of visual deficiencies in deaf children inasmuch as intersensory facilitation has been reduced.

The experimental work on sensory deprivation, which has revealed a relationship between lack of stimulation and function of the nervous system, has provided a frame of reference for understanding certain effects of deafness and blindness, especially when they occur congenitally. Snider[20] has found a high incidence of occipital lobe disturbances in the electroencephalograms of congenitally blind children. It is conceivable that investigation will disclose a similar disturbance in the temporal lobe for those having congenital deafness. Such findings, however, could not be interpreted as indicating the presence of brain lesions similar to those deriving from trauma or brain disease. Evidence from psychological studies and from experience educationally with the deaf and the blind have taught us that the brain does not deteriorate as a result of sensory deprivation. Although certain specific changes must be assumed, ostensibly the radiations in the brain, especially for hearing and vision, are sufficiently diffuse and overlapping so that deprivation of one does not leave wide cell areas totally without stimulation.

The work of Love,[12] who was studying this problem in the early 1900's, is most intriguing. He quotes a report of the autopsy of Laura Bridgman as follows:

> The examination of the brain showed that those portions which from youth up could not be brought into activity in the ordinary way through external impressions, viz., all the cerebral nerves, were small; the gustatory nerve, the auditory nerve, and a nerve that moves the eyeballs were stunted,

and this was specially true of the tract of the optic nerves. The cerebral hemispheres appeared somewhat flattened behind, and the occipital lobe, in fact, smaller on the right than on the left, and the right cuneus much less developed than the left. This difference in the region belonging to the visual centres is intelligible when we consider that Miss Bridgman from her second year was completely blind with the left eye, whereas with the right she retained some sensation of light until her eighth year, enough at any rate, to allow the development of the centres of the left side to go on.

Love comments on this report to the effect that, assuming correctness of the findings, absence of hearing or vision is accompanied by a shrivelling of the tracts leading to the brain and the parts of the brain which are connected. He speculated that greater reliance on the residual senses, when deafness or blindness was present, might result in a corresponding increase in the cortical areas related to these senses. It is interesting that recent experimental findings for lower animals are essentially in agreement with Love's interpretations, although there is no evidence that certain cortical areas are increased due to greater reliance on the residual senses. We can assume that the sensory deprivation experiments with lower animals as well as further study of central nervous system functioning in the deaf and the blind will add substantially to our knowledge concerning the vital question of relationships between deficiencies in hearing and in seeing.

Color Vision and Deafness

To evaluate further the visual capacities of deaf children we studied their ability to perceive color. The Ishihara Test[9] was administered to 199 children ranging in age from six to 21 years; all of the subjects were in attendance at a Residential School. An instruction card, not from the test, was used to demonstrate the task. The child responded by tracing the number on the card with his forefinger, assuring objectivity of scoring. The children enjoyed the test, and administration was accomplished readily. The results from this investigation are given in Table 93.

TABLE 93. The incidence of defective color vision in deaf children

Total	Normal		Defective	
N	N	%	N	%
199	186	93	13	7

Bartley[1] has described nine types of defects in color vision and the incidence of each found in the general population. While it can be assumed that the major defects in color vision are measured by the Ishihara Test, we did not treat each of these separately. Therefore, the results given in Table 93 include the various inabilities to perceive color. According to Bartley, the most common color defect is "green weakness" which occurs in five percent of the general population. The incidence of each type of defect varies from one to five percent. Our study disclosed that seven percent of the children having profound deafness from early life had some defect in color vision. Although the exact type of defect was not tabulated, making specific comparison with the normal impossible, these results do not suggest unusual color vision problems in relation to deafness. While auditory experience might enhance and enrich the experience of color, as far as the development of the capacity to perceive it is concerned, it is unlikely that deafness plays a significant role.

Eye Dominance and Deafness

For a number of years there has been a presumption that eye dominance was important in various aspects of visual behavior, particularly in learning to read. The concept included the opinion that eye dominance was an indication of cerebral dominance. The work of neurologists such as Penfield,[16] Nielsen,[15] and Cobb[4] has largely dispelled this view. However, eye dominance may have significance behaviorally, if not neurologically, and, therefore, we have included study of this factor in our research pertaining to sensory deprivation and language pathology.

Tests of eye preference were administered to 209 children in residence at a school for the deaf. Two such tests were used, sighting and looking through a hole in a card (The Key-Hole Test). The results are given in Table 94. Of the total number tested 54 per cent showed right eye preference and 46 per cent left eye preference. The difference between the groups was not statistically

TABLE 94.   The eye preference of deaf children

	Right Eye Preference		Left Eye Preference	
N	N	%	N	%
209	113	54	96	46

significant; an equal number showed right and left eye dominance. The incidence of left-eyedness was considerably greater than antici- pated, although the incidence of left-sidedness, as shown in Table 47, was greater than average in deaf children. Unfortunately, com- parison of our results with the normal is difficult because of the varying criteria and test procedures which have been used. How- ever, these data suggest that right eye dominance is markedly less typical of deaf children in comparison with the normal. Apparently lack of hearing from early life modifies the development of eyedness.

IMPLICATIONS FOR EDUCATION AND TRAINING

Although it would be premature to draw final conclusions re- garding the relationships between deafness and visual defects, evi- dence is accumulating that these sensory functions are conjoined. Profound hearing loss from early life per se seems to affect the development of visual processes. An inescapable implication is that deaf children, for their total welfare, must have careful study of their vision.

More broadly, investigation of the visual functioning of hear- ing impaired children seems to have important implications for the psychology of sensory deprivation and for the study of the nervous system organismically. There is evidence that lack of sensation, lack of sensory stimulation, results in deterioration of certain cell structures. Further knowledge of the relationship between sensory stimulation and the behavior of the nervous system can be expected to contribute to the understanding of the problems involved in the use of amplification as well as other aspects of educational training. The implication seems to be that unless sensory stimulation can be affected early, the prognosis for successful outcome may be greatly reduced.

This area of study offers great challenge and potential for the future, not only in terms of benefits to be derived by those having deafness but for the expansion of knowledge and understanding in general.

REFERENCES

1. Bartley, S.: Principles of Perception. New York, Harper, 1958.
2. Braly, K.: Incidence of defective vision among the deaf. West Trenton, New Jersey School for Deaf, Tech. Series, #4, 1937.
3. Brogden, W.: Tests of sensory pre-conditioning with human subjects. J. Exp. Psychol., 31, 505, 1952.

4. Cobb, S.: Borderlines of Psychiatry. Cambridge, Harvard University Press, 1948.
5. Gesell, A., Ilg, F. and Bullis, G.: Vision: Its Development in Infant and Child. New York, Paul B. Hoeber, 1949.
6. Harris, J. D.: Some Relations Between Vision and Audition. Springfield, C. C. Thomas, 1950.
7. Hartmann, G.: Changes in visual acuity through simultaneous stimulation of other sense organs. J. Exper. Psychol., 16, 393, 1933.
8. Hebb, D.: The Organization of Behavior. New York, John Wiley and Sons, 1949.
9. Ishihara Color Perception Test. Kannehara, Tokyo.
10. Jenkins, T.: Facilitation and inhibition. Arch. Psychol., 14, 1, 1926.
11. Kravkok, S.: Changes of visual acuity in one eye under the influence of the illumination of the other or of acoustic stimuli. J. Exp. Psychol., 17, 805, 1934.
12. Love, J.: The Deaf Child. New York, William Wood, 1911.
13. Myklebust, H. R.: The deaf child with other handicaps. Am. Ann. Deaf, 103, 496, 1958.
14. _____ and Brutten, M. A study of the visual perception of deaf children. Acta Oto-laryng., Suppl. 105, 1953.
15. Nielsen, J.: Agnosia, Apraxia and Aphasia. New York, Paul B. Hoeber, 1946.
16. Penfield, W. and Roberts, L.: Speech and Brain Mechanisms. Princeton, Princeton University Press, 1959.
17. Riesen, A.: Plasticity of behavior: Psychological Series, in Harlow, H. and Woolsey, C. Biological and Biochemical Bases of Behavior. Madison, University of Wisconsin Press, 1958.
18. Serratt, W. and Kerwoski, T.: An investigation of the effect of auditory stimulation on visual sensivity. J. Exper. Psychol., 19, 604, 1936.
19. Shoemaker, W.: Retinitus Pigmentosa. Philadelphia, Lippincott, 1909.
20. Snider, R.: Chicago, Northwestern University Medical School. Personal communication, 1960.
21. Stockwell, E.: Visual difficulties in deaf children. Arch. Ophthalmol. 48, 428, 1952.
22. Werner, H. and Wapner, S.: Toward a general theory of perception. Psychol. Review, 59, 324, 1952.
23. Worchel, P.: Space perception and orientation in the blind. Psychol. Monog., #332, 1951.

Suggestions for Further Study

Ammons, C., Worchel, P. and Dallenbach, K.: Facial vision, the perception of obstacles out of doors by blindfolded and blindfolded-deafened subjects. Am. J. Psychol., 66, 519, 1953.
Bartley, S.: Vision: A Study of its Basis. Princeton, Van Nostrand, 1941.
Beebe-Center, J. and Waddell, D.: A general psychological scale of taste. J. Psychol., 26, 517, 1948.
Burtt, H.: Auditory illusions of movement. J. Exper. Psychol., 2, 63, 1917.
_____: Tactual illusions of movement. J. Exper. Psychol., 2, 371, 1917.
Cotyzin, M. and Dallenbach, K.: Facial vision, the role of pitch and loudness in the perception of obstacles by the blind. Am. J. Psychol., 63, 485, 1950.

Geldard, F.: The Human Senses. New York, John Wiley and Sons, 1953.

Gibson, J.: The Perception of the Visual World. Chicago, Houghton Mifflin, 1950.

Hunter, I.: Tactile-kinesthetic perception of straightness in blind and sighted humans. Quart. J. Psychol., 6, 149, 1954.

Lashley, K. S.: Brain Mechanisms and Intelligence. Chicago, University of Chicago Press, 1929.

Lawson, L. F.: Current management of strabismus in childhood. J. Pediatrics, 52, 307, 1958.

Leeper, R.: A study of a neglected portion of the field of learning—the development of sensory organization. J. Genetic Psychol., 46, 41, 1935.

Riesen, A.: Effects of stimulus deprivation on the development and atrophy of the visual sensory system. Am. J. Orthopsychiatry, 30, 23, 1960.

_____: Vision, in Annual Review of Psychology, Vol. 5, 1954.

Vernon, J. and Hoffman, J.: Effect of sensory deprivation on learning rate in human beings. Science, 123, 1074, 1956.

Walls, G.: Land! Land! Psychol. Bulletin, 57, 29, 1960.

Chapter XIII

OTHER HANDICAPS

IMPAIRED HEARING OFTEN IS FOUND in conjunction with other handicaps. The opinion is expressed that the incidence of children with multiple disabilities is on the increase, with the presumption that improved medical practice causes children to survive who previously might have expired. While clinical experience tends to support this opinion, it is difficult to secure conclusive evidence. Nevertheless, educators of the deaf and the hard of hearing are aware of the need to provide specialized programs for children who present problems in addition to their hearing loss.

Psychologically and educationally multiple handicaps can be viewed as deterrents to learning, illustrated schematically in Figure 45. As indicated by this figure, deficits in learning can be classified into three major categories; those due to the malfunctioning of the central or of the peripheral nervous systems and those caused by emotional disturbance. Most individuals presenting difficulties with learning have only one of these disorders. For example, most persons having deafness do not also have central nervous system disorders or emotional disturbance. However, as suitable nonverbal

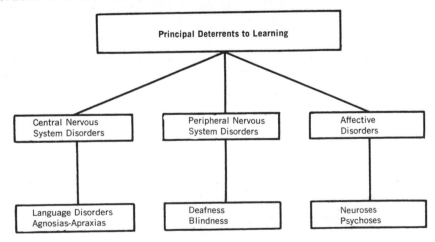

FIG. 45. Principal deterrents to learning.

techniques have become available, psychologists have demonstrated that individuals having deafness might have difficulties in learning which are unrelated to their hearing loss. In such instances, in addition to deafness usually there is a superimposed central nervous system disorder, a visual defect, or a pronounced emotional disturbance.

PSYCHONEUROLOGICAL LEARNING DISORDERS

Evaluation of hearing impaired children, especially by psychological, neurological, and electroencephalographic procedures, has manifested that some have learning disorders due to central nervous system deficits. Such learning disorders occur more frequently than has been assumed, whether or not sensory impairments are present. While it has been generally recognized that neurological disorders cause gross involvements such as cerebral palsy and mental deficiency, it has not been stressed that minimal neurological deficits might cause disabilities in reading, writing, spelling, arithmetic, and speaking; disabilities which are referred to as *psychoneurological learning disorders.* The learning disorders of this type, seen most commonly in children with deafness, are Speechreading Aphasia, Dyslexia, Dysgraphia, Dyscalculia, Dyschronometria, Disorientation, and Disturbance of Topographic Ability.

Speechreading Aphasia

As discussed in Chapter XI, speechreading is a language system. Therefore, through disorder of the central nervous system an individual might sustain an aphasia for this verbal symbol system just as he might for any other type of language. By aphasia is meant the inability to associate the appropriate unit of experience with the verbal symbol for that experience. *In the case of speechreading, it is an inability in relating the word (symbol) seen on the lips with its meaning; the child cannot associate the word and the experience.* Speechreading Aphasia is a receptive language disorder and is comparable to the aphasia seen in both children and adults who cannot associate the words heard with the appropriate meanings, the units of experience symbolized by the words. Aphasias are due to disorders of the central nervous system; inabilities to use language because of primary mental deficiency, neuroses, or psychoses are not designated as aphasias.

While we have studied many children who have speechreading aphasia and although our follow-up studies of some of them cover a period of more than a decade, it would be premature to come to definite conclusions regarding the extent and nature of this problem. Nevertheless, in regard to the extent of this language disorder, the incidence seems to exceed two per cent. Therefore, in a random population of 100 children having a significant degree of deafness, it might be expected that there would be at least two who have an aphasia for speechreading. The actual incidence in a given population is dependent on factors such as the criteria used for admission and exclusion and may vary from one to five per cent.

It can be assumed that there are degrees of speechreading aphasia. However, because diagnostic procedures still are relatively undeveloped, usually a diagnosis can be made only when the problem is severe. Perhaps the most obvious symptom of this condition, other than the lack of speechreading ability, is the marked incapacity to imitate speech positions and to speak; the rationale for the reciprocal involvement of the lack of speech was discussed in Chapter X. Unless the child can internalize the speech movements he observes on the lips, he cannot imitate them; hence, if he has a severe aphasia for speechreading he is devoid of the ability to speak. However, after he begins to read, he often shows progress in speech. Apparently now he has internalized the printed form of the word so this serves as the basis for the use of the word expressively in speech.

Intensive appraisal of children showing an inability to learn speechreading and of children with normal hearing who presented a similar disability in the perception of movements has indicated that learning disorders of this type derive principally from deficits in the parietal lobe of the brain. For some time we assumed that speechreading aphasia derived from damage to the occipital lobe, the area known to be chiefly involved when dyslexia is present. Such speculation was based on the presumption that the same area, or areas, of the brain responsible for integration of the printed word, reading, would also be responsible for reading words on the lips. Neurological, electroencephalographic, and psychological findings, however, do not support this supposition. Rather, the results suggest that speechreading aphasia occurs when there is a deficiency of function in the parietal lobe in the dominant cerebral hemisphere. The implication is that speechreading and reading of the printed word are not identical neurologically nor psychologically. The tasks are different in various respects, including the fact that one entails the perception of letters which remain stationary on the page, while the other entails perception of movements which are perceived only momentarily.

Another provocative problem is found in children, both deaf and hearing, who have parietal lobe lesions. Often they show obvious deficits in their interpersonal relationships. In some instances this is so marked that the child is erroneously classified as schizophrenic; his behavior superficially simulates childhood schizophrenia. Because of this behavioral concomitant of parietal lobe dysfunctioning, some neurologists and psychologists have speculated that body image, self-perception, and person-perception may be, at least partially, represented in the parietal lobe. In terms of speechreading it is apparent that this language function cannot be achieved without the ability to perceive other people, especially their faces. Some individuals having speechreading aphasia lack the ability to recognize faces; this condition is referred to as an *anosognosia*.[3] Also, infrequently they have an aphasia for gestures; the child cannot comprehend natural gestures or the manual sign language; this is referred to as *amimia*.

Experience with hearing impaired children having speechreading aphasia shows that they might be normally intelligent or even intellectually superior. Furthermore, if undue emphasis is placed on speech and speechreading, they usually develop an emotional disturbance. The best results have been secured when speech and speechreading have been minimized and when preference has been given to reading and writing at the proper age level. It is important that the child be permitted to gesture if he finds this is a satisfactory means of communication.

Dyslexia

The condition of being unable to read because of a brain disorder has been recognized for several decades. Orton[13] gave considerable impetus to the understanding of this condition in children. When, as a result of a lesion in the brain the individual lacks reading ability, it is referred to as *alexia,* whereas if he has a partial disability of this type, it is classified as a *dyslexia.* Dyslexia in children may be either exogenous or endogenous and is a type of agnosia. The results from one of our surveys of a normally hearing group of school children indicates that this condition is more prevalent on a congenital basis than has been assumed.

Dyslexia is a language disorder in which the individual cannot normally learn to relate the proper units of experience to the printed word. There are two primary types. In one the difficulty derives from an inability to learn the *sound* of the letters, while in the other the problem is caused by an inability to learn the *appearance* of the letters. In learning to read the hearing child associates what the letters sound like and what they look like simultaneously. Workers such as Krieg[8] and Nielsen[12] have stressed the neurological bases of these auditory and visual types of dyslexia. While the auditory aspects of the dyslexia might be ascertained in some of the hard of hearing, the effect of such an involvement in the deaf is unknown. Presumably, in those with profound deafness the dyslexia can be of the visual type only. When this condition is present, the child shows a marked inability in learning to read and to spell. Like other dyslexics usually he shows confusions in the identification of letters. In contrast to the dysgraphic he finds it possible to copy letters but may do so more slowly and with more errors than the child without dyslexia. Usually this reading disability is accompanied by other disorders, such as difficulties in learning arithmetic, time concepts, direction, right from left, and the significance of maps. Despite the presence of this *syndrome* of dyslexia, the child might have average or even superior intelligence. Although the incidence of dyslexia in hearing impaired children is not known, it is found frequently in those who show little progress in learning to read but who have good learning ability.

Dysgraphia

This language disorder is an inability to learn to write because of brain deficit. It is not due to a motor paralysis but derives from a deficiency in ability to relate the word (symbol) to the motor system for writing, referred to as an *apraxia*. In contrast to speech-reading aphasia and dyslexia which are receptive language disorders, it is a defect in expressive language. The child might speech-read, read, and speak but be unable to write. It must be stressed that the dyslexic child, too, cannot write normally, not because he is dysgraphic but because he cannot internalize the printed form of the word. His limitation in writing is reciprocal to his inability in reading. In dysgraphia the problem is markedly different psychologically and neurologically. Often the distinction can be made on the basis of dyslexic's being able to copy letters, whereas the dysgraphic usually cannot; this oversimplifies the diagnostic problem but illustrates the primary difference between these conditions.

Dyscalculia

Disorders in the learning of arithmetic also may be due to neurological involvement. These disabilities are of several types. In some instances the individual cannot recognize numbers in the written form while in others he cannot comprehend them when they are spoken. In either case usually he is limited in his ability to write numbers. Another type of dyscalculia is a disability in the learning of arithmetical principles; the individual executes the problem well *if* he is told that he is to add, subtract, multiply, or divide. His difficulty is in ascertaining the principle which is involved, not in the actual computation. Frequently this disorder is found in conjunction with a generalized deficit in arithmetical concepts. A third type of involvement is a disorder in the learning of the symbols which connote the principle to be followed, such as + for addition and × for multiplication. When this problem is present, the individual might do well in arithmetic, if he is not required to follow these symbols.

Achievement test studies disclose that children with profound deafness learn to do arithmetical computation more successfully than they learn to do other subjects requiring verbal facility; they do not show inferiority in computation. Therefore, if a hearing impaired child shows poor computational ability but otherwise good learning aptitude, a dyscalculia should be suspected. Inasmuch as this is a psychoneurological learning disorder, a diagnosis can be made only when all aspects of the problem have been adequately evaluated. The incidence of dyscalculia in children with deafness has not been determined. Often it occurs in normally intelligent children.

Topographic Disorder

Some persons who have sustained an involvement to the brain cannot relate experience to symbolic representations such as maps, globes, blueprints, and floor plans; this is referred to as a *topographic disorder*. Characteristically it causes a marked limitation in the learning of geography. A psychoneurological disorder of this type also may be seen in hearing impaired children who have a central nervous system deficit in addition to their deafness.

Disorientation

A learning disability which has been recognized for decades in individuals having brain disorders is the inability to distinguish right from left or one direction from another, referred to as *disorientation* and commonly occurring in association with dyslexia. Benton[1] has made an extensive analysis of this condition. It is found with some frequency in deaf children having psychoneurological learning disorders.

Dyschronometria

One of the most intriguing learning disorders found in those having deficits of the central nervous system is a defect in the sense of time, referred to as *dyschronometria*. It appears in several forms but often the deficiency is generalized, affecting all aspects of the time concept. The dyschronometric child cannot normally learn to tell time from the clock, learn the days of the week, months of the year, or the meaning of before, after, until, in a minute, next week, or tomorrow. This condition, too, is commonly associated with dyslexia, and can occur in children who are normal intellectually.

Summary of Psychoneurological Learning Disorders

In recent years there has been considerable discussion concerning children with deafness who have good learning ability but who make little progress academically. Such children have been studied especially by Birch and Birch,[2] Fiedler,[4] and Myklebust.[11] It is apparent that many of these children are not mentally deficient or primarily emotionally disturbed. Rather, they have sustained through disease, trauma, or heredity, a minimal disorder in the brain which markedly affects a specific type of learning; this has been designated as a psychoneurological learning disorder. The brain involvement neurologically may be inconsequential, but the effect psychologically is dramatic and of great importance. The incidence of these disorders in the total population of children who have deafness has not been fully determined. However, there is considerable need for diagnosis of these conditions in hearing impaired children who show special problems in learning. The diagnostic evaluation should be made early in life rather than after several years of frustrating school failure. Experience with these children shows that with proper education and training their learning disorders can be alleviated. The training program must include techniques and procedures designed specifically for both the learning disorders and the deafness, and the teachers must be trained in the educational techniques for those having psychoneurological learning disorders as well as for those having deafness.

THE MENTALLY RETARDED

The question of intellectual capacities in relation to deafness was discussed in Chapter V. Here our attention is directed to those children who have mental retardation in addition to hearing loss. However, we again raise the question of incidence in an attempt to clarify further this important problem. Frisina,[5] in a study of mentally retarded deaf children, concluded that 12 per cent of the population in schools for the deaf fell below an IQ of 80. From the discussion and findings presented in Chapter V, we can assume that the number of children showing retardation will vary according to the test or tests being used. However, as Frisina has shown, there is a significant correlation between various mental tests indicating retardation in the deaf child, including the Draw-a-Man Test, the test used in our National Study of children in schools for the deaf. Using the same criterion as Frisina, that is, a score below IQ 80, we ascertained by school, age, and sex the number who showed retardation. These data, presented in Table 95 are interesting in several respects. They closely parallel the intelligence

TABLE 95.   The incidence of children scoring below IQ 80 on the Draw-a-Man Test

	Day						Residential					
Years	Males		Females		Total		Males		Females		Total	
	N	%	N	%	N	%	N	%	N	%	N	%
7							48	14	27	0	75	9
9	51	14	45	13	96	14	36	8	41	20	77	14
11	37	3	50	10	87	7	82	15	59	34	141	23
13	51	33	43	16	94	26	35	14	43	30	78	23
15	22	0	19	16	41	7	47	23	44	30	91	26
17							25	8	26	8	51	8
Total	161	16	157	13	318	14	273	15	240	23	513	19

quotient results given in Table 16, Chapter V, where it was noted that there was a gradual decline in the scores from 9 to 13 years of age, after which there was an increase, again reaching normal levels at 15 and 17 years of age. *This pattern was found for both the deaf and the hearing and must be interpreted as a function of the test being used.* Therefore, the higher incidence, as shown in Table 95, of children scoring below 80 IQ at the 13 and 15 year age levels cannot be taken as an indication of the actual number having mental retardation. Rather, it is a reflection of the generally lower scores earned on this test at these ages. On the other hand, interesting differences appeared by School and by Sex. In the Day School twice as many males as females scored below IQ 80 at the age level of 13 years. This trend was reversed in the Residential School group, where twice as many females scored below the criterion point. However, except for the 13 year old male subjects, the incidence of below 80 scores in the Day School was highly similar to that reported by Frisina.

In the Residential School the females were clearly different from the total Day School group and from the Residential males. In agreement with the other analyses of intelligence test results, a considerably higher number of females in the Residential School scored as being inferior intellectually. Despite this the total 'number of children in Residential Schools who scored below the IQ level of 80 was only slightly greater than in the Day School. When the sexes were combined, 14 per cent in the Day School and 19 per cent in the Residential Schools fell below this criterion. When the decline at adolescence is considered and accounted for, the number showing actual mental retardation falls between 10 and 15 per cent, which is in close agreement with the findings of Frisina.

It must be stressed that this group includes slow learning children and should not be construed as the incidence of mentally deficient children. However, there is evidence that at least 10 per cent of children in schools for the deaf would be benefitted by special programs designed for those who are inferior mentally. It seems, therefore, that all large schools should provide a specialized program for the most effective training of this group. Another implication is that universities train teachers to work with children who have mental retardation in addition to deafness.

THE VISUALLY IMPAIRED

Although as indicated by the discussion of Vision in Chapter XIII, deaf children have more visual deficiencies in comparison with the hearing, in general, this cannot be viewed as an additional handicap. If the visual defect can be corrected through refraction so that the individual's capacities fall within normal limits, it is not considered a disability. Such correction is possible for most of the visual problems which occur in hearing impaired children just as it is in those who have normal hearing. Only when vision remains significantly reduced with correction does it constitute a significant handicap. On the other hand, because children with profound deafness have a greater incidence of visual impairment, they may have more difficulties in seeing that are of such severity that they cannot be brought within normal limits through refraction or other corrective measures. Unfortunately none of the studies which have been accomplished to date provide adequate information relative to this critical question.

In Chapter XII we presented data showing the number of children in our study who had one or more, and two or more visual deficiencies as determined by the Keystone Visual Survey Tests. While all children who show one or two defects on these tests should have the benefit of a complete visual examination, usually such involvement is not severe and is readily corrected. To ascertain the number who had more severe defects, tabulation was made of those showing marked visual disorders on the 11 tests administered. Of the 191 children, 25 per cent had four or more and 13 per cent had five or more deficiencies. The greatest number of defects found in a given child was seven, with several children having this extent of involvement. It seems, therefore, that 10 to 15 per cent is a conservative estimate of the number of deaf children in this sample who had marked visual deficiencies. It appears that all schools for the deaf, as well as other programs which include the hearing impaired, should make special provision for those who also have defective vision. Likewise, it seems imperative that emphasis be placed on the prevention of visual defects in those who have deafness.

It is interesting that further analysis of the group having four or more visual defects disclosed no differences on the basis of etiology. Moreover, there were no sex differences for the exogenous nor for those whose etiology was unknown. In contrast, in the endogenous there were twice as many females as males having more visual defects, a finding which is in agreement with the results for the total sample.

Deaf-Blind

In the psychology of sensory deprivation one of the most challenging problems is presented by the deaf-blind. An individual usually is so classified if he has profound deafness and a visual impairment exceeding 20/200. If he has profound deafness and a visual deficiency ranging between 20/70 and 20/200, he is classified as being deaf and partially sighted. Salmon[15] has reviewed the history of the education and training of deaf-blind persons. Through his efforts much has been learned concerning rehabilitation procedures for adults having this dual sensory deprivation.[14] The Perkins Institution for the Blind for decades has played a leading role in the education of deaf-blind children; this work has received considerable impetus through the efforts of Waterhouse, who provided an opportunity for a group of professional people to study the problems of diagnosis and training as they pertain to the deaf-blind child. A discussion of this work has been provided by Myklebust.[10]

The causes of deaf-blindness are various. The etiology in the case of Laura Bridgman[9] is reported as scarlet fever and for Helen Keller it is thought to be meningitis. A frequently reported etiology is retinitis pigmentosa, a disease which may occur later in the life of an individual who has congenital deafness. It was first studied extensively in a group of deaf children by Shoemaker,[16] who found it to be endogenous in many instances. Gilroy[6] has investigated the relationship of retinitis pigmentosa to the general problem of etiology in deaf-blind adults. In our work with those having this dual sensory deprivation, there have been a number in whom the indicated etiology was maternal rubella.

It is apparent that the needs of the deaf-blind can be met only through the cooperative efforts of educators, psychologists, physicians, and rehabilitation workers. Because the incidence of persons having this dual handicap is not large, we can assume that adequate diagnostic and educational facilities can best be maintained through regional centers. A critical implication is that teachers and psychologists be trained to work with this group.

In Chapter IV we presented a frame of reference for the psychology of learning when distance senses are seriously impaired. The impairment predisposes the individual to make a shift in his psychological perceptual organization. Helen Keller[7] has described the manner in which taction becomes the lead, the foreground sense when deafness and blindness are present. As shown in Figure 5, we assume that olfaction becomes the primary background sense, with gustation serving as the supplemental sense. This frame of reference provides a basis for the psychology of learning in the deaf-blind, as discussed by Myklebust.[10] It can be anticipated that through further experience with those having impairment of both distance senses, much will be learned concerning the psychology of sensory deprivation.

THE EMOTIONALLY DISTURBED

Emotional problems may be moderate or severe. They would be considered an additional handicap only when they are of a sufficient degree to be a primary problem. Examples are individuals with deafness who also have significant psychosis or neurosis. In daily life this may take many different forms, such as marked withdrawal, sexual perversion, stealing, or aggression. Although individuals having deafness, as seen from the discussion in Chapter VI, are in greater need of psychological and psychiatric assistance, a distinction must be made between the emotional disturbances accepted as being within the range of normal and those which require specialized treatment and management. It is those falling in the latter category which constitute another handicap when they occur in addition to deafness. Unfortunately, available statistics relative to the number of individuals with deafness who are mentally ill or have other marked emotional disturbances are inadequate. We have stressed the difficulty of interpretation of personality test data and have emphasized that those having profound deafness from early life might score deviately without having an emotional disorder. Nevertheless, we analyzed our personality test results for children and adults according to the degree of atypicality shown. This tabulation was made on the basis of the total protocol or profile, thus eliminating some of the loading of abnormal scores which might be normal for the deaf.

When this procedure was applied to the population of deaf college students, discussed in Chapter VI, approximately 25 per cent of the males and 15 per cent of the females fell into the category of having a marked emotional disturbance. These estimates must be considered tentative until further evidence becomes available. However, there can be little question that even in this selected sample there are a number of individuals who have the dual handicap of deafness and emotional disorder. Comparison with the hearing college population has been made in Chapter VI. When our total sample, males and females, was considered, approximately 20 per cent seemed to be in need of assistance with their emotional problems. This is the incidence of severe emotional problems usually given for the *average*, not the *selected*, hearing population. Ostensibly the incidence for the average unselected deaf population is above 20 per cent.

Using a protocol of test results and clinical evaluations, we attempted to ascertain in a given school population the number of children who had marked emotional disturbances. The sample consisted of 65 children in an advanced department of a residential school for the deaf; the mean chronological age was 16 years. This group was selected because language tests of personality for children were included in the battery. Clinical evidence was also considered; factors such as nailbiting, wholesome friendships, indulgence in phantasy, and sleep habits were studied. Each subject was interviewed by an experienced psychologist. On the basis of this "mental hygiene" survey we concluded that approximately one-third of these children had emotional problems of sufficient severity as to constitute a handicap in addition to deafness. It must be emphasized that the incidence which would evolve if the same survey were done on a population of hearing children is unknown. It is generally assumed that the estimate of one-fifth, used to indicate the incidence of emotional disorders in the average hearing population, pertains principally to adults; there is a possibility that the incidence for hearing children is lower. In any event there is sufficient evidence concerning the emotional problems which occur in both children and adults with deafness to indicate the need for specialized programs in schools, mental hygiene clinics, and in psychiatric hospitals. Perhaps the greatest need is for psychologists, guidance workers, and educators who have had specialized training and who would be prepared to inaugurate programs for the emotionally disturbed deaf; programs of this type are urgently needed. In some instances they might be established in schools for the deaf. Again, we see the implication that universities should provide opportunities for advanced training in the areas of psychology, psychiatry, education, social work, and rehabilitation as it pertains to those with the sensory deprivation of deafness.

MOTOR DISORDERS

Motor behavior in relation to deafness was discussed in Chapter VIII and the conclusion was that motor function might be altered by lack of hearing. However, it would be viewed as an additional handicap only when the individual has a cerebral palsy, a hemiplegia, an ataxia, an amputation, or some other obvious imposition on his motor capacities. No complete data are available covering the number of deaf and hard of hearing who are also motorically handicapped. Schools for the deaf characteristically do not admit children unless they are ambulatory and unless they can learn to care for themselves in dressing and feeding. Children who have a major motor involvement must be transported and given assistance which is not provided for the typical deaf child. Therefore, when there is a dual handicap of deafness and motor disability, the child usually is entered in a school for crippled children. While this facilitates his needs as far as the motor problem is concerned, his educational needs can be met only if the program also includes persons who are trained to work with the hearing impaired.

SUMMARY AND IMPLICATIONS

There are many children with deafness who have an additional handicap. While this problem has been recognized, there is need for the development of more special programs for these children with the concomitant necessity of providing training opportunities for the teachers and psychologists required to work with those having an additional disability. The greatest urgency is for programs for those having psychoneurological learning disorders, mental retardation, visual impairment, or emotional disturbance.

The adult deaf also would be benefitted by greater emphasis on these additional handicaps. Establishing treatment centers for the mentally ill is of paramount importance. Such programs to be most effective must include individuals trained in the psychology of deafness and skilled in dealing with the hearing impaired. There also is need for centers and programs especially designed for the aged deaf.

REFERENCES

1. Benton, A.: Right-Left Discrimination and Finger Localization. New York, Hoeber-Harper, 1959.
2. Birch, J. R. and Birch, J. W.: The Leiter International Performance Scale as an aid in the psychological study of deaf children. Am. Ann. Deaf, 96, 502, 1951.
3. Critchley, M.: The Parietal Lobes. Baltimore, Williams and Wilkins, 1953.
4. Fiedler, M. F.: Good and poor learners in an oral school for the deaf. Exceptional Children, 23, 291, 1957.
5. Frisina, D. R.: A psychological study of the mentally retarded deaf child. Evanston, Northwestern Universtiy, Unpublished Doctoral Dissertation, 1955.
6. Gilroy, R.: A study of primary degeneration of the retina, in Rehabilitation of Deaf-Blind Persons, Vol. 1. Brooklyn, Industrial Home for the Blind, 1958.
7. Keller, Helen: The Story of My Life. New York, Doubleday, 1905.
8. Krieg, W.: Brain Mechanisms in Diachrome. Evanston, Brain Books, 1955.
9. Love, J. K.: The Deaf Child. New York, William Wood, 1911.
10. Myklebust, H.: The deaf-blind child. Watertown, Perkins School for the Blind, Publ. #19, 1956.
11. _____: The deaf child with other handicaps. Am. Ann. Deaf, 103, 496, 1958.
12. Nielsen, J.: Agnosia, Apraxia and Aphasia. New York, Paul B. Hoeber, 1946.
13. Orton, S.: Reading, Writing and Speech Problems in Children. New York, W. W. Norton, 1937.

14. Salmon, P.: Rehabilitation of Deaf-Blind Persons, Vol. 1. Brooklyn, Industrial Home for the Blind, 1958.
15. _____: The deaf-blind, in Zahl, P. Blindness. Princeton, Princeton University Press, 1950.
16. Shoemaker, W.: Retinitus Pigmentosa. Philadelphia, Lippincott, 1909.

Suggestions for Further Study

Benton, A., Hutcheon, J. and Seymour, E.: Arithmetic ability, finger-localization capacity and right-left discrimination in normal and defective children. Am. J. Orthopsychiat., 21, 756, 1951.

Clark, W., and Russell, W.: Cortical deafness without aphasia. Brain, 61, 375, 1938.

Critchley, M.: Aphasia in a partial deaf-mute. Brain, 61, 163, 1938.

Hallgren, B.: Specific Dyslexia. Acta Psychiat. and Neurol., Suppl. 65, 1950.

Kanner, L.: Child Psychiatry. Springfield, C. C. Thomas, 1948.

Karlin, I.: Aphasias in children. Am. J. Dis. Child., 87, 752, 1954.

McCarthy, D.: Language disorders and parent child relationships. J. Speech and Hearing Disorders, 19, 514, 1954.

Myklebust, H.: Aphasia in children—language development and language pathology, in Travis, L. (ed.) Handbook of Speech Pathology. New York, Appleton-Century-Crofts, 1957.

_____ and Boshes, B.: Psychoneurological learning disorders in children. Arch. Pediatrics, 77,247, 1960.

Reinhold, M.: A case of auditory agnosia. Brain, 73, 203, 1950.

Strauss, A. and Lehtinen, L.: The Brain-Injured Child. New York, Grune and Stratton, 1947.

Thurston, J.: An empirical investigation of loss of spelling ability in dysphasics. J. Speech Hearing Disorders, 19, 514, 1954.

Wepman, J.: A theory of cerebral language disorders based on therapy. Folia Phoniatrics, 7, 223, 1955.

Weinstein, S.: Time error in weight judgment after brain injury. J. Comp. Physiol. Psychol., 48, 3, 1955.

Werner, H. and Carrison, D.: Measurement and development of the finger schema in mentally retarded children: relation of arithmetic achievement to performance on the finger schema test. J. Ed. Psychol., 33, 252, 1942.

Zangwill, O.: Agraphia due to left parietal glioma in left-handed man. Brain, 77, 510, 1954.

Chapter XIV

INTEREST PATTERNS, APTITUDES, AND SPECIAL ABILITIES

AN INDIVIDUAL'S VOCATIONAL LIFE is an integral part of his total abilities, interests, motivations, and personal adjustment. It is a manifestation, a projection ·of his total maturity. In Chapter VIII we considered the question of social maturity in relation to deafness; the question of whether deafness resulted in greater dependency. This consideration is inherently involved in study of the vocational abilities and adjustment of the hearing impaired. An independent life generally means being able to earn a living which assumes a matrix of factors often taken for granted. To some extent there must be integrity of physical and sensory capacities, of intelligence, and of personality. Because of the human being's plasticity and potential, considerable deficit may be present in any one of these areas without total dependency ensuing. Salmon[8] and his associates have shown that those who are both deaf and blind often can attain substantial independence. It is clear that those with mental retardation also can achieve a degree of self-care and a measure of vocational success. Evidence from psychology and psychiatry reveals that an individual may have considerable emotional maladjustment and maintain independent behavior socially and vocationally.

We have seen that deafness from early life results in a reduction of social competence, but what is the effect on vocational choice and success? When aptitudes are studied specifically do the deaf show inferiority as compared to the normal. Another question inherently related concerns their interests and motivations; does deafness influence basic interest patterns? What is the nature of their vocational goals and aspirations? These considerations are of importance in a discussion of the relationship between deafness and vocational adjustment. The psychologist, the rehabilitation counselor, the administrator, and the shop instructor concerned with the deaf are routinely confronted with such questions.

Handicaps make vocational choice and success more difficult; vocational choice becomes more critical. The basic nature of the activity must not be in conflict with the handicap which for the deaf means that the work must not entail normal hearing. Individuals with normal capacities have a much wider range of selection vocationally. There are many other factors which are indirectly involved but usually are not less important. Most of these are personal-social, such as being accepted *by* the co-workers and being accepting *of* the co-workers. It must be stressed that the deaf and hard of hearing as a group are employable, vocationally successful, and self-supporting. However, vocational stability may be less than average and the incidence of persons who are not successful vocationally may be above average. Conclusive evidence is difficult to obtain and programs for vocational guidance have been at a mimimum. Such programs are in great demand, as is research concerning this total area.

One of the major limitations of present approaches to the vocational guidance of the hearing impaired is the lack of scientifically verified body of knowledge. Frequently this is manifested through over-generalization and disregard of individual differences. While those having deafness have common problems, and apparently common characteristics psychologically, they also have marked individual differences. It is the responsibility of the educator, the guidance counselor, and the psychologist to assist the individual in using his *assets* most effectively. This entails realistic attitudes and understandings on the part of those providing guidance for the hearing impaired and their families.

We have emphasized that deafness, especially when onset is in early life, limits and impedes the development of potentials and aptitudes. This is true especially of communication, which has implications for guidance and often is of considerable significance even in childhood. An example is that because of the marked limitation imposed on language, most individuals having profound early life deafness do not attain higher education, hence, do not enter the professions. While improved methods of training can be expected to make such attainment possible for a larger number in the future, it is unlikely that the majority of such persons will achieve this level of competence in language. Stated positively, as is true for the normal population, most deaf people pursue the type of vocational work commonly referred to as the trades; this pertains primarily to males because of the differing roles of the sexes. Such comparison with the normal population may be misleading because deafness makes this type of vocational choice more mandatory. Proportionately more deaf persons *must* select the trades, which means that selection of the type of trade becomes more critical and consequential. Inasmuch as most deaf people must choose the trades, vocational training assumes major importance, but does not preclude other choices and the need for various types of training for both men and women. Our primary concern here is that those providing guidance and vocational counseling be informed and be realistically aware of the implications of deafness vocationally.

Similarly, it is of importance that the hearing impaired themselves have realistic attitudes. The major purpose of a well-founded guidance program is to assist the individual in being objective about himself. Such programs are dynamic and encourage the development of wholesome self-concepts. The counseling is based on rigorous, objective differential diagnosis. In addition to an appropriate history, there are eight major diagnostic areas of behavior which must be studied in a comprehensive guidance program for the hearing impaired. These are shown schematically in Figure 46. General health problems are not included. In previous chapters we have considered the areas of mental ability, emotional maturity, motor function, social maturity, linguistic abilities, and sensory

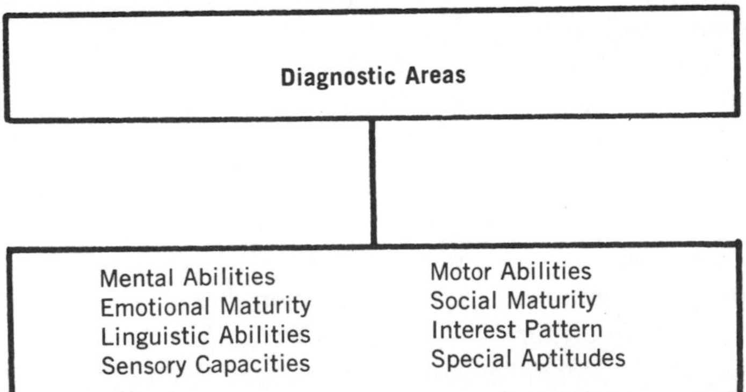

Diagnostic Areas	
Mental Abilities	Motor Abilities
Emotional Maturity	Social Maturity
Linguistic Abilities	Interest Pattern
Sensory Capacities	Special Aptitudes

FIG. 46. Diagnostic areas involved in counseling the hearing impaired.

capacity. In this chapter our major concern is with the individual's interest pattern and his special abilities.

To investigate each of these areas of behavior requires considerable time; the average is six to eight hours for an adult and four to six hours for younger persons. The approach is wholistic, with no single factor nor even two or three factors considered to be an adequate basis on which to base one's conclusions relative to an individual's aptitudes and needs. Moreover, no amount of information entitles the counselor to dictate goals or potential careers. On the other hand, in general, the more information he has the more effectively he can provide the situation from which the person can gain insight and make choices for himself. From experience we can state that deaf youth and adults do seek such services and are particularly curious as to what goals and vocational pursuits are suitable for them. When adequate information is secured, when fundamental principles of guidance are used, much can be done to assist with the decisions which are critical to them personally and to our society as a whole.

INTEREST PATTERNS

The study of interest patterns is an adjunct to the study of personality. It is difficult to conceive of interests and personality characteristics as being separate entities. The individual's interests often are a primary projection of his personality. Conversely, and perhaps more fundamentally, his interests are largely determined by the particular construct of his personality. Nevertheless, the study of interest patterns usually entails techniques and goals which differ from those associated with the study of emotional adjustment. Two widely used tests of interest patterns have been developed, one by Kuder[2] and the other by Strong.[12] There is a quantity of literature concerning both tests. We chose the Kuder for study of the interest patterns of deaf adults.

In Chapter VI we presented results from a study of personality of adults who sustained deafness in early life. The Kuder Preference Record,[2] which is a questionnaire-inventory type of test, was administered to this same population. Norms are provided for adults in a number of occupations, and the test provides an indication of the extent to which an individual's interests correspond with those engaged in various occupational pursuits. There are nine scales and an individual score is derived for each. These scales are:

1. *Mechanical:* enjoyment in working with machines and tools; repairman, engineer, etc.

2. *Computational:* interest in working with numbers; bookkeeper, accountant, etc.

3. *Scientific:* desire for discovering new facts; chemist, dietician, etc.

4. *Persuasive:* interest in dealing with people; salesman, minister, etc.

5. *Artistic:* liking to work with the hands in a creative way; sculptor, dress designer, etc.

6. *Literary:* interest in reading and writing; teacher, news reporter, etc.

7. *Musical:* a preference for music; musician, singer, etc.

8. *Social Service:* an interest in helping people; scout leader, vocational counselor, etc.

9. *Clerical:* a preference for office work; file clerk, secretary, etc.

For purposes of guidance an individual's profile of interests may be further classified according to whether he prefers being outside, being active in groups, working with ideas, avoiding conflict, or prefers directing others and stable situations. Because vocational choice is a critical factor in the total development of independence and in the adjustment of the deaf, a study was inaugurated to explore relationships between interest patterns and profound early life deafness. As indicated in Chapter VI, the sample consisted of a select group of deaf adults; having a select sample was one reason this type of study was considered useful. The results for the males by class in college are given in Table 96. Comparison by class was made to evaluate the influence of college experience on interests,

TABLE 96. Mean and percentile scores by college class for deaf males on the Kuder Preference Record

Scale	Freshman Mean	SD	%*	Sophomore Mean	SD	%*	Junior Mean	SD	%*	Senior Mean	SD	%*
Mechanical	68.8	16.6	32	72.7	16.9	42	70.5	23.4	34	72.3	21.8	37
Computational	38.3	10.6	60	32.9	13.0	31	41.3	9.7	70	35.5	8.5	50
Scientific	63.7	18.1	50	59.4	14.8	38	62.4	16.1	45	16.1	16.3	42
Persuasive	56.9	10.9	22	56.9	14.3	22	59.9	19.9	26	67.7	19.7	42
Artistic	49.0	13.7	62	50.5	15.6	66	50.5	10.4	65	44.5	23.0	47
Literary	59.1	21.3	82	50.9	17.2	62	51.6	19.0	65	54.0	18.2	70
Musical	13.0	10.2	42	5.5	4.0	8	9.2	6.7	23	8.1	6.8	18
Social Service	65.2	12.8	31	88.7	19.2	80	78.0	12.2	60	80.0	18.5	68
Clerical	54.5	14.3	60	54.7	8.6	64	51.8	14.8	50	53.6	11.4	57
	N=18			N=12			N=12			N=19		

*% Percentile.

as well as to study the changes which might occur by age in early adulthood. These scores show considerable stability. There was only one marked change: the Freshman males scored below the males in the advanced classes on Social Service. However, the scores on this Scale seemed to stabilize at the Junior and Senior level. While there were moderate changes in the interest patterns by class, it was the similarity of interests rather than the differences which was most striking. This is shown by Figure 47. Those areas in which the Freshman showed below average interest remained the lowest throughout the four year period. In no instance was there a shift in interest from very high to very low.

The results for the females by class in college are presented in Table 97. This analysis was hampered by an unusually small num-

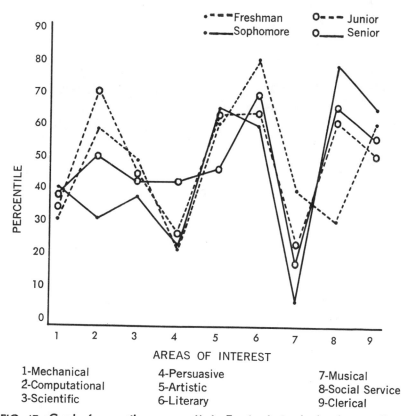

FIG. 47. Graph of percentile scores on Kuder Test for deaf males by class in college.

TABLE 97.   Mean and percentile scores by college class for deaf females
on the Kuder Preference Record

Scale	Freshman			Sophomore			Junior			Senior		
	Mean	SD	%*	Mean	SD	%*	Mean	SD	%*	Mean	SD	%*
Mechanical	58.5	11.0	70	55.0	12.7	61	52.0	21.8	54	56.2	6.0	63
Computational	33.5	7.8	60	35.4	10.9	63	33.5	10.0	55	39.6	19.3	78
Scientific	59.1	10.2	69	58.4	15.0	71	55.0	17.0	57	51.4	6.1	26
Persuasive	50.7	11.2	26	48.2	11.2	21	51.2	11.7	26	56.7	7.1	39
Artistic	54.2	5.4	56	51.2	20.4	50	56.1	15.2	61	58.6	15.8	63
Literary	53.0	15.1	55	59.7	15.4	71	55.5	15.4	61	45.8	16.3	39
Musical	11.3	7.9	12	9.3	7.2	8	13.7	9.9	22	6.7	6.4	5
Social Service	84.8	8.9	55	86.3	12.6	56	83.3	20.8	51	85.8	9.5	57
Clerical	63.7	11.4	52	59.0	14.8	41	63.1	11.9	50	66.5	8.3	58
	N=18			N=15			N=12			N=5		

*% Percentile.

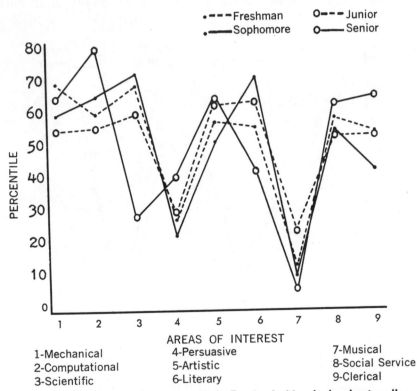

FIG. 48. Graph of percentile scores on Kuder Test for deaf females by class in college.

ber in the Senior class group. However, as in the case of the males,
the scores show marked stability for the four year period, shown
also by Figure 48. The only exceptions were the scores for the

Seniors on Scientific and Literary, which must be attributed to the limited sample. These data by class for the males and the females indicate a stability of interest pattern for this group of deaf college students.

Patterns of Interest by Sex

All research on the interest pattern of the hearing has disclosed variation by sex, which would be anticipated on the basis of interests being a manifestation of the total personality. Although we hypothesized that similar differences by sex would appear for the deaf, such variation has not been reported previously and in some respects deafness obscures such differences psychologically. It is apparent from the data given in Tables 96 and 97, and in Figures 49 and 50 that this is not true so far as interest patterns are concerned. Clear differences were revealed. The mean and percentile scores for both the males and females are given in Table 98.

TABLE 98.   Mean and percentile scores for deaf males and females on the Kuder Preference Record

Scale	Females			Males		
	M	SD	%*	M	SD	%*
Mechanical	55.3	12.9	61	71.2	19.9	35
Computational	35.2	10.8	63	37.1	10.8	56
Scientific	57.2	13.4	62	62.2	16.9	45
Persuasive	50.8	11.2	26	60.9	17.6	29
Artistic	49.9	16.7	46	45.9	13.9	54
Literary	55.0	16.1	60	54.8	19.6	71
Musical	11.2	8.9	12	9.2	7.9	19
Social Service	85.3	14.8	55	77.1	18.7	57
Clerical	62.5	13.0	50	55.1	11.0	63
	N=52			N=61		

*%Percentile

From these results we find that the males showed above average preference for areas of Literary, Clerical, Social Service, Computational and Artistic. They had below average interest in the areas of Scientific, Mechanical, Persuasive, and Musical. By comparison the females demonstrated above average preference for the areas of Computational, Scientific, Mechanical, Literary, and Social Service. They showed average interest in Clerical work, with below average preference for the areas of Artistic, Persuasive, and Musical. The profile of interests for each of the groups, males and females, is shown in Figures 49 and 50.

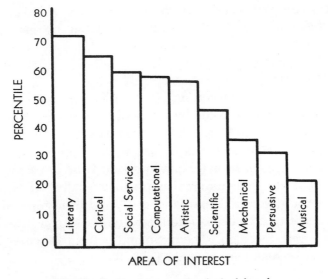

FIG. 49. Profile of interests for deaf adult males.

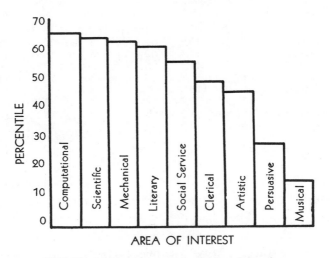

FIG. 50. Profile of interests for deaf adult females.

The comparison between the sexes is interesting in a number of ways. Both groups are lowest in the area of Persuasive and Musical, indicating the validity of the total findings. It would be unusual to find that this group had a strong interest in a musical career; realistically, they manifested virtually no preference for this area. The next lowest scores were for Persuasive, which is the category showing a desire for dealing with people, to sell, and to promote projects. Apparently deafness influences the development of this interest inasmuch as both sexes show a marked lack of preference for activities of this type. This, too, may be a realistic attitude deriving from the limitations imposed by deafness. Ostensibly the isolating effect of deafness, together with the inherent restriction on communication, make it difficult to deal with people in general, especially in terms of being persuasive. We find, therefore, as far as these results are concerned that those interests which assume normal hearing, or are the basis of a preference for influencing people, are lowest in this group of adults having profound deafness from early life.

On the seven remaining Scales there was considerable variation by sex. Both the males and females showed above average interest on five Scales while three of the five were the same for each sex group, Literary, Computational, and Social Service. However, the order of magnitude was different. As shown in Figures 49 and 50, the three areas of greatest interest in order of highest preference for the males were Literary, Clerical, and Social Service while for the females this order was Computational, Scientific, and Mechanical. This comparison suggests that neither group had a preference for directing others, for being active in groups, or for outdoor activities.

Perhaps one of the most provocative implications of these results is that the males tended to be most interested in activities which are not associated with feelings of masculinity, whereas the females showed high interest in such activities. In other words, the interest profile for the males emphasizes the less masculine preferences and for the females, the more masculine. This interpretation is based largely on the work of Terman[14] revealing a conjunction between interest patterns and the psychosexual aspects of personality. The suggestion that the males show femininity and the females masculinity in their interests as compared to the normal is in agreement with the results given in Chapter VI, where we noted that this trend was shown by the Masculinity-Femininity Scale of the MMPI. Apparently deafness from early life makes it more difficult to identify with the typical socio-cultural role for each sex. These findings are of general significance and further investigation of these possibilities is clearly indicated.

Interest Patterns in Relation to Other Factors

Several analyses were made to investigate the possible effects of specific factors relating to deafness. For example, the consequence of having deaf relatives in the home was studied. Those having deaf parents or siblings were compared to those deaf from meningitis; the sexes were compared separately. Two differences were found for the males; the meningitic males showed greater preference for the areas of Literary and Music. Likewise, there were two differences for the females; females having deaf relatives were much more interested in the area of Computational while the meningitic females were much more interested in the area of Literary. These findings can be summarized by stating that both sexes deaf from meningitis were more highly interested in literary activities than males or females who had deaf relatives in the home. The males deaf from meningitis were also more interested in Music. As shown in Table 48, the mean age of onset for the meningitic group was 6.63 years. The probabilities are great that those having deaf parents or siblings were congenitally deaf. While the similarities exceeded the differences for these groups, the variations which occurred are of interest. The total sample, males and females, showed above average preference for Literary activities. It is of considerable importance in this connection to emphasize that this category includes a preference for *teaching*, as seen in the Kuder Manual.[2] From the analysis of stated occupational preferences discussed below, we can conclude that those who sustained deafness from meningitis and thus had an advantage in language competence, manifested a preference for teaching, scoring higher on Literary than those having familial deafness.

It is interesting, also, that the males deaf from meningitis disclosed greater preference for activities pertaining to music, while the females having this etiology showed no such preference in comparison to the females having deaf relatives. In view of the finding discussed in Chapter VI that deaf males show inferior adjustment when compared to deaf females, we must infer that this is further indication of unrealistic attitudes on the part of the males. Although the females deaf from meningitis also had had the experience of hearing, with the possibility of recollection of this experience, in their interests they showed no evidence of a preference for musical activities, when compared to other deaf females. It must be stressed, however, that profound deafness sustained in early life results in a general similarity of interests, a similarity of interest pattern, irrespective of whether the deafness is primarily congenital or primarily acquired.

TINNITUS AND VERTIGO: In the study of personality discussed in Chapter VI, it was found that those having no vertigo or tinnitus were the better adjusted. Because these symptoms were associated with adjustment, they were studied also in relation to interest patterns. With the sexes separated, those having tinnitus were compared to the non-tinnitus group. Interesting trends appear. *Both males and females having tinnitus comparatively were much more interested in Music.* Furthermore, the females having tinnitus were much less interested in the area of Mechanical and Computational with somewhat less interest in the Scientific. While other important variations occurred for the females, the most intriguing disclosure was the preference of the tinnitus group for activities involving music. This should not be construed as a major interest of this group inasmuch as neither the males nor the females scored above average in this area. Rather, they showed significantly more preference for musical activities as compared to the other deaf adults. The psychodynamics of this relationship remain obscure. Undoubtedly these involvements are complex and do not necessarily reflect an association between sound, ringing in the ears, and music. Inasmuch as those having tinnitus showed greater inferiority in adjustment, their comparatively higher interest in music may simply indicate more unrealisticness generally. On the other hand, possibly they were projecting their problem of tinnitus and, thereby, disclosing more interest in auditory phenomena. Only further study will clarify this problem which may be of considerable consequence in the psychology of hearing impairment.

The number of subjects having vertigo and to whom the Kuder Test was administered was small, making the use of the statistical

analyses somewhat precarious. Nevertheless, the results were in
support of the personality test data for this group. There were no
significant differences between females having and not having
vertigo. In contrast the males having this condition were less interested in the areas of Persuasive and Literary but disclosed a
higher preference for the Scientific.

The appraisal of the interest patterns for the tinnitus and
vertigo groups in comparison to those not reporting these conditions,
raises intriguing questions. These findings, in addition to those
presented in Chapter VI, suggest that these factors are of importance in adjustment and may be of striking significance psychologically. In comparison to the other deaf adults those having tinnitus
or vertigo were more typical of the hearing, the males being more
masculine and the females more feminine in their interests. On this
basis we would expect that their emotional adjustment also would
be more typical, less deviate. However, the personality test findings
reveal that this is not the case. Our results can only indicate that if
tinnitus and vertigo are present, it is likely that attitudes and
interests will be different from those having comparable deafness
but who do not have the problems represented by these symptoms.

Interest Pattern and Speechreading

In Chapter X we reported on relationships between speechreading and factors of personality. To pursue this type of appraisal
further, interest pattern scores were analyzed according to self
ratings of speechreading ability. With the sexes separated, comparisons were made between those who rated themselves "good" and
those who rated themselves as "average" or "poor." As in the case of
the personality test scores, no differences appeared for the females
with an exception of a slight trend for the "good" group to show a
higher interest in the area of Persuasive. Two differences were found
for the males. Those in the "good" group were less interested in
Social Service. While the differences were not extensive, the variations which occurred warrant consideration because there was a
trend for both males and females who rated themselves as "poor" in
speechreading to manifest less interest in other people. In the male
group where this trend was statistically significant, the relationship
was manifested in two ways: those rating themselves as "good"

showed less preference for the Artistic, activities often not entailing other people, and those rating themselves "poor" had less preference for Social Service, activities not only entailing other people but involving specifically an interest in others. Although speechreading apparently presents a different problem to each of the sexes, it seems that as far as the males are concerned, self-estimates of speechreading ability are related to basic attitudes as they pertain to person-perception. Stated differently, one's self-perception and one's perception of others is related to one's estimate of his ability to speechread.

Interest Pattern and Estimate of Deafness as a Handicap

Evaluation of personality on the basis of subjective estimates of the extent to which deafness was a handicap revealed differences which were reported in Chapter VI. Interest scores also were analyzed according to estimates of no handicap, slight, and considerable. Mean scores were remarkably similar to those for the total groups. No statistically significant differences appeared. Subjective estimate of the degree to which a hearing loss is a handicap seems unrelated to measured interests.

Summary of the Interest Test Results

The study of interest patterns indicated the usefulness of this type of measure with deaf adults having adequate verbal facility. Moreover, the results disclosed that deafness was a factor in expressed interests in specific ways. For example, both sexes as a group showed a marked lack of interest in musical activities and in pursuits involving persuasion. In general, this group of deaf persons was most interested in activities which did not require direction of others or major group participation. In contrast to what might be anticipated, the males did not have primary interest in things or in activities involving working with their hands. However, the findings from the analysis of stated occupational preferences, discussed below, suggest that they had more such preference than revealed by the Kuder. The females showed somewhat greater interest in objective phenomena as disclosed by their having most interest in work involving computation, science, and mechanics. We may infer that their interests suggested less introversion and preoccupation with themselves. There was a trend also for each of the sexes to show an interest in activities more commonly associated with the opposite sex. The usefulness of such information for psychologists, educators, and guidance counselors is self-evident.

OCCUPATIONAL PREFERENCES

Often the task of the guidance counselor is to assist the individual in harmonizing his deliberate vocational choice with his measured interests and abilities. A deaf man may state that he wishes to be a teacher when his measured interests and aptitudes indicate that he is more suited and better equipped for work as a mechanic. In our studies of interests and abilities covering a period of time, we have asked the individual to list in order of preference three occupational choices. This was done also in the present study; the population of deaf adults was asked to "list the three kinds of work, in order of preference from most preferred to least preferred, that you want most to do when you finish college." The responses were tabulated and as much as possible were classified into the same vocational areas as those used in the Kuder Preference Test. It was necessary to vary the classifications slightly for the sexes inasmuch as the males listed "farming" and the females listed "housewife"; otherwise the same classifications were used for both sexes.

Analysis of these stated vocational preferences was made by sex, class in college, and on the basis of first, second, and third choice. No differences were found except for the comparison by sex. For example, Freshmen did not list "teaching" more often than Sophomores, or any other class; actually this was the most frequent choice of all the classes. As far as these data are concerned, it seems that college experience had remarkably little influence on vocational preference. Specific areas, such as teaching and trades, were listed most frequently by the preparatory class, and by all of the other classes.

Because no differences appeared on the basis of first, second, or third choice, or by class, the results are presented by sex only. The incidence scores represent the total number of times an area was listed, irrespective of the order of preference. These scores for males and females are given in Table 99. In addition to the vocational areas given in this table, 37 females gave "housewife" as their preference. As is done on the Kuder, teaching was included with

TABLE 99.   The number of times each vocational choice was listed by deaf adults

	Males	Females
Literary	95	77
Trades	75	19
Scientific	32	14
Business	22	2
Physical Education	21	7
Social Service	18	17
Artistic	18	13
Clerical	15	68
Farming	14	0

Literary. The high incidence of teaching as a choice by both sexes explains the area of Literary being the highest area of interest revealed by the Kuder Test. Very few chose a literary career such as being a writer. We find, therefore, that the measured interest of high literary and the high incidence of "teaching" as the stated choice are in agreement. It is clear that by teaching was meant a teacher of the deaf; this usually was stated specifically.

There seems not to be agreement between measured and stated interests in all respects. Trades, such as linotyping, carpentry, and machinist, was the second highest choice. It was not anticipated that this type of vocational work would be chosen frequently by this college group. A trade was often given as first choice by all five classes. This preference was not indicated by the Kuder although the area of Mechanical is measured. It is conceivable that the items on the Kuder are more suited to "white collar" vocational pursuits. In any event, as far as *stated* preferences are concerned this population of deaf males are highly committed to only two areas, teaching and trades.

The two most frequently listed choices by the females were teaching and clerical. Under Clerical the most common type of work indicated was typist. The classification of clerical as used here can be assumed to include activities defined as Computational on the Kuder. We find, therefore, that the choices of Literary and Clerical are in close agreement with the measured interests of the females as shown in Figure 50. On the other hand Mechanical, Scientific, and Social Service, all of which fell above average by measurement, were not listed frequently. For the females the three most common choices were teaching, clerical, and housewife.

The implication which is derived most clearly from this analysis is that the range of vocational choice was remarkably limited. Apparently there was a lack of knowledge about vocational possibilities. It seems also that as compared to the normal, the choices were unusually unimaginative for a college population. It must be recognized, however, that the choice of trades and typing may be realistic in many instances for those who have profound deafness from early life even though they have college training. These findings seem to be in agreement with those of Lunde and Bigman.[3] Their choices may reflect unconscious awareness that opportunities are limited or that deafness imposes a major limitation as far as many types of work are concerned. Nevertheless, an inference is that much more can be done to provide the information and guidance which is needed to make a wider choice of occupations possible.

SPECIAL APTITUDES

Information concerning aptitudes is especially necessary in the guidance of handicapped individuals. The various types of information required is shown in Figure 46. Specific study of aptitude in spatial relations, art, mechanical ability, and in other ways often provides clues to strengths and weaknesses in an individual's matrix of total potentials. However, the measures involved frequently entail normal verbal facility and are not suitable for use with many deaf persons. Tests must be chosen carefully according to their suitability. Accordingly, a study of the usefulness of mechanical aptitude tests in the guidance of deaf boys was made by Myklebust[5]; the major findings are given below. Stanton[10] made the only other such study. These two investigations are highly complementary and indicate the significance of appraisal of aptitudes.

The study by Myklebust included 80 boys between 12 and 21 years of age in attendance at a Residential School. The tests included were the Stenquist Mechanical Aptitude Test, Test I,[11] the Minnesota Paper Formboard, Series AA, the Minnesota Spatial Relations Test, Boards A and B, and the Minnesota Assembly Test, Sets I and II.[1] The results are presented in Table 100.

With the exception of the error score on the Minnesota Spatial Relations Test this group of deaf boys fell within normal limits in mechanical ability, which is in agreement with the findings of

TABLE 100. Scores for deaf boys on selected tests of mechanical aptitude

	Mean	SD	Percentile
Stenquist	55.2	12.3	41
Paper Formboard	34.3	12.2	50
Spatial Relations			
Time	556.2	129.9	50
Errors	30.3	12	15
Mechanical Assembly			
Set I	71.7	19.7	30
Set II	78.3	18.5	50

Stanton. In view of the inferiority of deaf children on various other abilities, this finding warrants emphasis. Presumably it provides at least a partial explanation for the fact that despite their limitations, the deaf are generally successful in vocational pursuits. Likewise, these results provide an objective basis for planning vocational training programs which capitalize the potentials of deaf children, youth, and adults. In other words, while attention must be given to areas in which the deaf show inferiority, it is of equal importance to give consideration to the development of those potentials on which they are not inferior. Presumably it is in these areas that they will attain their maximum success.

An attempt was made to ascertain the validity of these aptitude tests. This was done by having the shop instructor rate the subjects on the basis of their success in learning a specific trade. The trades included were printing, linotyping, metal work, photoengraving, and woodwork. The corelations between the test scores and ratings in these trades are presented in Table 101. With the exception of

TABLE 101. Correlations between scores on tests of mechanical aptitude and ratings of success in trade training

	Stenquist	Paper Formboard	Spatial Relations Time	Spatial Relations Errors	Mechanical Assembly Set I	Mechanical Assembly Set II
Printing	.60±.10	.56±.10	.18±.15	.16±.11	.42±.12	.23±.15
Linotyping	.09±.27	.78±.12	.00±.02	.27±.27	.11±.29	.05±.02
Metal work	.56±.14	.33±.19	.43±.17	.17±.20	.56±.14	.52±.15
Photoengraving	.51±.20	.27±.25	.42±.22	.31±.25	.32±.24	.25±.15
Wood Work	.50±.16	.34±.19	.34±.19	.13±.21	.39±.18	.41±.17

the error scores on the Minnesota Spatial Relations Test, all tests correlated with one or more ratings in trade training. It is interesting that no one test was found to correlate significantly with all of the trades rated. In fact these findings suggest that only through a battery of tests can the aptitudes required for various trades be properly appraised. These findings indicate further that such tests are valid for evaluation of mechanical aptitudes in deaf youth.

SPECIAL ABILITIES AND HOBBIES

The study of special abilities is not intended to convey the presence of endowments peculiar to those with deafness. Rather, the purpose is to highlight the need for appraising abilities in detail in order to ascertain information relative to all types of potential. Furthermore, as knowledge is gained it is conceivable that special abilities will include heightened memory ability and other psychological factors which derive from the fact of deafness. As indicated in Chapter V, there are psychological concomitants of deafness which might be exploited gainfully in the use of their potentials. More broadly, it might be hypothesized that areas of endeavor capitalizing visual abilities and not requiring high levels of verbal facility are the best possible areas for those having profound deafness from early life. If so, the question is whether such persons are inferior, average, or above average on abilities so defined. Pintner[7] raised this question directly and indirectly. This was his reason for studying the artistic appreciation abilities of deaf children through use of the McAdory Art Test.[4, 6]

To secure more information concerning this possibility, we, too, administered this test to a group of deaf children. In this test the individual rates pictures on the basis of their aesthetic qualities. Norms were established through the use of professional artists who made judgments of each picture. Our sample consisted of 177 students from nine through 19 years of age who were in attendance at a residential school for the deaf. The results are presented in Table 102. The data reveal progressive maturation of ability to make

TABLE 102. Scores by age for deaf children on the McAdory Art Test

Age	N	Males	Females	Total
9	8	89.5	68.5	79.0
10	11	93.2	88.5	90.6
11	18	79.0	83.0	81.1
12	17	86.6	88.5	88.5
13	16	87.0	108.5	97.7
14	23	106.0	127.5	116.7
15	14	115.3	144.3	129.8
16	19	120.0	136.7	128.3
17	24	132.4	150.5	141.5
18	12	114.0	141.0	127.5
19	12	137.5	147.3	142.4

artistic judgments, at least from nine through 17 years of age for both sexes. The females showed slightly more rapid maturation, and the level of ability attained by them tended to be higher than for the males.

In comparison with the normal, Pintner[7] found deaf females to be inferior to hearing females, while the deaf males approximated the norm for hearing males. The average range for Pintner's sample was from 11 to 21 years, whereas for our sample the range was from nine through 19 years. Interestingly, in our group those less than 14 years of age scored below the norm for deaf children as established by Pintner; above this age level the results were more comparable.

The McAdory Art Test scores were analyzed also by etiology and total sex groups; the results are given in Table 103. The

TABLE 103. Scores on the McAdory Art Test by sex and etiological group

	Exogenous	Endogenous	Males	Females	Total
Mean	113.3	113.2	110.7	120.3	115.0
SD	32.3	31.5	29.1	35.0	31.6

differences between the sexes and between the etiological groups were not statistically significant. According to the work of Siceloff,[9] sex differences are found for hearing children, the females being superior to the males in this type of artistic appreciation. At the upper age levels studied, our group of deaf females scored more closely to the norm for hearing females than was indicated by Pintner's findings.

These data suggest, in agreement with Pintner's conclusions that deaf children are not inferior in the artistic judgment involving pictorial material, that sex and etiology are not important influences, and that in deaf school children intelligence is not a major factor. It must be stressed that this test does not require verbal facility and measures ability to use *visual* aesthetic judgment only. Accordingly, this type of ability offers possibilities vocationally and avocationally, not in the sense that many deaf people would be expected to become professional artists but that various vocational pursuits may entail this aptitude. There is indication that this type of test could be developed and used to indicate special areas of competence and potential in various other ways.

Hobbies and Avocations

Authorities in the field of guidance emphasize the importance of avocations.[13] Perhaps as automation progresses this will become an increasingly significant aspect in the lives of everyone. In the lives of those having impaired hearing, it is apparent that hobbies might play an unusually important part. Study of deafness psychologically reveals an isolation effect and for this as well as for other reasons guidance and training in avocational activities is highly indicated. The stated vocational preferences as studied in the deaf college student group provided various clues accordingly. Analysis of these choices from this point of view disclosed that practical, earn-a-livelihood types of occupations were given as first choices, with more of the "I would like to" selections given last or as the third choice. Examples of third choices given by the males are cartoonist, aviator, gardener, sportswriter, poultry farmer, and photographer; for the females, gift shop operator, forestry, horse trainer, florist, library worker, and decorator were third choices. It is noteworthy that these preferences include mainly activities concerned with drawing, viewing, plants, animals, and books. A similar emphasis was noted in the autobiographical sketches of the hard of hearing presented in Chapter VI, where the importance of hobbies was mentioned frequently. These studies indicate a need for guidance programs, not only for the more practical purpose of direction relating to choice of occupation, but for the broadening of interests and for the enrichment of life in general for the hearing impaired.

IMPLICATIONS AND NEEDS

Earlier in this discussion we mentioned the need for most persons deaf from early life to earn their livelihood by working in the trades. This observation is supported by the fact that even most deaf college trained individuals stated a strong preference for this type of work. It seems, therefore, that through guidance and training programs excellent assistance could be offered in this regard. Such programs should not be concerned only with the trades, but concerted effort should be given to the diagnosis of various aptitudes and to the training which is indicated. The suggestion that deaf males are not inferior in mechanical ability is an example of how special assets might be capitalized.

There are other implications. These studies revealed that deaf persons lack knowledge about vocational opportunities. There seems to be a need for counseling in regard to specific areas of work which may be suitable and rewarding to the hearing impaired. Such training and guidance should include emphasis on avocational activities.

In the area of aptitude, as was noted in regard to intelligence, there seems to be some delay in maturation as compared to the normal. Growth was noted to continue until 18 to 21 years, the highest age levels studied. A number of investigations have shown that full potential is not attained until two to four years later than for the hearing. This must be considered when making a diagnostic evaluation as well as in the training program. Perhaps vocational training should begin somewhat later and continue to a later age than is typical for the hearing.

In general it would be advantageous to both the deaf and hard of hearing if technical study were made of their aptitudes, if guidance were given on the basis of broad findings from differential diagnosis, if the total influences of deafness were considered, and if total potentials were more fully exploited.

REFERENCES

1. Bennett, G. and Cruikshank, R.: A Summary of Manual and Mechanical Ability Tests. New York, Psychol. Corp., 1942.
2. Kuder, G.: Kuder Preference Record Vocational: Manual. Chicago, Science Research Associates, 1953.
3. Lunde, A. and Bigman, S.: Occupational Conditions among the Deaf. Washington, Gallaudet College, 1959.
4. McAdory, M.: The Construction and Validation of an Art Test. New York, Columbia University, T. C. Contrib. to Ed., #383, 1929.
5. Myklebust, H.: A study of the usefulness of objective measures of mechanical aptitude in guidance programs for the hypacousic. Am. Ann. Deaf, 91, 123, 1946.
6. Pintner, R.: Artistic appreciation among deaf children. Am. Ann. Deaf, 84, 218, 1941.
7. _____, Eisenson, J. and Stanton, M.: The Psychology of the Physically Handicapped. New York, F. S. Crofts, 1946.
8. Salmon, P.: Rehabilitation of Deaf-Blind Persons. Brooklyn, Industrial Home for the Blind, 1958.
9. Siceloff, M. et al.: Validity and Standardization of the McAdory Art Test. New York, Columbia University, Bureau of Publ., 1933.
10. Stanton, M.: Mechanical Ability of Deaf Children. New York, Columbia University, T. C. Contrib. to Ed., #751, 1938.
11. Stenquist, J.: Stenquist Mechanical Aptitude Tests, Manual of Directions, Yonkers, World Book, 1922.

12. Strong, E.: Vocational Interests of Men and Women. Stanford, Stanford University Press, 1943.
13. Super, D.: Appraising Vocational Fitness by Means of Psychological Tests. New York, Harper, 1949.
14. Terman, L. and Miles, C.: Sex and Personality. New York, McGraw-Hill, 1936.

Suggestions for Further Study

Bingham, W.: Aptitudes and Aptitude Testing. New York, Harper, 1942.
Blum, M. and Balinsky, B.: Counseling and Psychology. New York, Prentice-Hall, 1951.
Burtt, H.: Applied Psychology. New York, Prentice-Hall, 1948.
Fusfeld, I.: Counseling the deafened. Washington, Gallaudet College, Bulletin #2, 1954.
Lyon, V. W.: The use of vocational and personality tests with the deaf. J. Applied Psychol., 18, 224, 1934.
Maslow, A.: Motivation and Personality. New York, Harper, 1954.
Myklebust, H.: The clinical psychologist in the hearing clinic, in Rubenstein, E. and Lorr, M. Survey of Clinical Practice in Psychology. New York, International Universities Press, 1954.
Rogers, C.: Counseling and Psychotherapy. Boston, Houghton-Mifflin, 1942.
Thorndike, E.: The problem of classification of personnel. Psychometrika, 15, 215, 1950.

APPENDIX

Differences Found on Each of the Items on the Projective Personality Test*

Figure	Differences Found	Age Level
	Item 1. Size	
a. Man	No more than Deaf	9
Father	R more than D	13
Mother	DM more than DF	11
	DM Se more than DM Mo	9
Self	R more than D	13
b. Man	Deaf more than No	9
Father	RF more than RM	9
	R more than D	11
Mother	RF more than RM	9
	RM Se more than RM Mo	11
	RM Mo more than RM Se	15
	DF Mo more than DF Se	11
Self	RF more than RM	9
	RM more than RF	11
	Item 2. Position	
a. Man	R more than No	15
Father	None	
Mother	RM Mo more than RM Se	11
Self	None	
b. Man	No more than Deaf	9
	Deaf more than No	13
	R more than D	15
Father	None	
Mother	RF more than RM	15
	DM more than RM	15
Self	None	
	Item 3. Placement	
a. Man	None	
Father	None	
Mother	None	
Self	DM more than DF	9
b.	None	
c. Man	D more than No	13
	Deaf more than No	15
	RM Man more than RM Fa	13
Father	DM Mo more than DM Fa	15
Mother	RM more than RF	11
	RF more than RM	15
	DM more than DF	15
	DF more than RF	11
	DM more than RM	15
	RF more than DF	15
Self	RF more than RM	9, 15
d.	None	
e. Man	None	
Father	None	
Mother	None	
Self	R more than D	13
f.	None	
g.	None	
	Item 4. Physique	
a.	None	
b.	None	

Figure	Differences Found	Age Level
	Item 5. View	
a. Man	NoF more than NoM	13
	RM more than RF	9, 11
	NoF more than DF	13
Father	DF Fa more than DF Mo	13
Mother	RM more than RF	11, 17
	RM Mo more than RM Se	15
Self	None	
b. Man	RF more than RM	9
	DM more than RM	9
	NoM more than RM	9
Father	RF more than RM	7, 9
	DM more than RM	9
Mother	RF more than RM	9
	DM more than RM	9
Self	D more than R	11
	RF more than RM	9
	DM more than RM	9
c. Man	R more than D	11
Father	R more than D	11
Mother	R more than D	11
Self	R more than D	11
	RM more than RF	9
	RM more than DM	9
	Item 6. Transparency	
Man	Deaf more than No	15
	R more than D	11
	RF more than RM	9, 13
	DM more than RM	9, 13
	R more than No	11
	DM more than NoM	13
	Deaf F more than NoF	13
Father	R more than D	11
	RF more than RM	13
	DM more than DF	13
	DM more than RM	13, 15
Mother	RF more than RM	13
	DM more than DF	15
	DM more than RM	15
	RF more than DF	15
Self	R more than D	11
	RF more than RM	13
	DM more than DF	15
	DM more than RM	13, 15
	RF more than DF	15
	Item 7. Portrait	
	None	
	Item 8. Props Used	
a. Man	RM Fa more than RM Man	9, 15
Father	RM more than RF	9, 15
	RF Fa more than RF Se	17

*Father = FA, Mother = Mo, Self = Se; Normal = No,
Female = Fe, Male = M, Residential = R, Day = D.

Figure	Differences Found	Age Level
	RM Fa more than RM Se	15, 17
	RM Fa more than RM Mo	15
Mother	R more than D	15
	RF Se more than DM Mo	15
	RM Mo more than RF Se	17
Self	DM more than DF	15
	RM more than RF	13
	DM more than RM	15
Man	RM more than RF	9, 13, 15
	DM more than DF	13
Father	RM more than RF	9, 13, 15
Mother	RM more than RF	13
	DM more than DF	9
Self	RM more than RF	13, 17

Item 9.   Sex Characteristics

Figure	Differences Found	Age Level
a. Man	None	
Father	RM more than RF	7
	DF Fa more than DF Se	11
Mother	DM more than DF	9
Self	RM more than RF	9
	DM more than RM	9
	DM more than DF	9
b.1 Man	RF more than RM	7
Father	RF Fa more than RF Se	7, 9, 11, 13, 15, 17
	DF Fa more than DF Se	9, 11, 13, 15
	RF Fa more than RF Mo	7, 9, 11, 13, 15, 17
	RM Fa more than RM Mo	7, 9, 11, 13, 15, 17
	DF Fa more than DF Mo	9, 11, 13, 15
	DM Fa more than DM Mo	9, 11, 13, 15
Mother	RM Se more than RM Mo	7, 9, 11, 13, 15, 17
	DM Se more than DM Mo	9, 11, 13, 15
Self	DM more than DF	9, 11, 13, 15
	RM more than RF	7, 9, 11, 13, 15
b.2 Man	Deaf more than No	7
	No more than Deaf	15
	NoF more than NoM	9
	RM more than RF	9
	NoF more than Deaf F	17
Father	RM more than RF	9
	RF Fa more than RF Se	7, 9, 11, 13, 15, 17
	DF more than RF	9
	DF Fa more than DF Se	9, 11 13, 15
	RM Se more than RM Fa	15
	RF Fa more than RF Mo	7, 9, 11, 13, 15, 17
	RM Fa more than RM Mo	7, 9, 11, 13, 15, 17
	DF Fa more than DF Mo	9, 11, 13, 15
	DM Fa more than DM Mo	9, 11, 13, 15
Mother	RM Se more than RM Mo	7, 9, 11, 13, 15, 17
	DM Se more than DM Mo	9, 11, 13, 15
Self	DM more than DF	9, 11, 13, 15
	RM more than RF	7, 9, 11, 13, 15. 17
	RM more than DM	9
b.3 Man	No more than Deaf	7
	Deaf more than No	13
	RM more than RF	15
	Deaf M more than No M	15
Father	R more than D	9, 11
	DM more than DF	13
	RF Fa more than RF Se	9, 11, 13, 15, 17

Figure	Differences Found	Age Level
	DF Fa more than DF Se	9, 11
	DM Fa more than DM Se	11, 13
	RM Fa more than RM Se	11, 15, 17
	RF Fa more than RF Mo	9, 11, 13, 15, 17
	RM Fa more than RM Mo	7 9, 11, 13, 15, 17
	DF Fa more than DF Mo	9, 11
	DM Fa more than DM Mo	9, 11, 13, 15
Mother	None	
Self	RM more than RF	13
b.4 Man	No more than Deaf	7, 15
	NoF more than NoM	13
	R more than D	13
	DF more than DM	9
	Deaf F more than No F	9
	RM more than No M	13
	NoF more than RF	13
	No more than R	13
Father	DF more than DM	9, 11, 15
	RM more than DM	11
	DF more than RF	15
	RF Fa more than RF Se	9, 11, 13, 15, 17
	DF Fa more than DF Se	9, 11, 13, 15
	DM Fa more than DM Se	9, 13
	RF Fa more than RF Mo	9, 11, 13, 15, 17
	RM Fa more than RM Mo	9, 11, 13, 15, 17
	DF Fa more than DF Mo	9, 11, 13, 15
	DM Fa more than DM Mo	9, 11, 13, 15
Mother	RM Se more than RM Mo	9, 11, 13, 15, 17
	DM Se more than DM Mo	11, 13, 15
Self	DM more than DF	11, 13, 15
	RM more than RF	9, 11, 13, 15, 17
	RM more than DM	9, 11, 13
b.5 Man	RM more than RF	15
	DM more than DF	11
	RM Fa more than RM Man	9, 13
	RF Fa more than RF Man	17
Father	RM more than RF	13
	RF Fa more than RF Se	11, 13, 17
	DF Fa more than DF Se	9, 13
	RM Fa more than RM Se	9, 11, 13, 15
	RF Fa more than RF Mo	11, 13, 17
	RM Fa more than RM Mo	9, 11, 13, 15, 17
	DM Fa more than DM Mo	11, 13, 15
Mother	DM Se more than DM Mo	13, 15
Self	DM more than DF	13, 15
	DM more than RM	15
b.6 Man	No more than Deaf	9, 11, 13, 15
Father	RM Fa more than RM Mo	15
Mother	RM Se more than RM Mo	15
Self	RM more than RF	15, 17
b.7 Man	Deaf more than Mo	15
Father	DF more than DM	13
	RM more than DM	13
	RF Fa more than RF Se	9, 11
	DF Fa more than DF Se	13
	RF Fa more than RF Mo	9, 11, 17
	RM Fa more than RM Mo	11, 13, 15
	DM Fa more than DM Mo	9
Mother	RM Se more than RM Mo	11
	DM Se more than DM Mo	11
Self	None	
b. Man	RM more than RF	13

Figure		Differences Found	Age Level
8		RM more than DM	13
	Father	RM more than RF	13, 15
		RF Fa more than RF Se	9, 13, 15
		DF Fa more than DF Se	11, 13, 15
		RF Fa more than RF Mo	9, 11, 13
		RM Fa more than RM Mo	11, 13, 15, 17
		DF Fa more than DF Mo	9, 11, 13, 15
		DM Fa more than DM Mo	9, 11, 13
	Mother	RM Se more than RM Mo	9, 11, 13, 15, 17
	Self	DM Se more than DM Mo	9, 11, 13
		DM more than DF	9, 11
		RM more than RF	9, 13, 15, 17
		DM more than RM	11
b.	Man	RM more than DM	13
9		D more than R	11
		DM more than DF	15
		D more than No	11
	Father	RM Fa more than RM Man	9
		RM more than RF	9
		RF Fa more than RF Se	13
		DF Fa more than DF Se	11, 13
		RM Fa more than RM Se	9, 13
		RF Fa more than RF Mo	13
		RM Fa more than RM Mo	9, 11, 13, 15
		DF Fa more than DF Mo	11, 13
	Mother	RM Se more than RM Mo	11, 15
	Self	RM more than RF	11, 15
b.	Man	RM more than RF	13
10	Father	RM more than RF	13
		RF Fa more than RF Se	15
		RF Fa more than RF Mo	15
		RM Fa more than RM Mo	11, 13, 15
	Mother	RM Se more than RM Mo	11, 13, 15, 17
		DM Se more than DM Mo	13
	Self	DM more than DF	13
		RM more than RF	13, 15, 17
b. 11		None	
b. 12		None	
c.	Man	None	
1	Father	RF Se more than RF Fa	7, 9, 11, 13, 15, 17
		DF Se more than DF Fa	9, 11, 13, 15
		RF Mo more than RF Fa	7, 9, 11, 13, 15, 17
		RM Mo more than RM Fa	7, 9, 11, 13, 15, 17
		DF Mo more than DF Fa	9, 11, 13, 15
		DM Mo more than DM Fa	9, 11, 13, 15
	Mother	D more than R	9
		RM Mo more than RM Se	7, 9, 11, 13, 15, 17
	Self	DM Mo more than DM Se	9, 11, 13, 15
		DF more than DM	9, 11, 13, 15
		RF more than RM	7, 9, 11, 13, 15, 17
c.	Man	None	
2	Father	RF Se more than RF Fa	7, 9, 11, 13, 15, 17
		DF Se more than DF Fa	9, 11, 13, 15
		RF Mo more than RF Fa	7, 9, 11, 13, 15, 17
		RM Mo more than RM Fa	7, 9, 11, 13, 15, 17
		DF Mo more than DF Fa	9, 11, 13, 15
		DM Mo more than DM Fa	9, 11, 13, 15
	Mother	DF more than DM	9
		RM more than DM	9
		RM Mo more than RM Se	9, 11, 13, 15, 17

Figure		Differences Found	Age Level
		DM Mo more than DM Se	9, 11, 13, 15
		RF Mo more than RF Se	7
	Self	DF more than DM	9, 11, 13, 15
		RF more than RM	7, 9, 11, 13, 15, 17
c.	Man	None	
3	Father	RF Mo more than RF Fa	15
		RM Mo more than RM Fa	11
		DF Mo more than DF Fa	11
	Mother	RM Mo more than RM Se	11
		RF Mo more than RF Se	15
	Self	None	
c.	Man	None	
4	Father	RM Se more than RM Fa	7, 9, 11, 13, 15, 17
		DF Se more than DF Fa	9, 11, 13, 15
		RF Mo more than RF Fa	9, 11, 13, 15, 17
		RM Mo more than RM Fa	11, 13, 15, 17
		DF Mo more than DF Fa	9, 11, 13, 15
		DM Mo more than DM Fa	9, 11, 13, 15
	Mother	RF more than RM	9
		DF more than DM	9, 11, 13
		DF more than RF	11, 13
		RM Mo more than RM Se	11, 13, 15, 17
		DM Mo more than DM Se	9, 11, 13, 15
	Self	DF more than DM	9, 11, 13, 15
		RF more than RM	7, 9, 11, 13, 15, 17
9c.	Man	None	
5	Father	RF Mo more than RF Fa	11, 15
		RM Mo more than RM Fa	11, 13, 15, 17
		DF Mo more than DF Fa	11, 13
		DM Mo more than DM Fa	13
	Mother	RM Mo more than RM Se	11, 13, 15, 17
		DM Mo more than DM Se	13
		RF Mo more than RF Se	11, 15
	Self	None	
c.	Man	None	
6	Father	DF Mo more than DF Fa	11
	Mother	DF more than DM	9
	Self	None	
c. 7		None	
c.	Man	None	
8	Father	RF Se more than RF Fa	9, 11, 13
		DF Se more than DF Fa	11, 13
		RF Mo more than RF Fa	9, 11, 13, 15, 17
		RM Mo more than RM Fa	11, 13, 15, 17
		DF Mo more than DF Fa	9, 11, 13
		DM Mo more than DM Fa	9, 11, 13, 15
	Mother	RM Mo more than RM Se	11, 13, 15, 17
		DM Mo more than DM Se	9, 11, 13, 15
		RF Mo more than RF Se	11
		DF Mo more than DF Se	11
	Self	DF more than DM	9, 11, 13, 15
		RF more than RM	7, 9, 11, 13
c.	Man	None	
9	Father	RF Se more than RF Fa	9, 13, 17
		DF Se more than DF Fa	9, 13, 15
		RF Mo more than RF Fa	9, 11, 13, 15, 17
		RM Mo more than RM Fa	11, 13, 15, 17
		DF Mo more than DF Fa	9, 11, 13, 15
		DM Mo more than DM Fa	9
	Mother	RF more than RM	9
		DF more than DM	9
		RM Mo more than RM Se	11, 13, 15, 17
		DM Mo more than DM Se	13
		RF Mo more than RF Se	11, 15
	Self	DF more than DM	9, 11, 13, 15

Figure		Differences Found	Age Level
		RF more than RM	9, 11, 17
		DF more than RF	15
c.	Man	None	
10	Father	RF Se more than RF Fa	9
		RF Mo more than RF Fa	9, 11, 13, 15, 17
		RM Mo more than RM Fa	7, 9, 11, 13, 15
		DF Mo more than DF Fa	11, 13, 15
		DM Mo more than DM Fa	9, 11, 13
	Mother	R more than D	9
		RM Mo more than RM Se	9, 11, 13, 15
		DM Mo more than DM Se	9, 11, 13
		RF Mo more than RF Se	9, 11, 13, 15, 17
		DF Mo more than DF Se	11, 13
	Self	R more than D	9
		D more than R	15
		RF more than RM	7
c.	Man	None	
11	Father	DF Se more than DF Fa	13
		RF Mo more than RF Fa	13, 15
		RM Mo more than RM Fa	11, 13, 15
		DM Mo more than DM Fa	13, 15
		DF Mo more than DF Fa	11, 13
		RM Mo more than RM Se	11, 13, 15
		DM Mo more than DM Se	13, 15
		RF Mo more than RF Se	13
	Self	DF more than DM	13
c.	Man	R more than D	15
12		RF more than RM	11
	Father	RF more than RM	11
		R more than D	9
		DF more than DM	11
		RF Mo more than RF Fa	15
		RM Mo more than RM Fa	13
		DF Mo more than DF Fa	11, 13
		DM Mo more than DM Fa	11, 13
	Mother	RF more than RM	11
		RM Mo more than RM Se	13
		DM Mo more than DM Se	13
		DF Mo more than DF Se	11
	Self	DF more than DM	13, 15
		RF more than RM	11

Item 10. Mood

Figure		Differences Found	Age Level
a.	Man	None	
	Father	R more than D	13
	Mother	RM Se more than RM Mo	13
	Self	R more than D	13
b.	Man	D more than R	13, 15
		D more than No	11, 13, 15
	Father	RF more than RM	15
		D more than R	13
		DM more than DF	11
	Mother	RM more than RF	13
		RF more than RM	15
		DF more than RF.	13, 15
	Self	D more than R	13
		RF more than RM	9, 15
c.	Man	Deaf more than No	13
		D more than R	9, 11
		D more than No	9
		RM Man more than RM Fa	15
		RF Man more than RF Fa	15
	Father	D more than R	9, 11
		RM Se more than RM Fa	15
	Mother	D more than R	9, 11
	Self	D more than R	9, 13
		DM more than RM	9

Figure		Differences Found	Age Level
		DF more than RF	9
d.	Man	No more than Deaf	15
		R more than D	9, 13
		No more than D	9
	Father	RF more than RM	13
		R more than D	11
		RF more than DF	13
	Mother	R more than D	9, 11
		RF more than RM	13
	Self	R more than D	9
		RF more than RM	13
		RF more than DF	9, 13

Item 11. Clothing

Figure		Differences Found	Age Level
a.		None	
b.	Man	D more than R	9
		RF more than RM	11
		RF more than DF	11
	Father	D more than R	9
		RF Fa more than RF Se	7
		RM Fa more than RM Se	7
	Mother	DM more than DF	11, 13
		RF more than DF	11
	Self	R more than D	11
		RM more than RF	7
c.	Man	Deaf more than No	11, 15
		RF more than RM	7, 13
		Deaf F more than No	13
	Father	RF more than RM	7, 13
		R more than D	9
		RF Fa more than RF Se	7
		RM Fa more than RM Se	7
	Mother	RF more than RM	7
		RM more than RF	11
		DF more than DM	11
		RM more than DM	11
		DF more than RF	11
		DF Mo more than DF Se	11
	Self	RF more than RM	7
d.	Man	NoF more than NoM	13
		No more than Deaf	11
		RM more than RF	13
		DM more than Deaf F	15
		RM more than DM	13
		NoF more than Deaf F	13
		Deaf M more than NoM	15
		RF Man more than RF Fa	15
	Father	RF Se more than RF Fa	7
		RM Se more than RM Fa	7
		RF Mo more than RF Fa	15
	Mother	RM more than RF	13
	Self	DM more than DF	15
		RM more than RF	13
		RM more than DM	13
e.		None	
f.	Man	R more than D	13
		RM more than RF	11, 17
	Father	RM more than RF	11
		R more than D	13
		RM more than DM	13
		RF Se more than RF Fa	9, 11, 17
		DF Se more than DF Fa	9, 11, 13
		RF Fa more than RF Mo	9, 11
	Mother	None	
	Self	RF more than RM	15

Item 12. Head

Figure		Differences Found	Age Level
a.	Man	DF more than DM	9, 11, 15
		RM more than DM	11

Figure	Differences Found	Age Level
	NoM more than DM	11
Father	R more than D	11
	DF more than DM	9, 15
Mother	R more than D	11
	DF more than DM	9
Self	R more than D	11
b.	None	
c. Man	RF more than RM	9
Father	RF more than RM	7, 9
	DM Se more than DM Fa	9
Mother	RF more than RM	7, 9
	RM more than RF	11
	DM more than RM	9
	RM Se more than RM Mo	9
	DM Se more than DM Mo	9
Self	DM more than DF	13
	RF more than RM	9
	DM more than RM	9

Item 13.   Eyes

Figure	Differences Found	Age Level
a.	None	
b. Man	R more than D	11, 15
	RF more than RM	7
	R more than No	11, 15
Father	DF more than DM	11, 13
	RF Mo more than RF Fa	15
	RM Mo more than RM Fa	13
	DF Mo more than DF Fa	11
	DM Mo more than DM Fa	11, 13
Mother	RF more than RM	9, 11
	RM Mo more than RM Se	13
	DM Mo more than DM Se	13
Self	DF more than DM	9, 15
	RF more than RM	11
c. Man	D more than R	15
	No more than Deaf	7
Father	RF more than RM	7
	D more than R	9
Mother	RF more than RM	7
Self	RF more than RM	9, 13
d. Man	NoF more than NoM	9
	D more than R	11
	D more than No	11
Father	DF more than DM	13
Mother	D more than R	11
	DF more than DM	13
Self	None	
e. Man	D more than R	11
	R more than D	13
Father	DM more than DF	11
	DF more than DM	13
Mother	DF more than DM	13
Self	D more than R	11
	RF more than RM	13
	DF more than DM	13

Item 14.   Nose

Figure	Differences Found	Age Level
a.	None	
b. Man	NoM more than NoF	7
	R more than D	9
	RF more than RM	7
Father	RF more than RM	7, 9
	R more than D	15
Mother	RF more than RM	7, 9
	RF more than DF	9
Self	RF more than RM	7, 9
	RM more than DM	9
	RF more than DF	9

Item 15.   Mouth

Figure	Differences Found	Age Level
a.	None	
b. Man	RM more than RF	9
	RF more than RM	13
	DM more than RM	13
	DM more than NoM	13
Father	R more than D	15
	DM Se more than DM Mo	13
Mother	RF more than RM	13
Self	DM more than DF	9, 13
c. Man	None	
Father	RF Se more than RF Fa	9
	RF Mo more than RF Fa	9, 15
	DM Mo more than DM Fa	13
Mother	RF more than RM	7
	DF more than DM	9
	RM Mo more than RM Se	11
Self	DF more than DM	13
	RF more than RM	7, 17

Item 16.   Teeth

Figure	Differences Found	Age Level
Man	None	
Father	None	
Mother	None	
Self	RM more than RF	15
	RM more than DM	15

Item 17.   Hair

Figure	Differences Found	Age Level
a. Man	NoF more than NoM	7, 9,
	No more than Deaf	15
	Deaf M more than NoM	7, 15
Father	RF more than RM	13
	RF Se more than RF Fa	11, 15
	DF Se more than DF Fa	9
	RF Mo more than RF Fa	9, 11 15
	RM Mo more than RM Fa	11, 15
	DF Mo more than DF Fa	9, 11
	DM Mo more than DM Fa	9, 11
Mother	RM Mo more than RM Se	7
Self	RF more than RM	13
b. Man	RM more than RF	13
	DF more than DM	9, 15
	RM more than DM	13
	RM more than NoM	13
	NoM more than DM	13, 15
	NoF more than Deaf F	13
	DF more than RF	15
	NoM more than RM	15
	NoF more than RF	15
	DF more than NoF	15
	RM Man more than RM Fa	13
Father	RM more than RF	11, 13
	DF more than DM	9, 15
	DF more than RF	11, 15
	RM more than DM	13
	RF Se more than RF Fa	9
	DF Se more than DF Fa	9
	RF Mo more than RF Fa	9
	DF Mo more than DF Fa	9
Mother	RF more than RM	7
	RM more than RF	11, 13, 15
	DF more than DM	9, 15
	RM more than DM	11, 13
	DF more than RF	15
Self	DF more than DM	9, 15
	RF more than RM	7, 9
	RM more than RF	11, 13

Figure		Differences Found	Age Level
		DF more than RF	11, 15
		RM more than DM	13
		Item 18. Ears	
a.	Man	Deaf more than No	7
		DM more than DF	11
		DF more than DM	15
	Father	DM more than DF	11
		RF Fa more than RF Se	9, 11, 13, 15, 17
		RM Fa more than RM Se	13
		DF Fa more than DF Se	11, 13, 15
		RF Fa more than RF Mo	11, 13, 15, 17
		RM Fa more than RM Mo	9, 11, 13, 15, 17
		DF Fa more than DF Mo	11, 13, 15
		DM Fa more than DM Mo	9, 11. 13, 15
	Mother	DM more than DF	11
		RM Se more than RM Mo	9, 11, 13, 15, 17
		DM Se more than DM Mo	9, 11, 13, 15
	Self	DM more than DF	9, 11, 13
		RM more than RF	9, 11, 13, 15, 17
b.	Man	DM more than DF	11
		RF more than DF	11
	Father	DM more than DF	11
		RF Fa more than RF Se	11, 13, 15, 17
		DF Fa more than DF Se	11, 13
		RF Fa more than RF Mo	11, 15, 17
		RM Fa more than RM Mo	9, 11, 13, 15, 17
		DF Fa more than DF Mo	11, 13
		DM Fa more than DM Mo	13 15
	Mother	RM Se more than RM Mo	9, 11, 13, 15
		DM Se more than DM Mo	13
	Self	DM more than DF	11, 13
		RM more than RF	9, 11, 13, 15
		RM more than DM	13, 15
c.	Man	Deaf more than No	7, 11, 13, 15
	Father	RF more than RM	13
		DM more than DF	9
		DM more than RM	13
		RF Fa more than RF Se	11, 13
		DF Fa more than DF Se	11, 13
		RM Se more than RM Fa	15
		RM Fa more than RM Se	13, 15
		RM Fa more than RM Mo	11, 15
		DF Fa more than DF Mo	13
		DM Fa more than DM Mo	13
	Mother	RM Se more than RM Mo	15
		DM Se more than DM Mo	9, 11, 13
	Self	DM more than DF	9, 11, 13
		RM more than RF	9, 15
		DM more than RM	11
		RM more than DM	15
d.	Man	Deaf more than No	13, 15
		D more than R	11
		RF more than RM	7
		DM more than DF	9
	Father	RM more than RF	11
		D more than R	13
		DF more than RF	11
		DF Fa more than DF Se	13
		DF Fa more than DF Mo	11, 13
		DM Fa more than DM Mo	9, 13
	Mother	RM Se more than RM Mo	11, 13
		DM Se more than DM Mo	11, 13
		RF Mo more than RF Se	15
	Self	DM more than DF	9, 11, 13
		RM more than RF	11, 13, 15, 17
		DM more than RM	9

Figure		Differences Found	Age Level
		Item 19. Arms	
a.		None	
b.		None	
c.	Man	Deaf more than No	9, 11, 13, 15
	Father	RF Fa more than RF Se	17
	Mother	RF more than RM	7
		RM more than RF	13
		DF more than RF	13
	Self	RF more than RM	7
		RM more than RF	13
		Item 20. Hands	
a.	Man	RM more than RF	11
		DF more than RF	11
	Father	RM more than RF	11
		R more than D	13
		DF more than RF	11
		RF Fa more than RF Se	17
	Mother	RM more than RF	11
		DF more than DM	11
	Self	DF more than DM	11
		DF more than RF	11
b.	Man	None	
	Father	D more than R	11
	Mother	None	
	Self	RF more than RM	13
c.	Man	None	
	Father	R more than D	9
	Mother	R more than D	11
	Self	R more than D	11
		Item 21. Fingers	
a.	Man	Deaf more than No	7, 13
	Father	R more than D	11
	Mother	RF more than RM	7
		RM more than RF	13
	Self	RM more than DM	13
b.	Man	RM more than RF	13
		NoM more than Deaf M	13
		NoF more than Deaf F	13
	Father	None	
	Mother	RM Mo more than RM Se	15
		RF Mo more than RF Se	15
	Self	None	
		Item 22. Legs	
a.	Man	None	
	Father	None	
	Mother	D more than R	13
	Self	None	
b.	Man	None	
	Father	RF more than RM	7
	Mother	None	
	Self	None	
c.	Man	None	
	Father	R more than D	13
		D more than R	15
		RF Fa more than RF Mo	7
	Mother	R more than D	11
	Self	R more than D	11
		RM more than RF	13
		RM more than DM	13
		Item 23. Feet	
a.		None	
b.	Man	Deaf more than No	7
		D more than R	11, 15
		RF more than RM	9
		RF more than DF	9
		RF more than NoF	9

Figure	Differences Found	Age Level		Figure	Differences Found	Age Level
	D more than No	11, 15			DF Mo more than DF Fa	9
Father	D more than R	11		Mother	None	
Mother	D more than R	11, 13		Self	R more than D	13
	RF more than RM	7, 9, 15			DF more than DM	9
	DM more than RM	9, 15			RM more than DM	9
Self	D more than R	11, 15	e.	Man	R more than D	11
	RF more than RM	7, 9			RM more than RF	13
	DM more than RM	11			DF more than DM	9
c. Man	No more than Deaf	15			RM more than DM	13
	D more than R	9		Father	R more than D	9
Father	D more than R	9			RF Fa more than RF Se	9
Mother	DF more than DM	9		Mother	None	
Self	DF more than DM	9		Self	None	
	DF more than RF	9	f.	Man	None	
d. Man	R more than D	9, 13		Father	R more than D	13
	R more than No	9, 13		Mother	None	
Father	R more than D	9, 13		Self	None	

INDEX OF NAMES

SUBJECT INDEX